# Handbook of
# Clinical Skills
## Second Edition

# Handbook of Clinical Skills
## Second Edition

**Edited by**

**Peter Kopelman MD, DSc(Hon), FRCP, FFPH, FFacMEd(Hon)**
Emeritus Professor of Medicine and Vice Chancellor
University of London, UK

**Dame Jane Dacre BSc, MD, FRCP**
Professor of Medical Education, University College London
and Consultant Physician and Rheumatologist
Whittington Health NHS Trust, London, UK

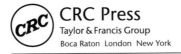
**CRC Press**
Taylor & Francis Group
Boca Raton London New York

CRC Press is an imprint of the
Taylor & Francis Group, an **informa** business

CRC Press
Taylor & Francis Group
6000 Broken Sound Parkway NW, Suite 300
Boca Raton, FL 33487-2742

© 2020 by Taylor & Francis Group, LLC
CRC Press is an imprint of Taylor & Francis Group, an Informa business

No claim to original U.S. Government works

Printed on acid-free paper

International Standard Book Number-13: 978-0-8153-6691-1 (Paperback)
978-0-8153-6696-6 (Hardback)

**Visit the Taylor & Francis Web site at
http://www.taylorandfrancis.com**

**and the CRC Press Web site at
http://www.crcpress.com**

# Contents

# Preface

The most important clinical skills required for day-to-day medical practice are the abilities to listen carefully, to observe, to take an appropriately comprehensive history, to examine a patient correctly and to perform simple procedures in the clinic or at the bedside. Mastery of these professional skills will enable clinicians to bring a reasoned approach to the possible diagnosis and management of their patients.

Such skills, combined with care and compassion, respect of the confidential nature of the interview, a constant awareness of infection control and the primacy of safe practice, provide the cornerstones of good medical practice. The acquisition and constant perfecting of clinical skills are a source of continuing enjoyment and challenge.

Although it is easy to request a long list of investigations, the good clinician is often able to resolve complicated clinical problems quickly, simply and satisfactorily after a thorough history and clinical examination and a small number of investigations focused on resolving a diagnostic hypothesis. Any request for an investigation should take account of potential discomfort and its cost against the likelihood of its result contributing to the patient's care. In short, competence in clinical method is a major contributor to excellence in practice.

Our objective for the second edition of this handbook is to provide a brief, readable introduction to these important skills, illustrated by videos accessed online to demonstrate how they can be mastered and how they may be applied. We continue to emphasise communication skills and a respectful approach to every patient, recognising that poor communication with patients and their relatives contributes to unsatisfactory clinical outcomes. This book is aimed primarily at those in the early stages of their training, but we appreciate its relevance to all those in medical practice.

The book begins with an overview of the general examination, followed by chapters on the examination of the cardiovascular, respiratory, gastrointestinal (including the urinary), locomotor and nervous systems. It includes chapters on the female and male reproductive systems, the endocrine system, the skin, child health and mental health. There is in addition a chapter on the general practice consultation, which collates the specialist clinical methods from previous chapters into a single chapter that considers their application within an abbreviated timescale.

The book is intended as a practical manual of clinical methods, designed to assist the learning clinician within every setting of patient care. It is our sincere hope that use of the book will instil the fascination for clinical practice that remains evident in all of the contributing authors.

The book's underlying message is that of Sir William Osler: 'The art of the practice of medicine is to be learned only by experience; 'tis not an inheritance; it cannot be revealed. Learn to see, learn to hear, learn to feel, learn to smell, and know that by practice alone can you become expert.'

**Peter Kopelman**
**Jane Dacre**

# Associate editors

**Claire Kopelman** BMedSc, MBChB, MRCGP
GP Partner, Holt Medical Practice, Holt, Norfolk; and Honorary
Senior Lecturer and Associate Tutor, Norwich Medical School,
University of East Anglia, Norwich, UK

**Iain MacPhee** DPhil, FRCP
Professor of Renal Medicine, St George's, University of London; and
Honorary Consultant Nephrologist, St George's University Hospitals
NHS Foundation Trust, London, UK

**Deirdre Wallace** MAEd
Lead for Clinical and Professional Skills and Leadership
and Management Development, University College London
Medical School, London, UK

# Contributors

**Julius Bourke** MBBS MRCPsych
Honorary Clinical Senior Lecturer in Neurophysiology and Clinical Psychiatry, Queen Mary, University of London; and Consultant Liaison Neuropsychiatrist, Nightingale Hospital, London, UK

**Stephen Brearley** MA, MB, MChir, FRCS
Consultant General and Vascular Surgeon, Whipps Cross University Hospital; Consultant Vascular Surgeon at the Royal London Hospital; and Honorary Senior Lecturer, Queen Mary, University of London, UK

**Dame Jane Dacre** BSc, MD, FRCP
Professor of Medical Education, University College London; and Consultant Physician and Rheumatologist, Whittington Health NHS Trust, London, UK

**Robert Klaber** OBE, MA, MBBS, FRCPCH, FHEA, FAcadMEd, MD
Consultant Paediatrician and Deputy Medical Director, Imperial College Healthcare NHS Trust, London, UK

**Claire Kopelman** BMedSc, MBChB, MRCGP
GP Partner, Holt Medical Practice, Holt, Norfolk; and Honorary Senior Lecturer and Associate Tutor, Norwich Medical School, University of East Anglia, Norwich, UK

**Peter Kopelman** MD, DSc(Hon), FRCP, FFPH, FFacMEd(Hon)
Emeritus Professor of Medicine, Vice-Chancellor, University of
London, London, UK

**Iain MacPhee** DPhil, FRCP
Professor of Renal Medicine, St George's, University of London; and
Honorary Consultant Nephrologist, St George's University Hospitals
NHS Foundation Trust, London, UK

**Clive Spence-Jones** FRCS(Ed), FRCOG
Consultant Obstetrician and Gynaecologist with special interest in
Urogynaecology, Whittington Health NHS Trust; and Honorary
Senior Lecturer, University College London, London, UK

## Acknowledgements

We are grateful to the following who so willingly and enthusiastically
contributed their valuable time to the making of the videos:

Deirdre Wallace – Clinical Skills Manager, UCLMS
Catherine Phillips – Senior Clinical Skills Tutor, UCLMS
Tina Nyazika – Senior Clinical Skills Tutor, UCLMS
Emma Thompsett – Clinical Skills Tutor, UCLMS
Dr Saniath Akbar – Gastroenterology Specialist Registrar, UCLMS
Dr Kanika Sharma – Clinical Teaching Fellow, UCLMS
Dr Anjali Rajendra Gondhalekar – GP Specialist Registrar, UCLMS
Dr Jonathan Mayhew – Clinical Teaching Fellow, UCLMS
Dr Natasha Malik – Clinical Teaching Fellow, UCLMS
Mr Richard Laing
and
Matt Aucott – Video Producer, University College London
Brian Barnes – Editor, Osmium Films

# Video resources

## Clinical examination

The cardiovascular, respiratory and musculoskeletal system chapters are accompanied by videos. The videos provide a step-by-step explanation of the physical examination procedure, demonstrating how each system examination is performed, what you are looking to elicit and what might be a positive or a negative finding. The videos should not be considered as an alternative to reading each chapter but a method of complementing your knowledge of underlying principles – they provide a demonstration of how the text is put into clinical practice.

The reader is encouraged to work through the chapters with colleagues and then test out the procedure for each system on one another prior to examining patients.

## Practical procedures

Videos demonstrating important practical procedures are included at the end of relevant chapters. For each procedure, you should know the indications and contraindications and be able to:

- Explain the procedure to patients, including possible complications, and gain valid informed consent.
- Carry out thorough hand washing and know how/when to use sterile gloves and, when appropriate, masks and protective clothing.
- Prepare the required equipment, including a sterile field.
- Position the patient and ensure their comfort.

- Adequately prepare the skin using aseptic technique where relevant.
- Administer local anaesthetic correctly for the procedure if required.
- Recognise, record and be able to undertake emergency management of common complications
- Safely dispose of equipment, including sharps.

## List of video resources

The videos listed below and referenced in the text can be accessed via the companion website that accompanies this text book by using the following link:

https://www.crcpress.com/cw/kopelman

It will take you to a webpage where you can click on Downloads/ Updates to access the resources themselves. From the ebook click on the above link to access the videos or use the link cited in the chapters.

## Chapter 1 History taking and examination

Video 1.1    Venepuncture using a vacutainer

Video 1.2    Venepuncture/phlebotomy using the butterfly system

Video 1.3    Preparing an intravenous infusion

Video 1.4    Preparing an antibiotic for intravenous infusion

## Chapter 2 The cardiovascular system

Video 2.1    The cardiovascular examination

Video 2.2    Measuring the blood pressure

Video 2.3    Recording an ECG

Video 2.4    Interpreting an ECG

## Chapter 3 The respiratory system

Video 3.1    The respiratory examination

Video 3.2    ABG sampling with a local anaesthetic

# Abbreviations

| | |
|---|---|
| ↑ | increased |
| → | deviated towards the right |
| ↓ | decreased |
| $A_2$ | aortic component of the second heart sound |
| AAA | abdominal aortic aneurysm |
| ACR/PCR | albumin:creatinine ratio/protein:creatinine ratio |
| ACTH | adrenocorticotropic hormone |
| ADH | antidiuretic hormone |
| AF | atrial fibrillation |
| ALP | alkaline phosphatase |
| ALT | alanine aminotransferase |
| aPTT | activated partial thromboplastin time |
| ASD | atrial septal defect |
| AST | aspartate aminotransferase |
| AVF/AVL/AVR | ECG leads looking from the right arm (AVR), left arm (AVL) and feet (AVF) |
| AVP | arginine-vasopressin |
| BCG | Bacille Calmette–Guerin – the vaccination against tuberculosis |
| BMI | body mass index |
| BNP | B-type natriuretic peptide |
| BP | blood pressure |
| bpm | beats per minute |
| BS | breath sounds/bowel sounds |
| C/O | complains of |

| | |
|---|---|
| **CCF** | congestive cardiac failure |
| **CCP** | cyclic citrullinated peptide |
| **CEA** | carcinoembryonic antigen |
| **CKD-EPI** | Chronic Kidney Disease Epidemiology (Collaboration) |
| **CMV** | cytomegalovirus |
| **CNS** | central nervous system |
| **$CO_2$** | carbon dioxide |
| **COPD** | chronic obstructive pulmonary disease |
| **CRP** | C-reactive protein |
| **CT** | computed tomography |
| **CVP** | central venous pressure |
| **CVS** | cardiovascular system |
| **CXR** | chest X-ray |
| **DVT** | deep vein thrombosis |
| **EBV** | Epstein–Barr virus |
| **ECG** | electrocardiogram |
| **EEG** | electroencephalogram |
| **eGFR** | estimated glomerular filtration rate |
| **ENA** | extractable nuclear antigen |
| **ESR** | erythrocyte sedimentation rate |
| **FBC** | full blood count |
| **FH** | family history |
| **FSH** | follicle-stimulating hormone |
| **γGT** | gamma-glutamyl transferase |
| **GALS** | gait, arms, legs, spine |
| **GFR** | glomerular filtration rate |
| **GI** | gastrointestinal |
| **GIS/GIT** | gastrointestinal system/tract |
| **GP** | general practitioner |
| **GTN** | glyceryl trinitrate |
| **Hb** | haemoglobin |
| **HbA1c** | glycated haemoglobin test |
| **HbeAg** | hepatitis B e antigen |
| **HbsAg** | hepatitis B s antigen |
| **HBV** | hepatitis B virus |
| **$HCO_3$** | bicarbonate |
| **HDL** | high-density lipoprotein |

| | |
|---|---|
| **HIV** | human immunodeficiency virus |
| **HPC** | history of the present condition |
| **HPV** | human papillomavirus |
| **Hx** | history |
| **ICE** | ideas, concerns and expectations |
| **Ig** | immunoglobulin |
| **INR** | international normalised ratio |
| **JVP** | jugular venous pressure |
| **kPa** | kilopascals |
| **LBBB** | left bundle branch block |
| **LDL** | low-density lipoprotein |
| **LMP** | last menstrual period |
| **LMN** | lower motor neurone |
| **LSD** | lysergic acid diethylamide |
| **LVF** | left ventricular failure |
| **LVH** | left ventricular hypertrophy |
| **MCV** | mean corpuscular volume |
| **MC&S** | microscopy, culture and sensitivity |
| **MDRD** | Modification of Diet in Renal Disease (Equation) |
| **MI** | myocardial infarction |
| **mmHg** | millimetres of mercury |
| **MMR** | measles, mumps, rubella |
| **MRI** | magnetic resonance imaging |
| **MSE** | mental state examination |
| **NHS** | National Health Service |
| **NSPCC** | National Society for the Prevention of Cruelty to Children |
| **NT-proBNP** | N-terminal pro-B-type natriuretic peptide |
| **O/E** | on examination |
| **OFC** | occipital frontal (head) circumference |
| **OS** | opening snap (heart sound) |
| **P$_2$** | pulmonary component of the second heart sound |
| **PA** | postero-anterior/pulmonary artery |
| **PaCO$_2$** | partial pressure of carbon dioxide |
| **PaO$_2$** | partial pressure of oxygen |
| **PEs** | pulmonary emboli |
| **PEFR** | peak expiratory flow rate |
| **PERLA** | pupils equal, react to light and accommodation |

| | |
|---|---|
| **PEWS** | Paediatric Early Warning Score |
| **PH** | personal history |
| **PMH** | past medical history |
| **PSA** | prostate-specific antigen |
| **PT** | prothrombin time |
| **PTT** | partial thromboplastin time |
| **QRS** | the wave form of the ECG |
| **RA** | rheumatoid arthritis |
| **ROS** | review of systems |
| **RS** | respiratory system |
| $S_1$ | first heart sound |
| $S_2$ | second heart sound |
| **SBE** | standard base excess |
| **SH** | social history |
| **SIADH** | syndrome of inappropriate antidiuretic hormone secretion |
| **SLE** | systemic lupus erythematosus |
| **SMA** | smooth muscle antibody |
| **SVC** | superior vena cava |
| **TIBC** | total iron binding capacity |
| **TSH** | thyroid-stimulating hormone |
| **TT** | thrombin time |
| **UMN** | upper motor neurone |
| **VDRL** | Venereal Disease Reference Laboratory |
| **VSD** | ventricular septal defect |
| **WBC** | white blood cell (count) |

# Chapter 1
## History taking and examination

The outcome of a consultation is different for doctor and patient because each has different objectives. The patient may have come simply to be given a diagnosis, may be in need of reassurance that all is well physically, or may have a more complicated psychosocial problem that needs to be assessed. The doctor's objective is to explore the patient's problems, decide whether or not there is a hidden agenda, make a diagnostic hypothesis, and offer advice on the next steps that need to be taken.

If the doctor recognises the pattern of the patient's illness, the diagnosis may be quick and simple. If not, there is a need to expand the history with repeated checking, confirmation and rejection of diagnostic hypotheses. In the majority of cases, the patient's problem becomes apparent during this process.

All patients must be examined. In some cases the diagnosis is only made after physical examination with the interpretation of clinical signs and/or with diagnostic test results and interpretation of investigations. During the examination procedure, the doctor is considering and confirming or refuting the diagnostic hypothesis that they have made.

The three sources of information that are helpful for evaluating a patient's problems and for making a diagnostic hypothesis are:

- The history – this is the patient's account of their illness or presenting complaint, including their reasons for visiting their doctor.
- The clinical signs – these include the abnormalities found on examination.
- The results of initial investigations, which may include biochemical, haematological and imaging results.

Throughout this book, we will draw attention to these three important areas. In most patients, the process of problem solving will involve the sequence 'history → signs → investigation', but this may not always be so. In some patients, it is immediately obvious that it will either be extremely difficult, or even impossible, to obtain a history (e.g. following a stroke). In such circumstances, it is appropriate to proceed to the examination, although it is always important to try to obtain a collateral history from someone – a relative, witness or the paramedics who have brought the patient to hospital.

There are some procedures that must be carried out routinely when examining every patient, and others that are used only when there is a special indication – these will be highlighted in the chapters of this book. In taking the history, there are a number of routine questions that must be asked of every patient, for example those which concern past illnesses, while the questions relating to the present illness will vary according to the problem. Similarly, certain examination procedures, for example measuring the blood pressure, should always be carried out during the clinical examination, whereas others, for example a rectal examination, are carried out only when certain abnormalities are anticipated. You will need to be able to identify the clues that may be provided from the history and the examination.

You will need to keep your wits about you as you progress through your assessment, making diagnostic hypotheses and refuting them. This will enable areas to be identified which may require closer analysis during the examination. You will learn best by witnessing as much as possible in the clinical setting and thereby learning from experience. Do not cut corners as you are learning to apply the techniques of clinical examination.

The practice of history taking (**Fig. 1.1**) and examination varies between clinicians, so you may see a number of slightly different techniques applied. It is a good idea to discuss any variability that you see, and decide on an appropriate method to fit in with your practice.

Finally, much of the basis of clinical medicine has evolved over several hundred years, so there is a wealth of experience but a limited evidence base for clinical method at the present time.

Remember – medicine is an art as well as a science. You may see experts take short cuts in their assessment of patients, but this is because experienced clinicians often work using pattern recognition – you need to have enormous experience before you can do this reliably.

**CLINICAL RECORD**

CONTINUATION SHEET

Surname ........ S – – – – –

Forename ........ J – – – – – –

Hosp No ........ 017652

PLEASE ATTACH LABEL HERE

| DATE Nov 18th | CONSULTANT'S NAME & DEPARTMENT |
|---|---|

9 pm Emergency admission via casualty

Mr JS Aged 75, Retired bus conductor from Hackney

%o Chest Pain

**HPC** Started whilst watching a football match on TV. Severe crushing pain — radiating to neck and jaw Never had it before ..... felt sweaty and dizzy --- Lasted 2 hours then lessened ..... Had angina diagnosed 1 year ago ...................................... - pain is still present now.

**ROS** CNS — No palpitations No chest pain ...........................................

**PMH** Jaundice as a teenager
Appendix aged 31 ............

**PH/SH** Smokes 20/day for >20 years.
21 u alcohol/week.
Widowed for 5yrs. Lives alone. copes well.

**FH** Father † MI aged 69
Mother † Old age. 96
Siblings still alive

**Treatment Hx** GTN only ....................................

**Summary** A 75 retired man with a 4 hour history of Chest pain ............

1583

Fig. 1.1 Handwritten history of a patient with chest pain.

## History taking

Several different processes should be going on in your mind while taking a history. The most obvious of these is forming a diagnostic hypothesis, as outlined, or an impression about the patient and their problems.

In taking a history, follow each line of thought; ask no leading questions; never suggest. Try to include the patient's own words in the complaint.

### BOX 1.1  HISTORY TAKING SKILLS

- Communication.
- Data gathering, assimilation and processing.
- Following an accepted structure.
- Forming a diagnosis and developing a plan of action.
- Writing it down.
- Presenting the history to others.

## Communication

The consultation is a time when you develop your relationship with the patient. You need to establish rapport and gain trust. You must make patients feel comfortable talking about themselves. Good communication, with careful formulation of questions and reflection of emotions, helps the patient to tell you all the information you need. The quality of your explanations helps the patient to trust your advice and decision making.

Prior to examining patients, you must thoroughly wash your hands with soap and warm water or apply an alcohol hand wash if a wash basin is not easily available. Also, it is advisable to seek a chaperone when examining a patient of the opposite sex.

### General advice

Introduce yourself to the patient – include your title if qualified, first name and surname. Address the patient by their title and name (Mr, Mrs or Miss Smith) and not by their first name unless the patient requests otherwise.

Always try to be polite – never talk to a patient without first introducing yourself, and then asking permission to perform an examination. Explain why you want to talk to them. Students are often embarrassed talking to patients because they feel they have nothing to offer. However, if the patient is told the purpose of the encounter, they very rarely object and often welcome the interest.

Be aware that most patients expect an appropriate appearance from a professional person. Make sure that you dress in a way which you believe a patient will expect of a doctor (i.e. neat, clean and conventional). Very fashionable clothing is often inappropriate. Avoid terms like 'dear'. Do not continue if the patient is tired – and do not embark on lengthy history taking sessions at mealtimes or when the patient has visitors. Find times when patients are free and come back. You will get a better history if they are not preoccupied.

The interviewer should guide the patient over the relevant areas of enquiry, striking a balance between the need to collect information in the time available and the wish to carry out the interview in a manner the patient finds most comfortable.

Be aware of non-verbal signals and body language. Good eye contact (i.e. looking at the patient as you speak to them), an appropriate space between you, and mirroring the patient's posture can encourage the patient to speak more freely and help develop trust. Adopt an 'open' posture (**Fig. 1.2**) so the patient is encouraged to talk to you.

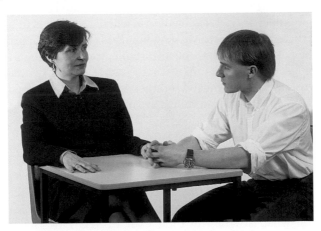

Fig. 1.2 An 'open' posture.

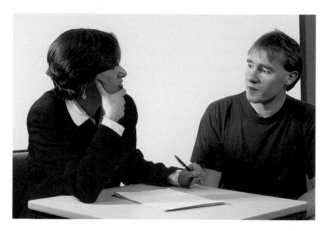

Fig. 1.3 A 'listening' posture.

Make it obvious that you are listening (**Fig. 1.3**) by perhaps occasionally leaning forward and putting your hand on your chin. Make sure
that you are sitting at the same level as the patient: it is intimidating
for the patient to be lying in bed with the doctor standing over them.
Make sure that you are at an appropriate distance – about an arm's
length away. Make use of touch – you must find the degree to which
you feel comfortable touching the patient – decide whether you are the
kind of person who wants to shake the patient's hand or put your hand
on their shoulder (**Fig. 1.4**). Recognise when a patient is indicating to
you that they do not regard shaking hands as culturally appropriate. If
you or the patient finds this uncomfortable, touch their hand or elbow
as this is less intimidating. Make eye contact regularly – do not just
look down at your notes – and interact with the patient by smiling or
by showing sympathy if sad things are discussed.

## Spoken communication

Always ensure that you speak clearly, and avoid the use of jargon.
Do not use technical or ambiguous wording. Encourage the patient to
talk about their problems. It is best to ask as many open questions as
possible, especially at the start of the interview, to enable the patient
to tell you what is wrong in their own words. This enhances trust
and confidence, as the patient will feel you are listening and therefore

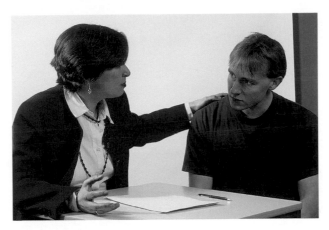

Fig. 1.4 Appropriate use of touch.

taking them seriously. Closed questions are needed to direct the interview and to explore abnormal experiences. Always try to open the question again to clarify the response, for example:

'Have you had the feeling, perhaps, that it is brought on by anything in particular?' (*Closed*)

'Could you tell me something about that?' (*Open*)

Leading questioning, in which there is an expectation of a particular response, should only be used to clarify an uncertain answer, for example: 'Your appetite's been poor, hasn't it?', or 'You've lost weight, haven't you?'

It is usually helpful to begin the consultation with an open question (*Table 1.1*), such as 'What exactly brought you into hospital/to the clinic/for surgery?' You should ensure that the patient replies by describing the presenting symptoms or worries and *not* an eventual diagnosis, for example angina or bronchitis.

It is useful in this context to use words such as 'How?' and 'Why?' For example, 'How can I help you?', 'How does it affect you?' In this way, it is difficult for the patient to give a one-word answer, and they have to describe the problem. If you use phrases such as 'Do you have a pain in your chest?', the patient may just say 'Yes' – and tell you nothing more.

## Table 1.1 Useful phrases in open questioning

| | |
|---|---|
| 'How can I help you?' | 'Can you describe it?' |
| 'What can I do for you?' | 'Where did ...?' |
| 'Why did you ...?' | 'What is it like?' |
| 'Tell me about ...' | 'When did ...?' |

Try not to interrupt at the beginning of the history. Use techniques like nodding and saying 'I see', or paraphrase the patient's last statement. Once you have the patient talking, you must listen to what they say, follow their story and explore the problem. Only then can you begin to concentrate on your own agenda and ask more direct or focused questions, either leading or closed. Begin by reiterating the patient's phrases and checking your understanding of them: 'You say the pain felt like a band – what sort of band?' Then move to direct questions to elicit more specific information: 'Did the pain go anywhere else?', 'Where?', 'Did it make you sweat?' Try to show respect, and be non-judgemental towards whatever the patient is telling you. Be careful not to stop listening.

## Data gathering and assimilation

It is important to keep your eyes open, as well as to listen attentively, when taking the history – and to remember that you are gathering information throughout the encounter. Physical signs may be observed while taking the history, or an unexpected finding during the later examination may require you to return to the history and reanalyse a particular area.

The diagnostic value of the history will vary from patient to patient, and is generally dependent on the patient's presenting complaint. A complaint of chest pain should trigger a series of questions related to the possible causes, whereas a complaint of tiredness may be less clear-cut. Some patients are naturally good historians, while others will find it difficult to describe the problems.

Be aware that some patients will inadvertently select information that they think you should know, and thereby present a somewhat false

## BOX 1.2 EMPATHIC STATEMENTS

These can convey an acknowledgement of the patient's problems and may enable an inhibited patient to expand on a topic which is difficult for them to discuss openly.

'I can understand that this may be difficult for you but …' (before asking a question).

'I can see that this is causing you distress.'

'I can see you've been under a lot of stress.'

### CLARIFICATION

'I'm not entirely clear what you mean by …'

'Could you tell me a little more about …'

### REMARKS ON BEHAVIOUR

Made during the interview, these can help explore important areas or, perhaps, defuse a difficult situation.

'You seemed quite sad/angry/distressed when you talked about …'

### ENABLING STATEMENTS

'It is not uncommon when under a lot of stress to experience intense or strange feelings or worries. Has anything like this been happening to you?' The patient may then be asked to elaborate.

### CONTROLLING

This can be done during natural silences or by gently interrupting at an appropriate point.

'I hate to interrupt, but can you tell me more about …'

'I'd like to move on, if I may …'

'I'm sorry, but I need to know more about this' (change topic).

*(Continued)*

> ## BOX 1.2 (*Continued*) EMPATHIC STATEMENTS
>
> ### SILENCES
> A brief and well-timed period of silence can allow a patient space to elaborate about a painful topic. Allow a patient time to gather their thoughts – and do not be afraid to interrupt and redirect them if they are getting away from the subject – but beware of allowing long, embarrassing silences. Once you feel confident with using this style and pattern of question, it is possible to concentrate on the next stage of history taking and data gathering.

picture of the complaints. Similarly, you may not pick up the clues provided by other patients, and may fail to ask the right questions. It is helpful to summarise your understanding of what you have been told, and relay it back to the patient:

'I understand the pain lasted about 2 hours, is that right?'

This checks for accuracy and completeness. It is always important when you are first taking a history to be prepared to go back to the patient after you have finished the history if you realise that you have omitted a vital point. Do not jump to conclusions during the history taking, and avoid rationalising the different parts in order to fit a specific diagnosis you have in mind. You must explore every possibility – even an apparently straightforward history may have a twist. This underlines the value of problem listing at the end of the history taking and examination.

You should always create time for history taking, whether you are a student or a doctor in training, and try to be as comprehensive as possible. Although you may see senior colleagues cutting corners, it is not advisable to do this yourself until you are experienced enough to know what to leave out. They are using their clinical experience to do this – it is not wise to follow that example until you have a similar degree of expertise. Only with experience is it safe and permissible to take a more focused history (see Chapter 11).

## Following an accepted structure

The ability to take an efficient and accurate history will come only with experience. *Table 1.2* provides general guidance to enable you to cover the important areas and collect the relevant data: you are advised to follow the order of the topics whenever you write out a history, although the information may not come from the patient in that order.

There will be occasions when it is not appropriate to take a comprehensive history at the time you first see the patient. The patient in cardiogenic shock will need immediate treatment, as will the patient with a perforated peptic ulcer. A good general knowledge of medicine is required to enable you to judge when it is important to take a detailed history and when it is sufficient to question simply about the immediate presenting complaint.

## History of presenting complaint

Begin by listening to the patient's own account, asking questions around particular areas. This account may already suggest to you possible causes for the patient's problem and likely reactions to your information and advice. Your intention with supplementary questions should be to analyse such possibilities and deal with reactions and responses. Once the patient has described the presenting problem(s), you should try to establish more precisely the exact nature, severity and timing of the symptoms.

### Table 1.2 Following an accepted structure

- Name, age, etc
- Presenting complaint
- History of the present illness
- Past medical history
- Systems review
- Personal and social history
- Family history and treatment history

You must enquire whether the patient has ever experienced similar symptoms in the past. If so, you must explore the relevant history.

Continuously analyse the patient's symptoms (*Table 1.3*) and answers to your questions, considering the various conditions that might account for them. This will lead you to ask additional specific questions. Guidance about such questions will be provided in the history sections of the following chapters, but be aware that some presenting symptoms may reflect the involvement of more than one body system (*Table 1.4*). Symptoms may reflect ill health in more than a single body system.

## Systems review

The next step is to ask questions about the presence or absence of symptoms relating to all systems (review of systems) that have not been touched on in the first part of the history. This routine enquiry is

## Table 1.3 Ways of encouraging the patient's description of their presenting complaint

| | |
|---|---|
| *Location* | Can you point to it? |
| *Radiation* | Does it spread anywhere? |
| *Duration* | How long has it been present? Have you had anything like this before? |
| *Timing* | Is it there all the time, or does it come and go? If it comes and goes, how long do you get it for? |
| *Nature* | What sort of pain is it? Is it burning, stabbing, gripping, etc.? |
| *Severity* | How bad is it? Does it stop you working, or keep you awake at night? |
| *Precipitating/ alleviating factors* | Is there anything that makes it better or worse? |
| *Associated symptoms* | Do you have any other associated symptoms? |

**Table 1.4 Symptoms that may result from an illness affecting one or more systems**

Remember that a symptom may not be specific to a system

- Pain
- Fatigue
- Fever
- Nausea
- Weight loss
- Cough
- Shortness of breath
- Abdominal pain
- Swelling

designed not only to reveal additional symptoms or problems related to the presenting illness, but also to uncover symptoms resulting from other unsuspected disorders. The checklist will usually include questions covering the points shown in *Table 1.5*. Some clinicians prefer to ask these questions at the end of the history – the timing is a matter of personal preference.

## Past medical history

Some aspects of the past medical history may have already been obtained. Nevertheless, try to obtain more detailed information about any serious illness or surgical operations in the past. It is helpful to record the dates of the illness/operation and the hospitals that the patient attended. It is also useful to check whether the patient has had any previous medical examinations for insurance reasons, and the outcome of those assessments. Finally, trips abroad and details of immunisations are sometimes relevant, particularly in the case of a suspected infectious disease. In a female patient, it is important to note, where relevant, menstrual history or year of menopause. The history of the presenting complaint may guide some specifically focused areas that need to be explored with closed questioning.

## Personal and social history

Ask about the patient's social circumstances – marital status, what is their occupation, and where do they live? An enquiry about the home in relation to heating, sanitation and other facilities may be relevant.

## Table 1.5  Systems review topics

Remember to ask these questions in language the patient can understand

| | |
|---|---|
| *General* | Body weight – has there been a recent change? Appetite, fever? |
| *Respiratory system* | Cough and sputum; haemoptysis; dyspnoea; chest pain? |
| *Cardiovascular system* | Dyspnoea on exertion; nocturnal dyspnoea; chest pain; ankle swelling; palpitations; pre-syncope? |
| *Gastrointestinal* | Indigestion; abdominal pain; nausea or vomiting; constipation or diarrhoea; passing blood in the motions? |
| *Urinary* | Frequency of micturition; pain on urination (dysuria); passing blood in the urine; nocturia; difficulty in passing urine? |
| *Nervous system* | Headaches; disturbance of consciousness (faints or fits); disturbance of vision or hearing; disturbance of limb function? |
| *Locomotion* | Pain or stiffness in muscles or joints? |
| *Menstrual function* | Usual rhythm (duration of each period and length of cycle); disturbance of rhythm; excessive blood loss; post-menopausal bleeding? |
| *Allergies* | Urticaria; hay fever; specific allergies, in particular to drugs? |
| *Drugs* | Any drugs or medicines currently being taken or taken in the recent past, including 'over-the-counter' medications and recreational drugs; abnormal reactions to drugs (e.g. reactions to antibiotics)? |

Always ask patients about smoking and drinking habits. Alcohol intake should be recorded as units per week, where 1 unit is 10 ml of ethanol. One glass of wine (175–250 ml) contains 2–3 units, 1 pint (500 ml) of beer contains 2.5 units, and 1 measure of spirits (25 ml) contains 1 unit.

It is also helpful to enquire about eating habits, particularly if you suspect a nutritional deficiency. It may sometimes be appropriate to enquire whether the patient uses or has used recreational drugs. A sexual history may be relevant in certain patients.

The social history often offers the interviewer an opportunity to get to know the patient better, but can obviously be a sensitive area of enquiry. It is important that you are aware of such sensitivities and use common sense when asking questions. However, do not be reluctant to enquire about the patient's current or past occupations – it is sometimes fascinating to learn of a patient's background and their skills. A suggested general line of questioning is shown in **Box 1.3**. You may begin, for example, with the patient's occupation.

Try to ensure that you use your communication skills to explore areas of concern, and follow the leads that the patient offers you.

While you are taking the history, you may become aware that the patient is very anxious or unduly depressed by their situation. It is appropriate to ask the patient whether they are worried about anything or depressed – refer to Chapter 12 for guidance about taking a psychiatric history.

## Family history and treatment history

You should enquire about the health of parents, partner and siblings – 'Are your parents still alive?' ... 'What did they die from?' – and whether there is any family history of particular illnesses. It is important to note whether there is a family history of death at an early age from heart disease. When you have completed taking the history, you should have elicited some clues to the main causes of the patient's problems. The history may have indicated the system(s) that will require particular attention during the examination. If no such clues have come to light, a more detailed general examination is essential.

> ### BOX 1.3 PERSONAL AND SOCIAL HISTORY: QUESTIONS TO ASK
>
> 'What is your occupation ... describe your job to me ... what do you do during a normal day ... can you manage it without any difficulty? Do you drive a car?'
>
> Then enquire about the patient's home life, to assess whether the illness has affected their ability to cope at home:
>
> 'Where do you live ... in a house or flat ... do you own it ... are you up to date with the rent ... how many stairs are there ... can you get up and down them OK ... can you cope with the house-work ... do you have any help ... who is it from ... do you have any social service support ... who is at home with you ... are they fit ... do they help you ... are any relatives near you ... do they help you out ... do you have local friends?'

## The routine physical examination

Details of the various examinations you should perform are described in the chapters of this book. This section will summarise a system for performing a routine physical examination (*Table 1.6*). While you are learning the system for clinical examination, it is important to perform a complete examination as often as possible. This will ensure that the scheme becomes second nature to you, and should prevent you making serious omissions. You are strongly advised to return to your patient if you find that you have omitted a part of the examination – most patients will not mind this, providing that you are honest. This will ensure that you remember that area of the examination next time.

In the routine examination of each system, only certain assessments are performed as a routine unless an abnormality is found. If anything abnormal is found, additional tests or analysis is needed: an example is the series of manoeuvres required if a heart murmur is heard (see Chapter 2). You will find that the time you take to perform the general examination will be within acceptable limits once you have perfected the technique.

## Table 1.6 Checklist for the routine physical examination

- General observations (inspection)
- Hands and arms
- Head and neck, including lymph nodes, breasts and thyroid
- Heart and chest
- Abdomen
- Legs, including joints
- Nervous system

## Scheme for the routine physical examination

Before you examine a patient, thoroughly wash your hands with soap and warm water or apply an alcohol hand wash if a wash basin is not easily available. In addition, it is advisable to seek a chaperone when examining a patient of the opposite sex.

Ensure that you maintain the patient's privacy as much as possible throughout the examination, and do not do anything without asking the patient first. Always be polite and considerate. Give clear instructions about what you want the patient to do – they are unlikely to be familiar with some of the actions that you request. It is conventional to perform the examination from the patient's right side.

Although it is possible to perform a full examination by considering each system in turn, this is not recommended as it causes unnecessary duplication. It is more logical to start by observing the patient's general appearance and then to examine the hands, the face and head, neck, chest, abdomen, joints and finally the nervous system. Within the systems, follow the scheme: inspection, palpation, percussion, auscultation.

## General observation

A key initial assessment is whether or not the patient is acutely unwell, as this will dictate the pace of assessment and management. You should observe the patient's gait and ability to perform coordinated movements. While taking the history, you should note the patient's mental alertness and intelligence. You should also observe the patient's body build, their muscularity and the condition of the skin (rashes, pigmentation, surgical scars, etc.). If the patient feels febrile, or gives a history of fever, the body temperature should be taken.

## Hands and arms

Look for finger clubbing and examine the nails – excessive brittleness may reflect iron deficiency, whereas white nails (leuconychia) is a sign of chronic liver disease. Look at the skin creases in the palms of the hands for evidence of anaemia or pigmentation and any other abnormalities. Note any wasting of the muscles of the hands or arms, and look for swelling of the joints and limitation of movement. Feel the radial pulse and note the rhythm and rate. Measure the blood pressure. Palpate the axillae and epitrochlear regions for enlarged lymph glands, and note the presence or absence of axillary hair. Ask the patient to hold their arms out in front of them, and check for a tremor of the outstretched fingers.

## Head and neck

Look at the sclerae of the eyes for jaundice and the conjunctiva for anaemia. Examine the teeth, the tongue and the mouth, and look at the fauces, noting the presence or absence of the tonsils. Look at the buccal mucosa for evidence of hyperpigmentation. Examine the neck for cervical and supraclavicular lymphadenopathy, and determine whether the thyroid is palpable. You should examine the breasts in women for any swellings, masses or tenderness.

## Chest and heart

Estimate the central venous pressure by inspection of the internal jugular vein. Locate the carotid arteries, and note their character and whether they are equal in pulsation. Feel for the apex beat, and then palpate and assess whether the left or right ventricle is enlarged. Listen to the heart sounds and the presence of any murmurs – use the flat of your hand to detect any palpable thrills.

Observe the movement of the chest, and use your hands to confirm its symmetry. Palpate the trachea and locate its position. Percuss over the lungs on the front and sides of the chest, and then auscultate over the front of the chest. Now sit the patient forward, looking for any deformities of the chest or spine. Percuss and listen over the back of the chest; concentrate particularly at the lung bases for any added sounds such as crackles, and listen for vocal fremitus. While the patient is leaning forward, you must examine the sacral region for any evidence of oedema.

## Abdomen

Observe the general appearance of the abdomen, looking for distension, peristalsis, dilated veins, any obvious enlargement of the viscera and abnormal masses. Palpate the abdomen gently and then more deeply, feeling for the spleen, liver and left and right kidneys. Look for enlargement of the inguinal glands and feel the femoral pulses. Examine the hernial orifices in men and women and the external genitalia in men. Listen to the bowel sounds and listen over the aorta and renal arteries. Consider a rectal examination.

## Legs

You should examine the legs, looking for abnormalities such as wasting, swelling of the ankles, varicose veins and tenderness of the calves. You should also examine the joints for swelling or limitation of movement. You should note the state of the circulation, feeling whether the limbs are warm or unduly cold – feel for the femoral, popliteal, posterior tibial and dorsalis pedis arterial pulses.

## Nervous system

You will already have noted the patient's appearance and intelligence – if you suspect confusion or an impairment of mental function, more detailed questioning is appropriate (see Chapter 6). Ask the patient whether they are right- or left-handed. Test the cranial nerves, and look at the fundi and eardrums. Test motor function in the upper and lower limbs, including the tendon and plantar reflex responses, and follow this by assessing sensation (pinprick and vibration sense). Finally, assess the patient's ability to perform coordinated movements and to stand and walk. Ideally, you should examine the nervous system in detail when you are learning because it is a useful way of gaining experience of the wide range of normality for the many signs elicited.

Examples of examination findings written in the patient's notes are shown in **Figs 1.5** and **1.6**. In some clinical services, the record will be entered into either a paper or an electronic integrated care pathway. Although this will cue documentation of specific pieces of information, it remains important that your full assessment is recorded.

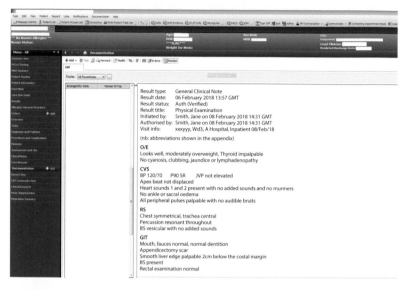

Fig. 1.5 Electronic medical records examination.

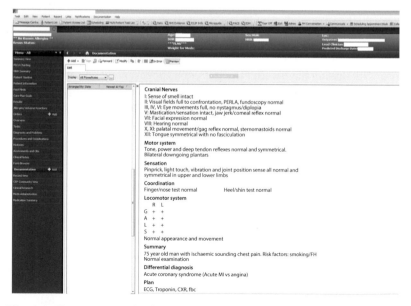

Fig. 1.6 Electronic medical records examination.

## Formulating a diagnosis

In some patients, the diagnosis is obvious. This is called a 'spot diagnosis', and it is based on pattern recognition, for example a child with a fever, a vesicular rash and a history of a brother with chickenpox. In these circumstances, the history and examination still need to be completed to help manage the case appropriately.

In a more complex case, a more detailed history is necessary to allow a diagnostic hypothesis to be formulated. For example, if a patient's joint pain is affecting several small joints, the diagnosis is more *likely* to be an inflammatory arthritis. If it affects a small number of large joints, it is *likely* to be degenerative. If the joints are stiff in the mornings, there is a *possibility* of inflammatory arthritis; if they are stiff in the evenings, the cause is *more likely* to be degenerative ... and so on. The diagnosis is made by matching the history from your patient with your knowledge of the pattern of the condition in your current diagnostic hypothesis. Eventually, you will come up with what you believe to be the most likely diagnosis. A scheme for this kind of thinking is shown in **Fig. 1.7**.

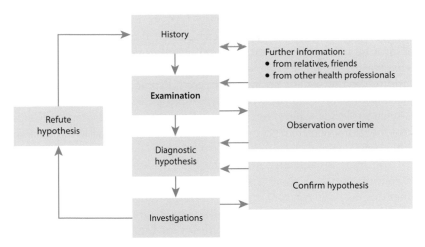

Fig. 1.7 Methods of clinical thinking to confirm or refute your diagnostic hypothesis.

## Writing it down

At the same time as taking the history, it is important to record the findings in an ordered way. Do not forget to put the date, year and time of the interview – this is a vital point of history recording that has considerable medico-legal importance. In addition, make sure the name of the patient is recorded at the top of every page. An example of this is shown in **Fig. 1.1** (see page 3). This enables you to use your notes to present the patient to your colleagues, and acts as a prompt aide memoire to you and a lead to others treating the same patient.

It is acceptable to use some abbreviations in your note keeping. A list of those more commonly used is in the Glossary.

Finally, remember that you should be considering and refuting diagnostic hypotheses throughout the history taking process – it is worthwhile recording some of this process as an 'impression' or 'summary' section in the notes before recording the physical findings. This helps you and your colleagues to understand your line of thought.

Remember always to sign and date all your entries at the end. Make sure that your writing is legible and that your status is documented.

## Presenting your findings to others

**Presenting findings to colleagues** You should speak clearly, and have a clear summary of the patient's problems in your head. Remember that body language and eye contact are as important in presenting your findings as they are in taking the history. People often have a problem with what to do with their hands while presenting a history. It is good advice to decide where you will put them beforehand – and perhaps use them to illustrate a point – or gesture towards the patient – or even hold your notes!

You must be able to reorder the information given to you in the structure outlined above and summarise the most important points, mentioning any relevant negative findings and all of your positive findings. Then present and discuss your diagnostic hypothesis. For example, from the history written down for **Fig. 1.1**, you might make a verbal presentation along the following lines:

## BOX 1.4 VERBAL PRESENTATION

'Mr JS is a 75-year-old retired bus conductor who has presented with his first episode of severe chest pain. It lasted for 2 hours and made him feel sweaty. It radiated to his neck and jaw. A diagnosis of angina was made a year ago. The pain was still there when he arrived. He has a past history of jaundice and an appendicectomy.'

- Then *continue* with a summary of the relevant risk factors:

  'He smokes 20 cigarettes per day, and has a family history of ischaemic heart disease. We do not know his cholesterol level, and he is not hypertensive.'

- *Continue with the findings:*

  'On examination, he looked well. His blood pressure was 120/80 mmHg. General examination was normal. In his cardiovascular system, his pulse was 80 beats per minute and in sinus rhythm, and he was not in heart failure ...'

- *Then mention your diagnostic hypothesis:*

  'I think he has acute coronary syndrome.'

## Problem listing in the medical records

The purpose of problem listing is to structure the medical case history to make it easier to interpret the relevant clinical information, and to provide a framework for planning diagnostic tests and therapeutic procedures. It will also help to remind you – the clinician – what is troubling your patient and how such problems may be resolved.

The emphasis is the compilation of a list of problems based on the clinical findings (history and examination). The diagnosis or diagnoses will only be made if *all* problems are considered. If used appropriately, problem listing will help you to make decisions about patient care; it will also provide a structure that is very helpful in correspondence about the patient to other health professionals involved in the patient's care, the patient's personal record and any medical audit.

## How to draw up a problems list

You should consider the presenting complaint, the pertinent aspects of the history and the examination findings.

First, list the problems to formulate a differential diagnosis. You should divide the problems into those which you consider to be 'active' and major contributors to the patient's current symptomatology, and those that are relevant to the patient's overall health. Such problems are likely to be 'historic' (part of the past history) and not considered relevant to the presenting complaint.

**Approach to problem listing** In the case of the Mr JS (see **Box 1.4**), the presenting problem is severe chest pain (problem 1, P1) and this should be listed as 'P1, Chest pain – past history of angina'. All the problems should be listed, irrespective of whether they are currently active or inactive, if you consider that they may have a bearing on the patient's well-being. For example, Mr JS is a cigarette smoker, which is contributing to his coronary artery disease – P2 is therefore 'Cigarette smoker'. These are both active problems. He has a past history of jaundice, which is important to document but is not relevant to the current presentation – so P3 is 'Past history of jaundice'.

## Progress notes

Electronic medical records provide a structure for documenting a patient's progress once a presumptive diagnosis has been made. Such records identify presenting problems and list them in automatically generated correspondence. The inclusion of both active and inactive problems is most helpful because it will alert a doctor to the entirety of past problems at each consultation with the patient. During a hospital admission, it is useful to follow the patient's progress by continually entering progress notes in a similarly structured fashion, addressing each of the patient's active problems in turn. These should be clearly written, signed and dated.

# Initial investigation plan

A diagnostic flow chart is shown in **Fig. 1.8**. The history, examination findings and clinic/bedside test results are used to create a problem list. The problems are then listed as active or past problems and applied to establishing the differential diagnosis. This, in turn, will determine the initial investigations.

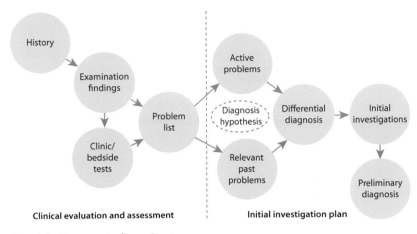

Fig. 1.8 Diagnostic flow chart.

**Figure 1.9** illustrates a scheme for investigating a patient. It starts with your diagnostic hypothesis, which usually will require testing using a number of investigations. Much can be potentially achieved in the clinic or at the bedside – measuring weight and height will enable the body mass index (BMI) to be calculated, which tells you about the patient's nutritional status. BMI is the weight in kilograms divided by the height in metres squared ($Kg/M^2$); the healthy adult range is 20–25. The blood pressure should always be measured, and a urine sample tested for glucose, blood and protein. Any suspicion of a cardiac lesion requires an electrocardiogram (ECG); airways diseases require a peak flow reading.

In some instances, a diagnosis can be made using these findings. However, it may be necessary to request additional tests – selection of a test should be based on the probability of the result contributing to either confirming or refuting the diagnostic hypothesis. It should never be based on ticking a request box. The potential discomfort to the patient and the financial cost of the investigation should also always be considered.

**Figure 1.10** provides examples of possible general investigations, more specific tests and highly specific investigations. Imaging may be required but, again, it is important to consider the likelihood of a positive finding from a specific imaging format (plain radiography,

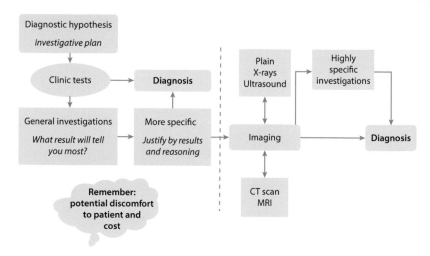

Fig. 1.9 Scheme for investigating a patient.

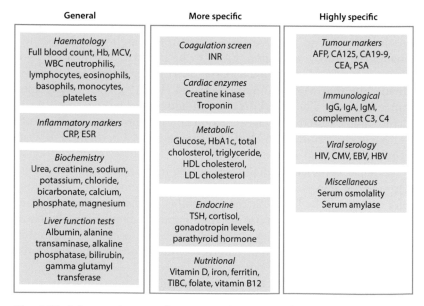

Fig. 1.10 Scheme showing the approach to general investigations, more specific tests and highly specific (blood) tests.

ultrasonography, computed tomography [CT] or magnetic resonance imaging [MRI]). Requests for highly specific investigations will be justified by narrowing down a differential to one or another diagnosis. The best clinicians continually test their hypothesis step-wise following investigation results.

## General therapeutic and technical skills

Before watching the videos given below, it is worthwhile thinking about the issue of informed consent (see **Box 1.5**). No procedure may be attempted on a patient unless they agree to have it carried out. With a conscious adult patient who is able to think rationally, the procedure must be discussed before it is attempted. Before larger procedures such as endoscopy or surgery, the patient is required to sign a form documenting their consent. With smaller procedures, verbal consent is adequate.

*Only when the patient understands this information are they in a position to decide whether or not they wish the procedure to be carried out.*

There are several instances of medical litigation relating to patients' lack of understanding of procedures and their outcomes ... so be careful.

### BOX 1.5 INFORMED CONSENT MEANS THE PATIENT NEEDS TO KNOW

- The procedure to be undertaken.
- The name of the person who will perform the procedure.
- The likely effects of the procedure (i.e. how will they feel when they wake up; whether there will be drainage tubes, catheters, etc.).
- The possible adverse (but unlikely) effects of the procedure.
- Any likely adverse effects of the procedure.

## Phlebotomy

Always introduce yourself and explain what you are going to do, and why. Outline how you will perform the procedure, and ask the patient if they have any questions. Make sure that you have the patient's verbal consent before you start.

Always check that the patient is not allergic to the drugs/solutions you are going to use. Before beginning any procedure, ensure that all the necessary equipment is there. Check the request form, and make sure you have the correct equipment, in a disposable tray, before you start (i.e. syringes, needles, blood bottles, cotton wool, an alcohol swab and a plaster).

Needles should be carefully disposed of either by clicking the needle off the syringe by using the keyhole-shaped opening in the top of the sharps bin, and disposing of the syringe in a yellow clinical waste bin, or by disposing of the waste needle and syringe in the sharps container, whichever is appropriate. If this is not possible, for example at the bedside, put all your instruments in the cardboard tray and dispose of them as above at the nearest sharps bin. *Never re-sheath needles.*

In most healthcare settings, blood will be collected directly into the bottle using a vacuum-based or other closed system. Check that you have filled the bottle to the line, and invert the bottle gently a few times to ensure the blood is mixed with any anticoagulant in the bottle. Finally, ensure that you label the bottle correctly. When taking blood for microbiological culture, ensure that you follow specific local guidelines for sample collection.

Use the links below for venepuncture using a vacutainer, and venipuncture/phlebotomy using a butterfly system.

▶ **VIDEO 1.1 Venepuncture using a vacutainer**

https://www.crcpress.com/cw/kopelman

▶ **VIDEO 1.2 Venepuncture/phlebotomy using the butterfly system**

https://www.crcpress.com/cw/kopelman

## Preparing an intravenous cannula

Intravenous cannulas are used for patients in whom constant venous access is required. This is because they require frequent intravenous injections or may need urgent resuscitation. The cannula is left *in situ* but sealed off with a rubber bung through which access is possible at any time.

Always introduce yourself to the patient and explain what you are going to do and why. Outline how you will perform the procedure, and ask if the patient has any questions. Make sure that you have the patient's verbal consent before you start, and remember to wash your hands and wear sterile disposable gloves.

This can be a painful procedure, so you need the patient's full cooperation if possible. Only attempt cannulation three times at one sitting, as it hurts and you may lose the patient's cooperation. If you think it will be a difficult cannulation, spend a long time locating the best vein, use topical local anaesthetic cream applied at least 1 hour beforehand and, if possible, get expert help.

## Setting up 'the giving set' for intravenous administration

This is a useful skill, seldom taught to doctors. The aim is to set up a bag of fluid attached to an intravenous line containing no bubbles.

> ▶ VIDEO 1.3 Preparing an intravenous infusion
>
> https://www.crcpress.com/cw/kopelman

## Preparing an antibiotic for intravenous infusion

Intravenous antibiotics are used to treat severe bacterial infections. This video demonstrates the procedure to be followed.

> ▶ VIDEO 1.4 Preparing an antibiotic for intravenous infusion
>
> https://www.crcpress.com/cw/kopelman

# Chapter 2
## The cardiovascular system

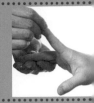

Cardiac problems are among the most common causes of acute admission to hospital. They also form a large part of a general practitioner's workload. Patients are generally knowledgeable about the symptoms of heart disease, so it is frequently a cause for anxiety. It is essential that all medical practitioners are aware of the patterns of presentation of heart disease, and take the patient's symptoms seriously.

The most common problem relating to the cardiovascular system is coronary artery disease – and many patients still die within the first few hours of a myocardial infarction (MI), or of heart failure after several years of ill health. The number of deaths caused by coronary artery disease in the UK has declined in recent years, but it remains a significant cause of premature death in both men and women. Overall mortality rates related to heart disease have reduced by 68% since 1980, with much of this reduction being attributed to a decrease in cigarette smoking, the use of statins and earlier intervention through angiography (angioplasty and stenting).

Several factors influence predisposition to coronary artery disease – the 'coronary risk factors'. These are shown in *Table 2.1*, and should form the basis of questions put to patients presenting with chest pain.

## Table 2.1 Coronary risk factors

- Increasing age
- Male gender
- Family history of coronary artery disease
- Hypertension
- Obesity
- Smoking
- Diabetes
- Hyperlipidaemia
- A diet high in saturated fat

# THE HEART

## Applied anatomy and physiology of the heart

All cardiac muscle has the intrinsic capacity for rhythmic excitation. The atria contain specialised fibres that are easily provoked into spontaneous rhythmic contraction, starting from the sinoatrial node. Ventricular muscle fibres can also contract on their own at a slow rhythm, but are usually excited through the specialised conducting tissues.

In isolation, the heart of a young adult will contract at an intrinsic rate about 110 beats/min (bpm). This intrinsic rate falls with age, to about 80 bpm at the age of 70 years. The intrinsic rate is modified by the central nervous system, which can slow the heart by means of impulses transmitted in the vagus nerve, and speed it up by impulses via the sympathetic nerves and by adrenaline from the adrenal medulla. In a young adult, the heart is under predominantly vagal influence at rest and contracts at about 70 bpm. However, it may accelerate to 200 bpm or more during exertion. By the age of 60 years, the maximum heart rate is about 170 bpm.

**BOX 2.1 THE HEALTHY HEART**

The healthy heart obeys Starling's law, which states that the force of cardiac contraction increases with stroke volume, so is dependent on cardiac filling.

- At a heart rate of 70 bpm in a young adult, each ventricle contains about 120 ml of blood at the end of diastole, 70 ml of which is expelled during systole. The resting cardiac output is therefore approximately 5 L/min.
- The force of cardiac contraction is continuously modified by the ionic environment, especially by the concentration of potassium and calcium in the blood.
- The normal mean pulmonary capillary pressure is probably only a few mmHg above the mean alveolar pressure. Therefore, little extra pressure is needed to drive blood into the lungs.
- The right ventricular pressure is usually 20/0 mmHg and the pulmonary artery pressure about 20/8 mmHg, with a mean of 12 mmHg.
- The mean left atrial pressure is about 4 mmHg, the left ventricular pressure about 120/5 mmHg, and the aortic pressure 120/80 mmHg, with a mean of about 93 mmHg.
- Most of the work of the heart is done by the left ventricle: the contraction of the left atrium makes only a small contribution to ventricular output.

Any change in intrathoracic pressure has a large influence on venous return, and hence on cardiac filling and cardiac output, due to the small pressure gradient available to fill the heart. During a deep inspiration, the intrathoracic pressure may be –25 mmHg, and during diastole most of this pressure is transmitted to the lax right ventricle, which sucks in blood. The diastolic volume of the right ventricle therefore increases, and the ventricle has to raise a greater amount of blood to a greater effective pressure during deep inspiration.

Expiration, on the other hand, squeezes blood out of the lungs so that output from the left heart increases. Right ventricular contraction begins before, but finishes later than, left ventricular contraction, so that the pulmonary second heart sound (marking pulmonary valve closure) follows the aortic second sound. During inspiration, the increase in right ventricular volume prolongs the time taken for the right ventricle to expel its contents. Thus, the gap between the aortic and the pulmonary second sound becomes wider.

## Assessment and diagnosis of cardiovascular disease

### Taking the history

Assessment of a patient with cardiovascular disease follows the same sequence and structure as for general history taking. The most frequent symptoms are chest pain and shortness of breath. These are both unpleasant and worrying symptoms, so it is important to recognise that the patient may be extremely anxious (and also possibly worried about dying). This may manifest itself in several ways.

The patient may appear angry, anxious or reticent. It is the doctor's job to deal with these emotions effectively in order to take a full history. This is achieved by appearing confident, competent and compassionate. Explore and reflect on their problems. Put the patient at ease before you start – remember that eye contact is important in establishing a rapport – and finally, make sure you listen (and *look* as if you are listening) to the patient's answers.

- Remember to start your history with an open question to encourage the patient to describe the symptoms more fully:

    'Tell me about your pain … How did it begin? … What is it like?'

- Then move to more closed areas of enquiry such as:

    'What were you doing when it started? … How long did it last?'

In general, it is better to encourage patients to describe the character of their symptoms in their own words.

#### The presenting complaint

**Chest pain** This is the main presenting symptom of angina or an MI, although it can be caused by respiratory system or musculoskeletal problems. It is important to have a clear idea of what the pain is like. Cardiac pain is frequently described as crushing, heavy or 'like a tight band around the chest'. Ask what the patient was doing when the pain came on, as angina is characteristically provoked by exercise. Find out if the pain goes anywhere else: cardiac pain often radiates to the left or both arms, or into the jaw. Ask about nausea, vomiting and belching. Encourage the patient to estimate how long the pain lasted.

**Breathlessness** This is a common manifestation of cardiac disease, and it may be mentioned as a decrease in exercise tolerance or a shortness of breath on climbing hills. Remember to ask how far the patient can walk before these symptoms appear:

'How far can you walk before feeling short of breath?'

Breathlessness may be at its worst at night. Ask the patient whether they can lie flat, or how many pillows they need, and whether they are woken at night by shortness of breath:

'Can you lie flat? … How many pillows do you use? … Do you ever wake at night with shortness of breath?' … Dyspnoea on lying flat is termed orthopnoea, and waking at night breathless is referred to as paroxysmal nocturnal dyspnoea.

If so:

'What do you do?'

Patients often feel that they need to go to the window for some air. In association with breathlessness, patients may have other symptoms of heart failure, so enquire directly about swelling of the ankles:

'Have you noticed whether your ankles are swollen?'

**Arrhythmias** Patients with heart disease may suffer from arrhythmias, which may cause fainting (syncope). Ask:

'Have you ever had any blackouts? … Tell me about them.'

Arrhythmias may also present with palpitations – a feeling of awareness of the heartbeat. Most people understand this term. It is

## Table 2.2  Important areas of enquiry

- Chest pain
- Breathlessness
- Ankle swelling
- Syncope
- Palpitations
- Claudication

## Table 2.3  Examples of different kinds of chest pain

| | |
|---|---|
| *Angina* | Central tight pain on exercise, usual relieved by rest |
| *Oesophageal pain/dyspepsia* | May be indistinguishable from angina |
| *Pleuritic pain* | Sharp pain at the periphery of the chest, made worse by breathing |
| *Pericarditic pain* | Like pleuritic pain, but relieved by leaning forward |
| *Musculoskeletal pain* | May be related to previous unaccustomed exercise<br>Tender to touch, and may be worse on movement |
| *Trauma* | History of excess alcohol or falls |

helpful to define whether the beats are 'regular or irregular', 'fast or slow', by asking the patient to tap out the beat of the palpitations on a table top.

Important areas of enquiry in cardiac patients are shown in *Table 2.2*. *Table 2.3* shows different kinds of chest pain.

## Other important points from the history

Patients with ischaemic heart disease may also have symptoms of vascular disease in other parts of the body. The most common of these is intermittent claudication, a cramp-like pain in the legs on walking, which is relieved by rest. Ask the patient how far they can walk before having to stop, what stops them, how long it lasts and whether they can continue walking after resting for a few minutes. Ask exactly where the claudication pain is located.

## Past medical history

When asking about past medical history, it is important to enquire specifically about rheumatic fever, as this may predispose to valvular disease. The importance of this condition is, however, diminishing because it has become uncommon since the routine use of antibiotics for sore throats. Nevertheless, elderly patients, and those brought up in developing countries, may still have been affected.

You must also ask about any history of hypertension and diabetes, or previous episodes of the cardiac symptoms outlined above. Enquire about previous chest pain and/or heart attacks.

## Personal and social history

This is an important part of the history in cardiovascular disease, as it will show you the effect that the patient's symptoms are having on their life. It also helps you to look for predisposing factors for cardiovascular disease in the patient's lifestyle.

Ask whether they take any exercise, and what kind of activity they are able to perform before developing symptoms. This may overlap with the presenting complaint.

At this stage, you may feel that a sexual history is relevant. If the patient has had a straightforward MI, it may not be important. However, in some circumstances it may be necessary to ask, for example, an older man whether he gets angina during intercourse, as this may be affecting his relationship with his partner.

## Family history and treatment history

A family history of heart disease is a significant coronary risk factor. It is essential therefore to establish whether any close relatives have had chest pain or heart attacks – or have suffered a sudden death. It is important to establish the age of the relative when these events occurred, as MI runs in families.

## Table 2.4 Checklist for cardiovascular history taking

- General approach: introduce yourself, establish rapport. Remember eye contact
- Assess the present complaint and its history (previous attacks, nature of the pain, etc.). Do not forget the coronary risk factors
- Ask about past medical history, particularly in relation to heart disease
- Ask about smoking/drinking/drugs
- Ask about social history (e.g. how many stairs in the home)
- Ask about family history: does anyone have heart disease or chest pain?
- Systematic enquiry

**Listen to the answers!**

Patients with cardiac conditions are often taking multiple medications. Ask specifically if the patient has tried GTN (glyceryl trinitrate), whether it relieves their pain and how long it usually takes for relief to occur (GTN usually acts within 5 minutes for ischaemic chest pain). It is important to note down the medications and doses, as well as what has been tried in the past and any known reasons for stopping drugs.

You can include tobacco and alcohol here. Ask whether the patient smokes; if the answer is 'no', find out if they have ever smoked, and how much. Also ask why the patient gave up smoking. Remember to include e-cigarettes and 'vaping'. Follow exactly the same line of enquiry for alcohol.

A checklist for cardiovascular history taking is given in *Table 2.4*.

## Examination of the patient (Video 2.1)

In order for you to perform a thorough cardiovascular examination, the patient should be comfortable and relaxed. Make sure that the room is not too cold. First, look at the patient's hands, check the neck, pulses and blood pressure, and then follow the scheme 'inspection, palpation, auscultation'.

> ▶ VIDEO 2.1 The cardiovascular examination
> ...........................................................................
> https://www.crcpress.com/cw/kopelman

## General observations

Begin the examination with an assessment of the patient's general condition:

- Do they look well or ill – are they comfortable or short of breath at rest?
- Do they have central cyanosis? Take the body temperature.

Then look at the patient's hands. In the cardiovascular system, you are looking for peripheral cyanosis, clubbing (**Fig. 2.1**) and splinter haemorrhages. Next look for anaemia in the conjunctiva, and re-check for central cyanosis. Patients undergoing acute MI typically look pale, sweaty, peripherally shut down and anxious.

## Arterial pulses

The radial pulse should be palpated, as illustrated (**Fig. 2.2**). The pulse should be confirmed as being equal and synchronous in both wrists, and the rate, rhythm, volume and should be character noted.

The radial pulse is usually counted over 15 seconds, and the rate (bpm) calculated. The rhythm of the pulse should be regular, apart

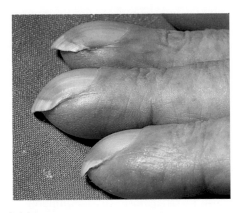

Fig. 2.1 Finger clubbing.

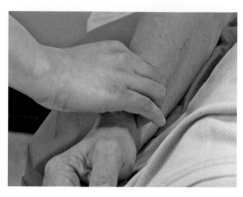

Fig. 2.2 Feeling the radial pulse.

from normal inspiratory speeding (sinus arrhythmia). You should ask yourself the following questions if the pulse is irregular:

- Is the pulse basically regular but with occasional irregularities (extra beats, or pauses)? This suggests the presence of ectopic beats (i.e. beats arising from some focus other than the sinoatrial node). Ectopic beats may arise either in the ventricle or at a supraventricular site (atrium or atrioventricular node). If they are ventricular in origin, they are usually followed by a compensatory pause.
- Is the pulse totally irregular both in timing and volume? This suggests atrial fibrillation. It can sometimes be difficult to analyse the cardiac rhythm simply by feeling the pulse – the rhythm may be resolved by auscultation. You may hear the terms 'irregularly irregular pulse' or 'regularly irregular pulse'. This is confusing terminology – it is easier to state that a pulse is either 'irregular' or 'regular'.

The volume of the pulse should be checked next – does the amplitude feel small or large? A small-volume pulse suggests a low stroke volume and reduced cardiac output, while a large-volume pulse may signify a large left ventricular stroke volume. Avoid the terms 'a weak' or 'a strong' pulse, particularly in front of patients.

In aortic incompetence, the stroke volume is high because a significant amount of blood regurgitates back into the left ventricle and has to be pumped again. Furthermore, the incompetent valve will let the arterial pressure fall markedly in diastole. Hence, a bounding, dynamic

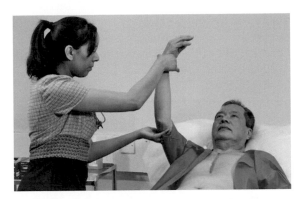

Fig. 2.3 Examining the radial artery to detect a collapsing pulse.

pulse collapses to give a very wide pulse pressure. The collapse of the pulse pressure can be felt with even greater effect if your hand is placed around the patient's wrist over the radial artery, and the patient's hand is raised above their shoulder so that the radial artery is palpated at a level above the heart (**Fig. 2.3**).

### BOX 2.2 PULSES AND THEIR IDENTIFICATION

- The *brachial pulse* (see **Fig. 2.38**) is best felt in the patient's right arm by applying the fingers or thumb of your right hand to the front of the elbow just medial to the biceps tendon, with the fingers supporting the back of the elbow.
- The *carotid pulse* (see **Fig. 2.34**) is best felt on the patient's right side: locate the mid-point of the anterior border of the sternomastoid muscle with the fingers or thumb of your left hand (this is often the site of a skin crease) and press firmly backwards. Do not feel both carotid pulses at the same time, as you will temporarily obstruct the cerebral blood flow, especially in elderly patients. Three main abnormalities are slow-rising, collapsing and bisferiens.

Auscultate over both carotid pulsations – a high-pitched 'blowing' systolic murmur, a carotid bruit, is associated with carotid stenosis on that side, or is referred from aortic stenosis and heard bilaterally.

The character of the pulse refers to the shape of the pulse wave. This is better assessed at the brachial pulse or, more particularly, at the carotid because of its size and its proximity to the heart. The pulse wave is greatly altered by transmission through the arterial tree, and certain abnormalities may be much more easily detected at one site than another.

Sinus arrhythmia results from the normal physiological changes in heart rate during inspiration and expiration due to changes in vagal tone. On inspiration, the heart rate quickens; on expiration, the pulse rate slows. Absence of this variation is a feature of autonomic neuropathy.

Pulsus paradoxus is the term applied when the pulse is felt to reduce in volume on inspiration. During the respiratory cycle, the intrathoracic pressure becomes more negative as the lungs expand during inspiration. As a direct result, blood pools in the pulmonary vessels, and the filling of the left ventricle is reduced (see 'Applied anatomy and physiology of the heart', page 33). Although this pressure difference can be palpated, it is usually quantified by measuring the difference in systolic blood pressure that occurs between inspiration and expiration. This is done by deflating the sphygmomanometer cuff very slowly and listening to the sounds appearing and disappearing as the level of mercury falls.

This reduction of left ventricular stroke volume can be exaggerated, as in pericardial tamponade or asthma, and is detectable by palpating the peripheral pulses or when measuring the blood pressure. The pulse volume feels less on inspiration and greater on expiration (the 'paradox').

## Peripheral arterial pulse examination

See 'Examination of the arterial system', page 75.

## Jugular venous pressure

In assessing the jugular venous pressure (JVP), the cervical veins form a blood-filled manometer connected to the right atrium and, as such, can be used at the bedside to measure the mean right atrial pressure (central venous pressure, CVP). In addition, the cervical veins can provide information about the wave form in the right atrium.

## BOX 2.3 MONITORING THE JVP

The internal jugular vein should be inspected with the patient resting on a pillow at 45° (**Fig. 2.4**). It is sometimes helpful to direct a light onto the root of the neck. Gentle pressure over the right upper quadrant of the abdomen (liver area) causes the JVP to become more obvious. This may be a useful aid to make the venous pressure more evident at the bedside. Venous pulsations can be distinguished from arterial pulsations in the neck in the following way:

- They are usually abolished by gentle pressure on the veins at the root of the neck.
- They often vary with respiration and can be made to rise by firm pressure over the upper abdomen.
- A rapid flickering and inward movement is the usual component, whereas arterial pulsations are typically outward pulses.

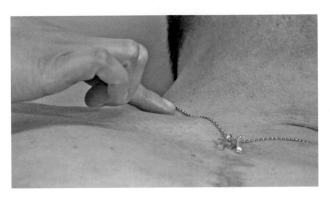

Fig. 2.4 Inspect the JVP with the patient resting at an angle of 45°.

Whenever possible, the right internal jugular vein is used for the assessment because it is in direct communication with the superior vena cava (SVC) and the right atrium – the pressure in the left internal jugular vein may be raised spuriously as a consequence of partial obstruction of the innominate vein by the arch of the aorta. Observation of the JVP is a difficult skill, so has been covered in some detail here. It is easier to see if you know what you are looking for!

The mean level of the venous pressure should be measured with reference to the sternal angle (**Fig. 2.5**). Generally, it is at the level of the angle – if it is 3 cm or more above this with the patient at 45°, the pressure is definitely raised (**Fig. 2.6**).

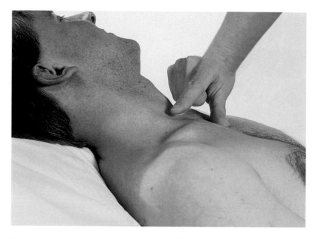

Fig. 2.5 Measure the venous pressure with reference to the sternal angle.

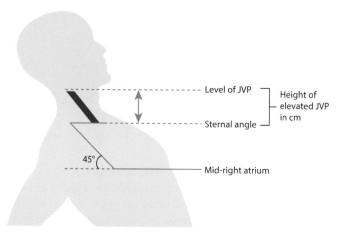

Fig. 2.6 The level of the JVP in relation to the sternal angle.

Conditions associated with a raised JVP include heart failure, volume overload, cardiac tamponade, pericardial effusion and pulmonary hypertension.

A raised JVP reflects a raised end-diastolic pressure in the right ventricle. If the JVP is grossly elevated but the cervical veins show no pulsation, obstruction of the SVC should be suspected.

It is often possible to identify the 'a' and 'v' waves of the normal venous pulse. The waves of the venous pulse are most easily identified by timing them against the carotid pulse, which provides a convenient indication of ventricular systole. They may occur either just before the carotid pulse (= 'a' waves, pre-systole) or approximately at the same time as the carotid pulse (= 'v' wave, systole) (**Fig. 2.7**).

Abnormally large 'a' waves are associated with right ventricular hypertrophy and tricuspid stenosis. The 'a' wave is absent in atrial fibrillation.

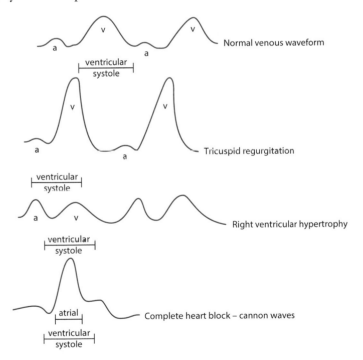

Fig. 2.7 Venous waveforms seen in the JVP in normal tricuspid regurgitation, right ventricular hypertrophy and complete heart block.

Abnormally large systolic 'v' waves may be caused by tricuspid regurgitation with reflux of blood during systole from the right ventricle.

Cannon wave results from contraction of the atrium against a closed tricuspid valve in complete heart block.

## Measuring the blood pressure

Blood pressure is recorded by writing the systolic pressure over the diastolic pressure with some notation of the position of the patient (*Table 2.5*). A normal blood pressure is approximately as shown. Because automated devices may not measure blood pressure accurately if there is pulse irregularity (e.g. due to atrial fibrillation), it is important to palpate the radial or brachial pulse before measuring the blood pressure. If pulse irregularity is present, you should measure the blood pressure manually using direct auscultation over the brachial artery.

## Table 2.5 Blood pressure

| | |
|---|---|
| 120/80 mmHg | Lying |
| 115/80 mmHg | Standing |

### BOX 2.4 MEASURING THE BLOOD PRESSURE (VIDEO 2.2)

The sphygmomanometer cuff should be smoothly applied around the patient's unclothed upper arm (**Fig. 2.8**), with the left hand supporting the patient's arm. If the arm is exceptionally thick or thin (e.g. extreme obesity, or in children), the standard cuff will give inaccurate readings and one appropriate for the arm size must be used. Modern cuffs use Velcro to secure them. Make sure you put it on with the airbag underneath, or the cuff will come apart when you blow it up.

- Once the cuff is in position, close the screw valve and pump it up to a level above your estimation of the systolic blood pressure (approximately 130 mmHg).

*(Continued)*

## BOX 2.4 (*Continued*)  MEASURING THE BLOOD PRESSURE

- As the pressure in the sphygmomanometer cuff increases above the systolic pressure in the brachial artery, the artery is compressed, and the radial pulse becomes impalpable.
- As the pressure in the cuff is then gradually lowered, blood can force its way past the obstruction for part of the cardiac cycle, creating sounds that can be heard with the diaphragm of the stethoscope placed over the brachial artery (Korotkoff sounds). As the pressure in the cuff is further lowered, the Korotkoff sounds become louder and more ringing in nature, and then suddenly become muffled. Very shortly afterwards, the sounds usually disappear altogether.
- The point at which you first hear the sound is the systolic measurement; the diastolic blood pressure is conventionally measured as the point of disappearance of the sound. The pressure always varies to some extent, so it is acceptable to round the measurement off to the nearest 5 mmHg.
- It is good practice to check the systolic pressure approximately by palpation of the radial artery before applying the stethoscope; this helps you to confirm the reading you hear. When there is considerable beat-to-beat variation in pressure (as in atrial fibrillation), the average level of the systolic and diastolic pressure must be judged by ear.
- When the blood pressure is seriously reduced and it is difficult to hear the Korotkoff sounds, it may be easier to measure the systolic blood pressure by palpation, noting the value at which the pulse is felt first as the cuff is deflated – diastolic pressure cannot be recorded satisfactorily by palpation.
- In situations where it is impossible to record blood pressure in the arms, for example if there has been damage to both radial arteries from surgery, blood pressure can be measured in the leg with an appropriately sized cuff on the thigh and auscultation over the popliteal artery.
- Systolic blood pressure should not usually fall by more than 10 mmHg when the patient moves from lying to standing. A fall greater than this suggests either hypovolaemia or autonomic neuropathy.
- In a patient presenting with chest pain, lower blood pressure in the left arm than the right is suggestive of aortic dissection.

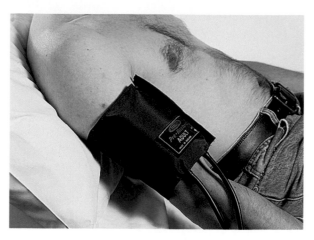

Fig. 2.8 The sphygmomanometer.

▶ VIDEO 2.2 Measuring the blood pressure

https://www.crcpress.com/cw/kopelman

## Inspection of the precordium

Inspection of the precordium is usually unhelpful; however, the apex beat is occasionally visible. It is also important to note any scars such as that of a mitral valvotomy under the left breast, or a sternal split for a valve replacement or coronary artery bypass graft.

## Palpation of the precordium

The apex beat is the point furthest to the left and downwards at which a definite cardiac impulse is felt; this should be located by palpation using the flat of the hand and the fingertips with the patient lying at 45°. A normal cardiac impulse is felt as a brief outward thrust; it usually lies within the fifth intercostal space and within the mid-clavicular line. If the apex beat is felt further out, it usually means there is enlargement of one or both ventricles, or displacement of the heart to the left by a chest deformity or disease of the lungs.

Now assess the quality of the impulse. A forceful apex beat usually indicates increased cardiac output: in left ventricular hypertrophy the apex beat is distinctive, with a sustained and forceful heave compared with the usual short, sharp impulse. In mitral stenosis, the apex beat is often described as tapping – this is due partly to displacement of the left ventricle nearer to the examining hand by an enlarged left ventricle, and partly to a palpable first heart sound.

Right ventricular hypertrophy is detected by firm pressure with the flat of your hand over the left sternal edge. In adults, the normal right ventricle does not produce a definite impulse, while in right ventricular hypertrophy a definite parasternal heave may be felt. Occasionally, the right ventricle enlarges anteriorly to replace the left ventricle in forming the apex of the heart. It is important to confirm the impulse felt by using bimanual examination, placing the flat of the left hand against the sternal border with the right hand feeling the apical impulse – two separate impulses are detectable where both ventricles are enlarged. During palpation of the precordium, thrills may be felt: these are the low-frequency components of loud murmurs that are more easily confirmed by auscultation.

## Percussion

In the examination of the cardiovascular system, it is not usually helpful to percuss over the precordium, except to locate the position of the mediastinum. This is useful in cases where it may be displaced, for example chronic airflow limitation or right lung collapse. If you do not suspect mediastinal shift from the history or the tracheal position, do not percuss the position of the mediastinum.

## Auscultation

The stethoscope has two principal functions: to transmit sounds from the chest wall with exclusion of extraneous noises, and to emphasise the sounds of certain frequencies. The bell of the stethoscope is best for listening to low-pitched sounds, whereas the diaphragm filters out low-pitched sounds and accentuates high-pitched ones. You should initially listen with the bell and diaphragm at the apex (**Fig. 2.9**) for the low-pitched diastolic murmur of mitral stenosis and the pansystolic murmur of mitral regurgitation. Then, using the diaphragm, listen

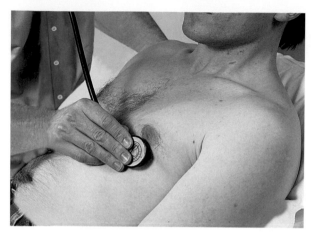

Fig. 2.9 Listen with the bell at the apex.

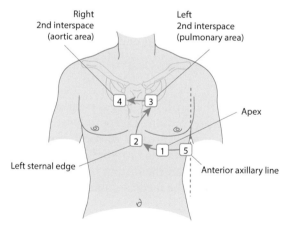

Fig. 2.10 Classical areas for listening to heart sounds.

over the classical areas shown in **Fig. 2.10**. These are the left sternal edge (for tricuspid murmurs) (**Fig. 2.11**), the left second interspace (for pulmonary murmurs) (**Fig. 2.12**) and the right second interspace (for aortic murmurs) (**Fig. 2.13**).

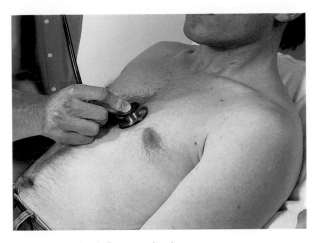

Fig. 2.11 Listening at the left sternal edge.

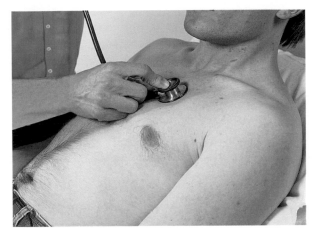

Fig. 2.12 Listening at the left second interspace.

## Heart sounds

It is impossible to listen critically to more than one sound at any one time, so try to train yourself to listen for single components of the heart sounds.

**First heart sound** This is produced mainly by mitral and tricuspid valve closure, and caused by the sudden tensing of the valve as it

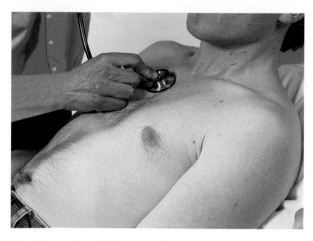

Fig. 2.13 Listening at the right second interspace.

halts after ballooning back into the atrium at the beginning of systole. The loudness of mitral closure, which is usually the main component of the first heart sound, depends on the force with which it is thrust back into the atrium, and this may be altered, for example in mitral stenosis. The length of the interval between atrial and ventricular systole also influences the loudness of the first heart sound. The sound is loudest when the PR interval is short. A soft first heart sound is characteristic of severe mitral stenosis due to the restricted mobility of the mitral valve. A loud first heart sound is heard in pulmonary hypertension, generally as a result of pulmonary veno-occlusive disease.

**Second heart sound** This is produced by closure of the aortic and pulmonary valves. If the valve cusps lose their mobility, as in calcific aortic stenosis, the sound produced at the affected valve is reduced and may be completely lost. The second heart sound splits into two components during inspiration, and these come together in expiration. This physiological splitting is due to minor changes in the stroke volume of the left and right ventricles during the normal respiratory cycle. During inspiration, the venous return to the right side of the heart is increased, thus increasing the right ventricular stroke volume and delaying closure of the pulmonary valve. At the same time, pooling of the blood in the pulmonary veins reduces the filling of the left ventricle and makes aortic valve closure slightly earlier than in expiration. This process is reversed in expiration (**Fig. 2.14**). The split may be widened by other factors that delay right ventricular contraction; examples are listed in **Fig. 2.15**.

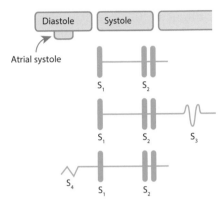

Fig. 2.14 The relationship between heart sounds and diastole and systole; the lower portion of the figure denotes the usual way to record heart sounds.

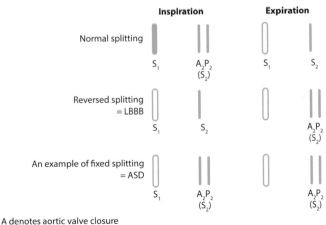

A denotes aortic valve closure
P denotes pulmonary valve closure

Fig. 2.15 Abnormal splitting of the second heart sound. ASD = atrial septal defect; LBBB = left bundle branch block.

**Third and fourth heart sounds** A third heart sound is usually a low-frequency sound best heard with the bell and occurring just after the second heart sound. It is caused by sudden distension of the ventricle at the end of the rapid filling phase in early diastole. A soft third heart sound may be heard at the apex in most normal children and adults less than 30 years of age: in older people it is abnormal and signifies unusually abrupt filling of the ventricle. This may arise from an abnormally large stroke volume or from increased ventricular filling pressure due to left ventricular failure (LVF).

A fourth heart sound is also a low-frequency sound. It is best heard immediately before the first heart sound and signifies that atrial systole is abnormally forceful. The presence of an atrial (fourth) sound implies that the end-diastolic pressure is raised in the ventricle concerned, for example in the left ventricle in systemic hypertension.

**Gallop rhythm** A gallop rhythm means that there are three heart sounds to the cycle, and that the extra one is either a third sound or an atrial (fourth) sound. The noises heard sound rather like Kentucky ('ken-tuc-kee'). At rapid heart rates, the third heart sound and atrial sounds may coincide, and a summation gallop is then heard – the noise suggests Tennessee ('ten-nes-see'). In clinical practice, this suggests impaired ventricular function.

The usual way to record heart sounds is shown in **Fig. 2.15**.

### BOX 2.5 FACTORS THAT MAY CAUSE MURMURS

- Increased velocity of flow.
- Localised constriction of the lumen through which the blood is flowing, with turbulence developing where the lumen widens out again.
- Roughening of a surface past which the blood is flowing (e.g. atheromatous plaque).
- Decreased viscosity of the blood.

## Murmurs

Cardiac murmurs result either from abnormal turbulence of blood flow or from vibrations in structures adjacent to an area of turbulent flow.

Factors favouring the development of turbulence giving rise to murmurs are shown above. Commonly, more than one of these factors is involved.

When a murmur is heard, it is essential to note:

- The site of maximum intensity and the direction of radiation.
- The timing of the murmur.
- The loudness.
- The quality – is it high- or low-pitched, or musical?
- The presence or absence of a palpable thrill.

**Timing of the murmur**  A murmur produced at a particular valve has a characteristic timing, as it may only occur when there is a pressure gradient across the valve. Timing of the murmur is of great help in its recognition. In relation to timing, it is important to decide whether the murmur occurs in systole or diastole – if there is doubt, the murmur should be timed against the carotid pulse. The timing of the murmur is then analysed in relation to the heart sounds. The usual sites and radiation of the common cardiac murmurs are shown in **Fig. 2.16**.

**Systolic murmurs**  Systolic murmurs are due to one of three factors:

1  **Pansystolic murmur:** leakage of blood through a valve structure that is usually closed during systole. The intensity of the murmur is therefore very similar throughout the length of systole.
2  **Ejection systolic murmur:** the flow through a valve that is usually open in systole but that has become abnormally narrowed. The murmur typically starts quietly, rises to a crescendo in mid-systole, and then becomes quiet towards the end of systole.
3  **Increased blood flow through a normal valve:** a physiological flow murmur; the character is identical to that heard in an ejection systolic murmur.

A mid-systolic click is heard shortly after the first heart sound, with radiation to the axilla. It is best heard with the diaphragm of the stethoscope over the apex with the patient in the left lateral position.

| Timing | Shape | Area best heard | Common cause |
|---|---|---|---|
| Ejection systolic | $S_1 \diamond S_2$ | Aortic radiating to carotid | Aortic stenosis |
| | | Pulmonary area, louder with inspiration | Pulmonary stenosis |
| Pansystolic | $S_1 \Box S_2$ | Apex radiating to left axilla | Mitral regurgitation |
| | | Fourth intercostal space at left sternal edge to right sternal edge, increasing with inspiration | Tricuspid regurgitation |
| | | Fourth to fifth intercostal spaces | VSD |
| Late systolic | $S_1 \triangleleft S_2$ | Apex radiating to left axilla | Mitral valve prolapse |
| Early diastolic | $S_1 \quad S_2 \triangleright$ | Left sternal edge (aortic area) | Aortic regurgitation |
| | | Pulmonary area on full inspiration | Pulmonary regurgitation |
| Mid-to-late diastolic | os $\diamond S_1 \quad S_2$ | Mitral area with patient in left decubitus position (os = opening snap) | Mitral stenosis |
| | | Fourth intercostal space at lower left sternal edge | Tricuspid stenosis |
| Continuous | Machinery like | Left upper chest | Patent ductus |

Fig. 2.16 Sites and radiation of the common cardiac murmurs.

The click corresponds to the sudden tensing of the chordae tendinae of the mitral valve that results from mitral valve prolapse.

A 'trap' in haemodialysis patients with an arteriovenous fistula for dialysis access is radiation of the bruit from the fistula to the precordium, mimicking a systolic murmur.

**Diastolic murmurs** Diastolic murmurs can be divided into early diastolic and mid-diastolic (see **Box 2.6**). An explanation for the murmurs associated with mitral stenosis, mitral incompetence, aortic stenosis and aortic incompetence is shown in **Fig. 2.16**.

## BOX 2.6 IDENTIFYING DIASTOLIC MURMURS

- An **early diastolic murmur** is nearly always caused by incompetence of either the aortic or the pulmonary valve. It is maximum at the beginning of diastole when aortic or pulmonary pressure is highest, and rapidly becomes quieter as the pressure falls. The murmur of aortic incompetence can be amplified by getting the patient to sit forward, placing the diaphragm of the stethoscope over the left sternal edge, and then asking the patient to hold their breath at the end of expiration (**Fig. 2.17**). Remember to give them permission to stop holding their breath when you have listened to the sounds. The sound can be difficult to separate from the second heart sound and can be thought of as an 'absence of silence' immediately after the second sound.

- A **mid-diastolic murmur** is usually the result of blood flow through a narrowed mitral or tricuspid valve, and the murmur is characteristically low-pitched and 'rumbling', and audible throughout the remainder of diastole. A mid-diastolic murmur may be made more obvious by having the patient lie on their left side, and for you to listen with the bell of the stethoscope over the apex.

In tricuspid regurgitation, the murmur characteristically gets louder on inspiration and is best heard over the left sternal edge in the fourth intercostal space.

The murmur of a ventricular septal defect (VSD) is a high-pitched pansystolic murmur, best heard in the fourth to sixth intercostal spaces, that does not radiate to the axilla and does not alter with inspiration.

**Pericardial rub** is a grating or scratching sound heard on auscultation throughout the cardiac cycle that is associated with pericarditis.

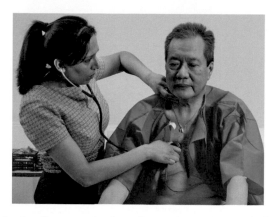

Fig. 2.17 Listening for an early diastolic aortic murmur with the patient sitting forward having exhaled and held their breath.

## Examination of the chest and ankles

It is important to sit the patient forward at the end of the examination of the cardiovascular system to examine the lung bases for crackles and/or a pleural effusion. The ankles must also be examined for evidence of pitting oedema – press firmly over the tibia, and see whether an indentation remains after the finger has been removed (**Fig. 2.18**). If the patient has been bed-bound for any length of time, peripheral oedema may have moved from the ankles to the sacrum, which can be palpated while the patient is sitting forward for examination of the lung bases.

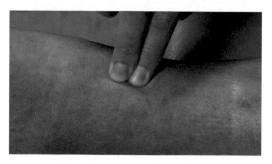

Fig. 2.18 Firm pressure of the fingers above the ankle shows indentation of the soft tissue indicative of oedema.

## Illustrated physical signs

**LVF or pulmonary oedema** is characterised by shadowing on the chest X-ray (CXR) in a bat's wing distribution (**Fig. 2.19**).

Peripheral oedema (**Fig. 2.20**) is also a sign of predominantly right-sided heart failure. There may be indentation after the examiner has removed their finger from the surface of the tibia after applying mild pressure.

A patient with **ischaemic heart disease** may have an arcus senilis in the eye, suggesting a chronically high level of plasma cholesterol (**Fig. 2.21**).

The examination findings in a normal patient are shown in *Table 2.6.* Important aspects of care of the cardiovascular patient are shown in *Table 2.7.*

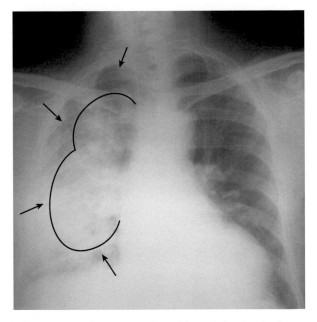

Fig. 2.19 Pulmonary oedema on a chest X-ray (a bat's wing), more pronounced on the right.

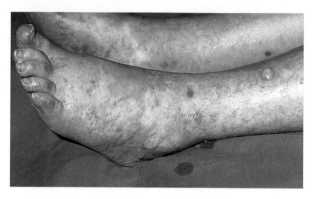

Fig. 2.20 Peripheral oedema with blistering.

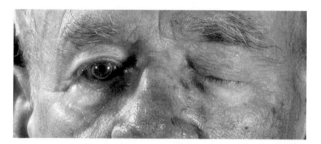

Fig. 2.21 Arcus senilis in a patient with ischaemic heart disease.

## Table 2.6 Normal cardiovascular examination

| | |
|---|---|
| *Hands and face* | No cyanosis, pallor, clubbing, etc. |
| *Pulses* | Radial, brachial, carotid: normal character, sinus rhythm, normal volume, rate 60–90 bpm |
| | No audible bruits over arterial pulses |
| *JVP* | Visible at the sternal angle or 2 cm above, with visible 'a' and 'v' waves |
| *Apex beat* | In the fifth intercostal space, mid-clavicular line |
| | No thrills or heaves |

*(Continued)*

## Table 2.6 (*Continued*)  Normal cardiovascular examination

| | |
|---|---|
| *Heart sounds* | Normal $S_1$ followed by physiologically split $S_2$ and no added sounds |
| *Lung bases* | No crackles |
| *Ankles* | No ankle oedema<br>No sacral oedema |
| *Blood pressure* | Do not forget to check the blood pressure yourself<br>Normal systolic pressure is usually 100–150 mmHg, but depends on the person's age<br>Normal diastolic pressure is usually 70–90 mmHg, but depends on the person's age |

## Table 2.7  Care of the patient with cardiovascular disease

- Appreciate the patient's anxiety
- Bed rest – use a cardiac bed (resting until pain-free in MI/angina)
- Keep the patient sitting up in bed at 45° or on at least 3–4 pillows (to prevent dyspnoea)
- No added salt in the diet (to minimise water retention)
- Oxygen always available (to maximise tissue oxygenation)
- Think about anticoagulation (many patients may require this)
- Cardiac monitoring may be necessary (to check arrhythmias)
- May need daily weight check if in heart failure (best indication of fluid retention)
- Frequent ECG monitoring

## Therapeutic and interventional skills

An electrocardiogram (ECG) and a CXR are two important investigations that are required to complete the clinical assessment of the cardiovascular system.

### The ECG

The ECG must be used as part of the diagnostic process alongside the clinical history. If the history is suggestive of a MI, the patient should be treated as if they are having an infarct, even if the ECG is normal. A patient with chest pain and a normal ECG may be in the very early

---

### BOX 2.7  PERFORMING AN ECG (VIDEO 2.3)

Before taking the ECG recorder to the patient, make sure you have all the parts. These are shown in *Table 2.8*. Explain the procedure to the patient: 'I am going to do an electrical recording of your heart; it is not painful, and should only take a couple of minutes'. Check that the patient agrees (gives verbal consent) to the tracing.

---

### ▶ VIDEO 2.3 Recording an ECG

https://www.crcpress.com/cw/kopelman

---

### Table 2.8  The ECG machine

| Four limb leads | Right arm | RED |
|---|---|---|
| | Left arm | YELLOW |
| | Right leg | GREEN |
| | Left leg | BLACK |
| One chest lead | Six sticky or suction electrodes | |
| Electrode jelly | (Alcohol swabs will do) | |

stages of a MI; this is when there is the greatest risk of death. In a patient with chest pain, it may be necessary for the ECG to be repeated later in the day to see if there have been any changes. The ECG pattern is recorded in a single lead during one heartbeat. Each individual pattern is called an ECG complex; its components are shown in **Fig. 2.22**. (An example of the evolution of the changes in an ECG during an MI is shown in **Fig. 2.23**.)

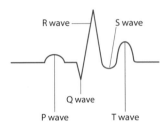

Fig. 2.22 ECG pattern of a single heartbeat in a single lead. P = atrial depolarisation; QRS = ventricular depolarisation; T = repolarisation.

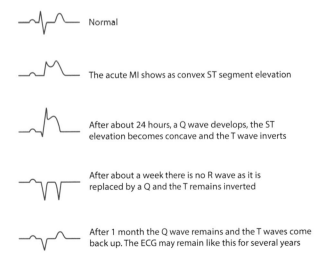

Normal

The acute MI shows as convex ST segment elevation

After about 24 hours, a Q wave develops, the ST elevation becomes concave and the T wave inverts

After about a week there is no R wave as it is replaced by a Q and the T remains inverted

After 1 month the Q wave remains and the T waves come back up. The ECG may remain like this for several years

Fig. 2.23 ECG changes over time following an MI. Note: it is possible to tell where the MI is located by noting which leads show the features most clearly (e.g. II, III and AVF reflect inferior damage).

**Interpretation of the ECG (Video 2.4)**  When examining the trace, remember that the different leads of the ECG are looking at the heart from different directions. These directions are in a sagittal plane for the limb leads and a coronal plane for the V leads (**Fig. 2.24**). This allows you to work out where an abnormality is coming from. If the trace is abnormal in leads II, III and AVF, the problem is inferior, as in **Fig. 2.23**; if the trace is abnormal in leads I, AVL and V6, the problem is lateral and on the left.

It is useful to develop a system for interpreting the trace to ensure that nothing is overlooked. A practical system is outlined in *Table 2.9*.

▶ VIDEO 2.4 Interpreting an ECG

https://www.crcpress.com/cw/kopelman

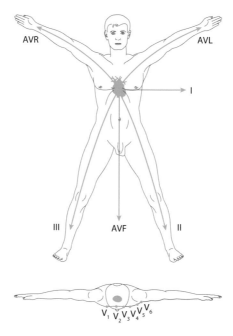

Fig. 2.24 The ECG leads, looking at the heart from different directions.

## Table 2.9 ECG interpretation

| | |
|---|---|
| *Rate* | Count the number of 5 mm squares between the R waves, and divide this into 300 to give the beats per minute (bpm) |
| *Rhythm* | Is it regular? Are P waves followed by a QRS? |
| *Axis* | Look at two perpendicular leads (e.g. I and AVF), and count the number of squares – the tallest R wave indicates the main line of depolarisation (axis) |
| *Complexes* | The P wave and PR interval |
| | The QRS complex |
| | The T wave |

## Key laboratory tests

In angina and the early stages of an MI, the haemoglobin and white blood cell values are normal. As an infarction evolves, there may be a neutrophil leucocytosis, although this settles as the condition settles.

**Cardiac enzymes** A diagnosis of acute coronary syndrome is supported by the measurement of changes in the blood concentration of cardiac troponin.

**Chest X-ray** A good quality postero-anterior (PA) X-ray of the chest will provide considerable information about both the heart and the lung fields. The cardiac silhouette in the PA view usually appears as shown in **Fig. 2.25**.

The right border of the normal cardiac shadow consists of:

• A slightly curved portion = outer edge of the SVC with the ascending aorta.
• A more convex portion = outer border of the right atrium, the lower margin of which lies at the diaphragm.

The left border of the cardiac shadow comprises:

• A prominent knuckle produced by the arch of the aorta as it passes backwards.

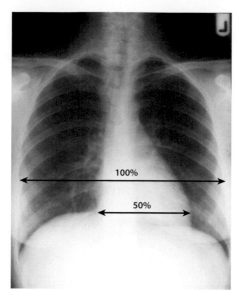

Fig. 2.25 A normal PA chest X-ray.

- A straighter line of the pulmonary artery.
- The left atrial appendage.
- The wide sweep of the left ventricle, ending at the apex where it rests on the diaphragm.

The site of the heart as a whole can be assessed by measuring the cardiothoracic index – the ratio of the maximum width of the cardiac silhouette to the maximum width of the thorax, measured from rib to rib (**Fig. 2.25**). The ratio can only be assessed on a PA film. In normal circumstances, it is less than 50%. Enlargement of the left ventricle and right atrium are usually easily identified. Enlargement of the left atrium is often seen as an area of added density within the cardiac outline.

The following illustrations depict the key features of common cardiovascular conditions: ischaemic heart disease (**Fig. 2.26**), mitral incompetence (**Fig. 2.27**), mitral stenosis (**Fig. 2.28**), aortic stenosis (**Fig. 2.29**), aortic incompetence (**Fig. 2.30**) and pulmonary emboli (**Fig. 2.31**).

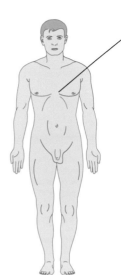

**History**

Crushing chest pain generally relieved by rest in angina but not in MI

**Examination findings**

The patient may be in pain

There is usually little to find but look for evidence of risk factors – tar stains, xanthelasma, corneal arcus

Always measure the blood pressure and examine the fundi for hypertensive changes

There may be evidence of peripheral vascular disease

Examine the peripheral pulses

Fig. 2.26 Ischaemic heart disease.

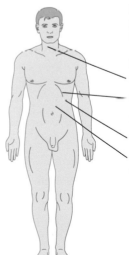

**History**

Symptoms of biventricular (congestive) cardiac failure. May present acutely as LVF

**Examination findings**

JVP raised in biventricular failure and tricuspid incompetence

Left parasternal heave. Apex beat displaced towards the axilla

Pansystolic murmur radiates to the axilla

Fine basal crepitations in LVF

Enlarged liver in biventricular failure; may be pulsatile if there is associated tricuspid regurgitation

Blood pressure may be normal or low

May be a low-volume pulse

Fig. 2.27 Mitral incompetence.

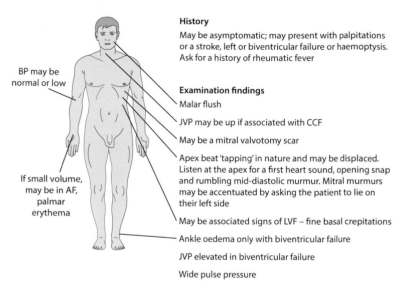

### History

May be asymptomatic; may present with palpitations or a stroke, left or biventricular failure or haemoptysis. Ask for a history of rheumatic fever

BP may be normal or low

### Examination findings

Malar flush

JVP may be up if associated with CCF

May be a mitral valvotomy scar

Apex beat 'tapping' in nature and may be displaced. Listen at the apex for a first heart sound, opening snap and rumbling mid-diastolic murmur. Mitral murmurs may be accentuated by asking the patient to lie on their left side

If small volume, may be in AF, palmar erythema

May be associated signs of LVF – fine basal crepitations

Ankle oedema only with biventricular failure

JVP elevated in biventricular failure

Wide pulse pressure

Fig. 2.28 Mitral stenosis. AF = atrial fibrillation; BP = blood pressure; CCF = congestive cardiac failure.

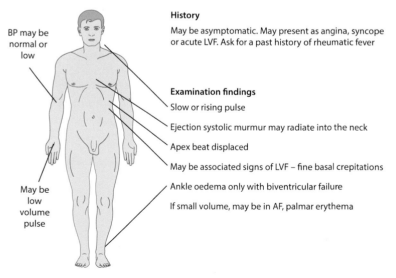

### History

May be asymptomatic. May present as angina, syncope or acute LVF. Ask for a past history of rheumatic fever

BP may be normal or low

### Examination findings

Slow or rising pulse

Ejection systolic murmur may radiate into the neck

Apex beat displaced

May be associated signs of LVF – fine basal crepitations

Ankle oedema only with biventricular failure

May be low volume pulse

If small volume, may be in AF, palmar erythema

Fig. 2.29 Aortic stenosis. AF = atrial fibrillation; BP = blood pressure.

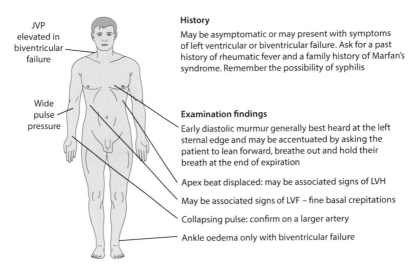

JVP elevated in biventricular failure

Wide pulse pressure

### History

May be asymptomatic or may present with symptoms of left ventricular or biventricular failure. Ask for a past history of rheumatic fever and a family history of Marfan's syndrome. Remember the possibility of syphilis

### Examination findings

Early diastolic murmur generally best heard at the left sternal edge and may be accentuated by asking the patient to lean forward, breathe out and hold their breath at the end of expiration

Apex beat displaced: may be associated signs of LVH

May be associated signs of LVF – fine basal crepitations

Collapsing pulse: confirm on a larger artery

Ankle oedema only with biventricular failure

Fig. 2.30 Aortic incompetence. LVH = left ventricular hypertrophy.

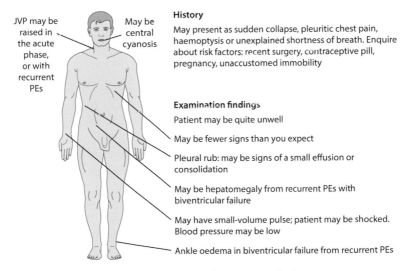

JVP may be raised in the acute phase, or with recurrent PEs

May be central cyanosis

### History

May present as sudden collapse, pleuritic chest pain, haemoptysis or unexplained shortness of breath. Enquire about risk factors: recent surgery, contraceptive pill, pregnancy, unaccustomed immobility

### Examination findings

Patient may be quite unwell

May be fewer signs than you expect

Pleural rub: may be signs of a small effusion or consolidation

May be hepatomegaly from recurrent PEs with biventricular failure

May have small-volume pulse; patient may be shocked. Blood pressure may be low

Ankle oedema in biventricular failure from recurrent PEs

Fig. 2.31 Pulmonary emboli. PEs = pulmonary emboli.

## THE ARTERIAL SYSTEM

Disease of the arteries may conveniently be divided into dilating disease (aneurysms) and occlusive disease (blocked arteries). Aneurysms may be divided into true aneurysms and false (or pseudo-) aneurysms. Blockage of the arteries can most usefully be divided into acute and chronic.

A true aneurysm is a localised dilatation of an artery resulting from a degenerative process in its wall. The combination of the degenerative process and the pressure of blood pulsating within the artery means that dilatation is progressive and the affected artery may ultimately rupture, with life- or limb-threatening consequences. A false aneurysm is effectively a hole in the wall of an artery communicating with a cavity whose wall is made up of connective tissue surrounding the artery and thrombus. Nowadays, most false aneurysms are iatrogenic in origin, resulting from arterial punctures made by radiologists, cardiologists, surgeons or anaesthetists for diagnostic or therapeutic purposes; they may also result from penetrating injuries (stabbings, shootings, shrapnel injuries, etc.). The term 'dissecting aneurysm' (of the aorta) is sometimes encountered, but this is a misnomer. An aortic dissection is a split that develops in the media of the vessel. Although dilatation may result, the pathology, natural history and treatment of aortic dissection are different from those of true aneurysm formation.

Chronic arterial narrowing (stenosis) or blockage (occlusion) is almost invariably the result of atherosclerosis, and develops slowly and insidiously. Acute arterial occlusion may also result from atherosclerotic disease, but in a minority of cases it is due to embolism, and in a smaller minority, due to trauma. An embolism is solid matter, almost always thrombus, that has formed at one site in the cardiovascular system, has broken free and has travelled in the bloodstream until it has reached vessels that are too small to allow its onward passage; here it causes a blockage. The most common source of peripheral embolisation is the left atrium, in patients who have atrial fibrillation, which is why most patients with atrial fibrillation are prophylactically anticoagulated. Aneurysms are also liable to accumulate thrombus within them, and this may embolise distally.

Arterial stenosis and occlusions result in ischaemia of (lack of blood supply to) the downstream tissues. The resulting symptoms are much more dramatic, and more likely to lead to loss of life or limb, following an acute, as opposed to a chronic, arterial occlusion.

## Applied anatomy and physiology of the arterial system

The most common site for an aneurysm to develop is in the infrarenal abdominal aorta, with or without extension to the common iliac arteries. The second most common site is one or other popliteal artery, with the common femoral artery coming third. Aneurysms of the ascending and descending thoracic aorta are less common, and aneurysms elsewhere are uncommon.

The complications of aneurysms are principally rupture, distal embolisation and thrombosis. Abdominal aortic aneurysms (AAAs) larger than 5.5 cm in diameter carry a substantial risk of rupture, occasionally embolise (causing acute leg ischaemia) but virtually never thrombose. Popliteal aneurysms rarely rupture but commonly embolise to the calf arteries and may thrombose, giving rise to acute limb ischaemia. The behaviour of femoral aneurysms falls somewhere between that of aortic and of popliteal aneurysms.

Chronic atheromatous arterial narrowing, which may ultimately lead to arterial occlusion, most commonly affects the superficial femoral artery, quite frequently affects the iliac arteries and may also affect the calf arteries (see **Fig. 2.39**, page 85). It is also common in the carotid arteries, especially at the origins of the internal carotid arteries, and is responsible for about 30% of all strokes. It is remarkably uncommon in the upper limb arteries and visceral arteries.

Slow and insidious atherosclerotic narrowing of the arteries leads to a gradual diminution of the blood supply to the tissues distally. If mild, this may not give rise to any symptoms. It most commonly presents as intermittent claudication: muscle pain felt in the calf or thigh or buttock brought on by walking and relieved by rest. As the disease progresses, the patient may experience pain even at rest, in the foot: ischaemic rest pain. Patients with severe peripheral arterial disease are at risk of developing soft tissue necrosis, ulceration or gangrene, usually affecting the toes, feet or ankles. Patients with rest pain or tissue loss are at risk of minor or major limb amputation.

As major arteries narrow and block, other smaller arteries running in parallel with them tend to dilate, forming what may be regarded as a 'natural bypass' and to some degree mitigating the effect of the major vessel disease. This is known as the development of a collateral circulation. If arteries block suddenly, there is no time for a collateral circulation to develop, and the consequences are correspondingly more severe. Acute arterial blockage, whether due to atherosclerotic disease, embolism or trauma, therefore carries a much greater risk of limb loss than chronic stenosis or occlusion.

## Aneurysms

### Assessment and diagnosis of aneurysms

Aneurysms do not usually give rise to symptoms unless and until they rupture, embolise or thrombose. Most AAAs are discovered by chance, as a result of the patient undergoing abdominal imaging for unrelated symptoms. Others are now being detected by screening. In the UK, all men are now invited for AAA screening by ultrasound scanning on or around their 65th birthday. (Women are not screened because the incidence of AAA is eight times lower than in men.) Occasionally, a slim man will consult a doctor after noticing marked abdominal pulsation. Rupture of an AAA typically results in the sudden onset of abdominal and/or back pain followed by circulatory collapse. It carries an overall mortality of 80%.

Popliteal and femoral aneurysms may present as a pulsatile swelling behind the knee or in the groin. They may also present with claudication, as a result of embolisation of arteries distally, or as acute limb ischaemia.

#### Taking the history

**Presenting complaint** Most patients referred to a vascular surgeon with an AAA will have no idea, or only a sketchy idea, of why they have been referred. They are unlikely to have any symptoms referable to the aneurysm. A few report awareness of abdominal pulsation. Some will complain of abdominal or back pain but, unless these symptoms are very recent, they are likely to be 'non-specific' or due to some other condition.

**Past/concurrent medical history** Treatment of AAAs, whether by open surgical or endovascular means, is a major undertaking that carries significant risk. It is therefore essential to obtain a detailed history of all concurrent and significant past medical conditions, illnesses and operations. Some patients will prove to be so frail and/ or unwell that the risk of treating the aneurysm exceeds the risk of complications from it. Those who seem fit enough to be considered for treatment require assessment in a high-risk pre-admission clinic before a final decision regarding intervention is taken.

## Examination for aneurysms

Abdominal palpation is a very insensitive way of detecting AAAs – only about 30% of AAAs can be detected by palpation. This is because not only the abdominal wall, but also the omentum and intestines separate the aorta from the examiner's hands. In addition, obesity is common.

The left border of an aneurysm is invariably easier to palpate than the right. With the patient supine and the whole abdomen exposed, examination should begin with the examiner's right hand pressing downwards and medially on the left side of the patient's abdomen above the level of the umbilicus. The aorta bifurcates at the level of the umbilicus, so AAAs are situated in the epigastrium. Quite firm pressure is needed if an aneurysm is to be felt. Although this must be applied with consideration for the patient, the belief that an aneurysm can be ruptured by palpation is untrue.

Keeping their right hand in place, the examiner next presses firmly with the left hand downwards and medially on the right side of the patient's upper abdomen, so that the two hands approach each other like a pair of calipers (**Fig. 2.32**). It may then be possible to feel an aneurysm as a pulsatile swelling in the epigastrium and to judge its size. Detection of AAAs, and assessment of their size and extent, by clinical means is, however, unreliable. Any patient suspected of having an AAA requires cross-sectional imaging, initially with ultrasound and then with computed tomography (CT) in order to plan treatment.

Femoral aneurysms are generally easy to detect by palpation at the level of the groin crease. A popliteal aneurysm may be palpable as a pulsatile swelling behind the knee (see 'Pulse palpation', pages 76–81).

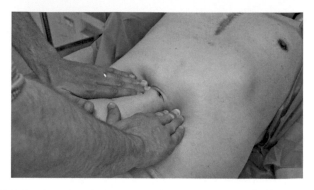

Fig. 2.32 Palpating the abdomen to detect aneurysmal dilatation.

## Care of the patient with an aneurysm

Patients with aneurysms require an explanation of what an aneurysm is and what the treatment options are. Drawing a simple diagram is likely to help. The risk of complications from aneurysms increases with increasing size; treatment is generally considered for AAAs measuring 5.5 cm or more, in order to prevent rupture. Smaller AAAs are kept under surveillance with serial ultrasound scans. Symptomatic popliteal and femoral aneurysms should be treated by exclusion bypass. Asymptomatic popliteal aneurysms are usually treated by exclusion bypass if they measure 2.5 cm in diameter or more, and femoral aneurysms if they measure 3 cm or more.

## Chronic arterial occlusive disease

### Assessment and diagnosis

Patients with mild chronic arterial occlusive disease may have no symptoms. Those who do develop symptoms usually present with intermittent claudication. The pain of intermittent claudication is most commonly felt in the calf muscles because the most common site for chronic arterial occlusive disease is the superficial femoral artery, which provides the blood supply to the calf; however, occlusive disease of the iliac arteries, or even the aorta, may give rise to claudication pain in the thighs or buttocks. Ischaemic rest pain is felt in the foot, is typically worst in bed at night, causes sleep deprivation and may make the patient hang the leg out of bed or get up and hobble about. Patients presenting with ulceration or soft tissue necrosis on the foot or ankle often have a history of claudication and/or rest pain. The onset of rest pain or tissue loss indicates that the survival of the limb is threatened.

## Taking the history

There are many causes of leg pain. Intermittent claudication is almost unique among them in that the patient does *not* have pain at rest, does *not* have pain on weight-bearing and does *not* even have pain walking very short distances, for instance from room to room. The pain only comes on, at a largely predictable distance, when the patient walks out of doors. It is, moreover, felt in *muscle*, and not bones, joints or ligaments, and it goes off *quickly* (within a minute or two) when the patient rests. The history must focus on determining whether or not these diagnostic criteria are fulfilled.

The principal risk factors for atherosclerotic arterial disease are smoking, diabetes, hypertension, high blood cholesterol and lipid levels and a family history of early-onset peripheral, coronary or carotid arterial disease. These risk factors should be enquired about systematically (although patients may not know what their cholesterol and lipid levels are). Details of all previous cardiovascular events, significant co-morbidities and medication should be obtained. The patient's social circumstances also need to be determined. The impact of intermittent claudication on quality of life and functional capacity, and therefore on the need for intervention, is greatly affected by such factors as the patient's type of work, level of support at home, need to climb stairs, access to a car and general fitness.

A very similar history needs to be taken from patients with suspected ischaemic rest pain or with tissue loss on the foot/ankle. Most of these patients will have a preceding history typical of intermittent claudication, but some who, for whatever reasons, have done very little walking for a considerable time may not. They are likely to have at least one and often several risk factors for atherosclerotic disease. The typical features of ischaemic rest pain, which should be enquired about, are described above.

## Examination of the arterial system

Upper limb arterial disease being uncommon, the section that follows describes examination of the arterial system in the legs. The same approach, with little adaptation, can be applied to the arms if necessary.

**Look** for signs of ischaemia. Ulceration or gangrene on the toes, feet or ankles is strongly suggestive of ischaemia. More subtle signs are pallor or cyanosis or dusky redness of the feet, especially if asymmetrical. Loss of hair from the legs is not a common or reliable finding. Chronic ischaemia does not typically cause peripheral oedema, although oedema may develop if the patient is very immobile.

If one or both feet are cyanosed or dusky red, it is useful to test for Buerger's sign. With the patient supine, elevate the leg(s) to about 45°. In the presence of severe arterial disease, the foot is likely to turn pale. Then ask the patient to sit on the edge of the couch with the feet dependent. In patients with severe arterial disease, the feet will slowly become dusky red. These colour changes result from loss of autoregulation of the microcirculation resulting from ischaemia, and do not occur in normal individuals.

**Feel** and compare the temperature of the feet. This does, of course, depend to some degree on the environmental temperature, but the foot on the patient's symptomatic side being cooler than its twin is a significant finding.

**Feel** for the pulses. Many medical students and many qualified doctors find pulse palpation difficult. It is, indeed, not straightforward and needs to be taught, learned and practised. It is common for inexperienced observers to fail to feel pulses that an experienced observer can easily detect. Much more worryingly, it is equally common for inexperienced observers to convince, or delude, themselves that they can feel pulses that are not, and could not possibly be, present. This is dangerous because it leads to a failure to diagnose ischaemia that may be limb-threatening. Limbs are lost on a regular basis because of false-positive pulse palpation and late diagnosis of limb-threatening ischaemia.

There is a simple rule that will protect against this grave error: 'If you can feel a pulse, you can count it; if you can't count it, you are not feeling it.' To add an extra layer of defence, check that the rate and rhythm of the pulse you have just counted are the same as those felt in the patient's radial or carotid artery.

Pulse palpation
See **Figs 2.33–2.38**.

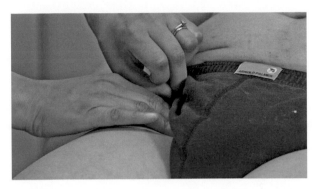

Fig. 2.33 Feeling the femoral pulse.

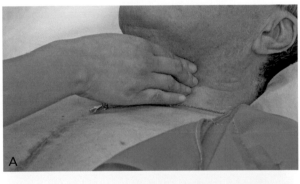

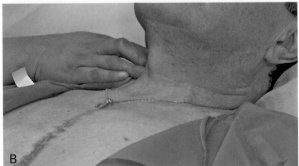

Fig. 2.34A, B Feeling the carotid pulse (**A**, left; **B**, right).

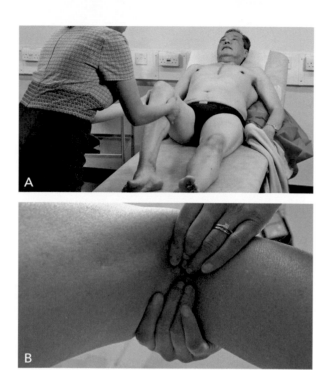

Fig. 2.35A, B Feeling the popliteal pulse.

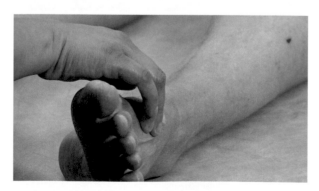

Fig. 2.36 Feeling the dorsalis pedis pulse.

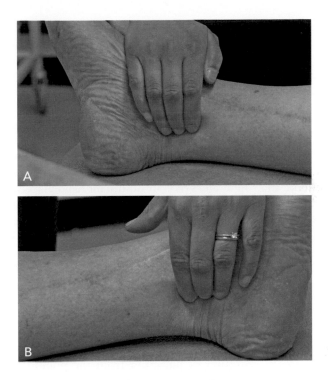

Fig. 2.37A, B Feeling the tibialis posterior pulse.

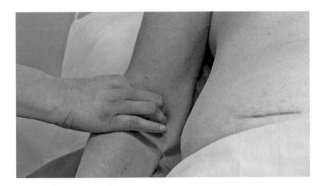

Fig. 2.38 Feeling the brachial pulse.

**The femoral pulse** Difficulty in feeling pulsation in the common femoral artery may result from patient obesity or from calcification of the artery, but it often results from seeking it too low down. Remember that the inguinal ligament lies parallel to but some 3 cm above the groin crease. The femoral pulse should be sought, with the patient supine, between the groin crease and the level of the inguinal ligament, not in the groin crease or below. The artery lies medial to the rectus femoris muscle and lateral to the medial border of the adductor muscles.

Even when the artery is not pulsatile, it is often palpable as a cylindrical structure akin to a stick of chalk. Feel for this structure with the index, middle and ring fingers of your dominant hand placed along the line of the artery, pushing upwards towards the inguinal ligament as you do so. You will probably need to increase and decrease the pressure you apply with your fingertips in order to detect the pulse. The right femoral pulse can usually be easily felt from the right-hand side of the bed or couch, but it may be more difficult to feel the left femoral pulse from there. If it is, and if you can get to the opposite side of the bed/couch, move there and feel for the left femoral pulse from that side.

**The popliteal pulse** This is generally the most difficult pulse to feel because it is deeply situated. Intervening soft tissues damp the pulsation, so the sensation of pulsation from the popliteal artery is more like a 'heave' than a 'tap'.

Flex the patient's knee by 5–10° to relax the muscles. Flexing the knee by more than this, however, makes the popliteal artery retreat deeper into the popliteal fossa and makes it more difficult to feel. Place one thumb either side of the tibial tuberosity, extend your fingers around both sides of the top of the calf, and feel for the popliteal pulse in the midline posteriorly, between the heads of the gastrocnemius muscle, compressing the artery against the top end of the tibia. (Pulses are always easier to feel if there is solid support behind them.) Use the index or middle finger of your dominant hand, supported by the equivalent finger of your non-dominant hand, to do this. You will have to squeeze quite hard, almost to the point of causing discomfort to the patient, in order to feel the pulse. Count the pulse, if you believe you have detected it, to prove to yourself that you really are feeling it.

**The dorsalis pedis pulse** This may be felt on the back of the foot about half way between the ankle and the bases of the toes, just lateral to the first metatarsal/extensor hallucis tendon. Rather light pressure is required here. If you press too hard, you will occlude the artery and it will therefore not pulsate. Count the pulse to prove to yourself that you really are feeling it.

**The tibialis posterior pulse** This may be felt behind the medial malleolus. Place your thumb on the lateral malleolus and extend your fingers across the front of the ankle. Use the index or middle fingertip to compress the soft tissues behind the medial malleolus, providing counterpressure with your thumb (a 'claw-like' grip). You may need to vary the site of palpation and the pressure applied a little in order to detect the pulse. Count the pulse to prove to yourself that you are feeling it.

## Care of patients with atherosclerotic peripheral vascular disease

There are three treatment options for patients with atherosclerotic arterial disease irrespective of where in the body it is detected: medical management, endovascular procedures and open surgical procedures. All patients should be given medical treatment as outlined in *Table 2.10*.

| Table 2.10 Medical management of atherosclerotic arterial disease | |
| --- | --- |
| *Smoking cessation* | The patient should be told of the strong causal link between smoking, their disease and its prognosis, and all possible help towards quitting should be given |
| *Diabetes control* | The link between diabetes and arterial disease should be explained, and all possible help should be given to obtain optimal control of the diabetes |
| *Hypertension* | The importance of good blood pressure control should be emphasised, and all possible help should be given to achieve this |
| *Weight loss* | Weight loss improves exercise tolerance and has a beneficial effect on other risk factors. This should be encouraged and support given if the patient is obese |

*(Continued)*

**Table 2.10 (*Continued*)  Medical management of atherosclerotic arterial disease**

| | |
|---|---|
| *Exercise* | Patients should be encouraged to go for regular walks, trying to increase the distance they can walk. Some medical centres offer physiotherapist-supervised walking classes |
| *Cholesterol/ lipid reduction* | Patients should be prescribed a statin, irrespective of their actual cholesterol and lipid levels, unless there is a strong contraindication |
| *Antiplatelet agents* | Patients should take an antiplatelet agent provided there is no contraindication |

## Acute limb ischaemia

Sudden blockage of a major limb artery may occur as a result of thrombosis against a background of atherosclerosis, embolism or trauma. It commonly results in limb-threatening ischaemia and constitutes a vascular surgical emergency. The symptoms and signs of acute limb ischaemia have since time immemorial been taught as six 'Ps': pain, pallor, pulselessness, paraesthesia, paralysis and 'perishing with cold'. Despite this, the diagnosis of acute limb ischaemia is frequently missed, or delayed until it is too late for the limb to be saved, resulting in avoidable limb loss. It is at first sight surprising that a condition with six characteristic symptoms and signs should so often be missed. The reasons for this include the following:

**Pain**  All patients with limb-threatening ischaemia have pain, which is often severe. There are, however, many causes of acute leg pain. Many failures to diagnose acute leg ischaemia result when this diagnosis is not considered. All patients, of any age, who present with acute leg pain must undergo a thorough assessment of the blood supply to the limb.

**Pallor**  Ischaemic limbs may be pale or cyanosed or dusky red or mottled. Often, however, the colour change is subtle and not necessarily noticeable under artificial light or behind blue curtains. Healthy patients may have pale extremities in cold environments. Discoloration is most likely to be noticed if the light is good and the foot on the symptomatic side is carefully compared with the opposite one. Buerger's sign (see page 76) may be present.

**Pulselessness**  Reference has been made above to the danger of false-positive pulse palpation. In patients with acute limb ischaemia in whom the diagnosis has been considered yet still missed, it is invariably the case that at least one health professional has purported to feel pulses that were not, and could not possibly have been, present.

**Paraesthesia**  This means abnormal sensations. Patients with acute limb ischaemia may have tingling sensations as well as pain, but usually they have reduced sensation. In the most severe or advanced cases, this amounts to frank numbness but, in less severe or earlier cases, the reduction in sensation may be mild and may be missed by a cursory assessment. Systematic testing of the sensory system to light touch and pin-prick, comparing the symptomatic limb with the opposite one, should be undertaken.

**Paralysis**  Ischaemia results in reduced muscular power and, ultimately, in total paralysis, but it may be subtle in milder or early cases. Doctors may attribute a patient's inability to demonstrate normal muscular power to pain rather than to ischaemia. They may fail to compare the muscular power in the symptomatic limb with the power in the opposite one.

**Perishing with cold**  Patients lying on trolleys in an emergency department or in other cold environments often have cold peripheries. It is not so much the absolute temperature of the symptomatic foot as the difference between its temperature and that of its twin that is important. Comparison of the temperature of the two feet is crucial.

The key to making the diagnosis of acute limb ischaemia and not missing it is, first of all, to consider the diagnosis in every patient presenting with acute limb pain and, second, to carry out a competent and thorough physical examination focusing on the six Ps. Assessment with a pocket Doppler machine may be helpful but only insofar as Doppler signals at the ankle are usually undetectable in patients with acute limb ischaemia.

## Care of the patient with acute limb ischaemia

At its most severe, acute limb ischaemia can result in death of the limb in as little as 6 hours. The diagnosis therefore needs to be made very quickly and the patient needs to be transferred immediately to specialist vascular surgical care.

# VARICOSE VEINS AND VENOUS INSUFFICIENCY

## Applied anatomy and physiology of the venous system in the legs

The anatomy of the venous system in the legs is shown in **Fig. 2.39**. It comprises: superficial veins, situated deep to the skin but superficial to the investing deep fascia (the long saphenous vein, the short saphenous vein and their tributaries); deep veins, situated deep to the deep fascia, between the muscles of the calf and thigh; and perforating veins, which link the superficial veins to the deep system. All these veins contain valves, which permit the flow of blood towards the heart but not in the opposite direction. The valves in perforating veins permit flow from superficial to deep.

The pressure in the leg veins is normally kept low by activity of the calf muscle pump. When the calf muscles contract, the deep veins are compressed and blood is propelled towards the heart. When the muscles relax, low pressure in the deep system encourages blood to move from superficial to deep via the perforating veins. Activity in the calf muscle pump is capable of reducing resting blood pressure in the foot veins from about 100 mmHg in an individual standing still to about 20 mmHg on exercise.

Failure of the calf muscle pump results in chronically raised pressure in the leg veins and may give rise to symptoms and signs of chronic venous insufficiency. Calf muscle pump failure is usually caused by (acquired) incompetence of the valves in the superficial venous system, deep venous system or both.

Varicose veins are dilated, tortuous, subcutaneous veins. They should be distinguished from other types of superficial venous blemish, such as thread veins, spider veins, telangiectases and intradermal venules. These conditions are of purely cosmetic significance and do not impair venous function.

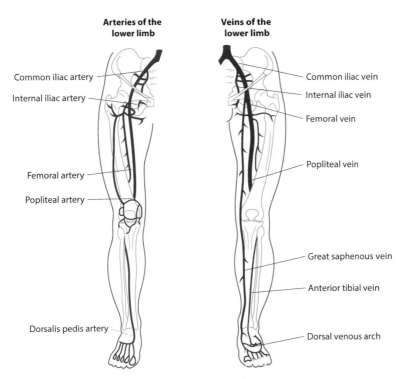

Fig. 2.39 The arterial and venous systems of the leg.

Varicose veins result from a degenerative process in vein walls that is, to a substantial degree, genetically determined. As veins dilate and become varicose, the cusps of the vein valves are liable to separate, rendering the valves incompetent and permitting retrograde flow of blood (reflux). Reflux may also develop in the deep venous system, but here it is usually a consequence of damage to the deep veins resulting from deep venous thrombosis (DVT). In about two-thirds of patients who suffer a DVT, the thrombus is more or less completely reabsorbed and venous function returns to normal. In one-third, the thrombus is converted into scar tissue, and this may render the vein valves incompetent, resulting in deep venous reflux.

In the presence of valvular incompetence in either system, blood that has been pumped up the leg during calf muscle contraction refluxes back down when the calf muscles relax, compromising the effectiveness of the calf muscle pump. It should be noted that the calf muscle pump is composed of both venous and muscular elements, and failure of either will give rise to chronic venous hypertension. Severe immobility (due to paresis, arthritis, obesity or other causes), as well as venous reflux, may thus be a cause of chronic venous insufficiency.

Chronic venous insufficiency may result in aching or heaviness of the affected leg(s), leg swelling, inflammation of the skin and subcutaneous tissues (varicose eczema) and, ultimately, leg ulceration.

## Assessment and diagnosis of varicose veins

### Taking the history

**Presenting complaint** Patients with varicose veins (**Fig. 2.40**) often have no symptoms other than concern about the appearance of their legs. Those whose varicosis is associated with superficial venous reflux may complain of aching or 'heaviness'. A few will have developed leg swelling or patches of eczema, or will have had one or more episodes of superficial thrombophlebitis. Brown staining of the skin around

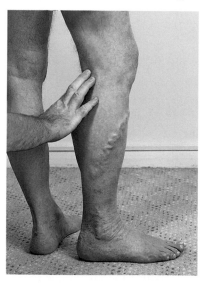

Fig. 2.40 Severe varicose veins.

the ankle (due to haemosiderin deposition) is a benign phenomenon. Severe chronic inflammatory skin changes (varicose eczema, **Fig. 2.41**) and leg ulceration (**Fig. 2.42**) are uncommon in patients with varicose veins, as is bleeding, except in a small minority of patients in whom the varicosities appear to be eroding through the skin.

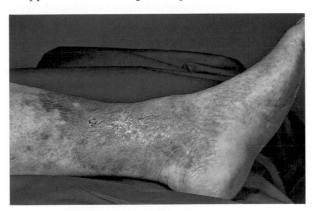

Fig. 2.41 Varicose eczema.

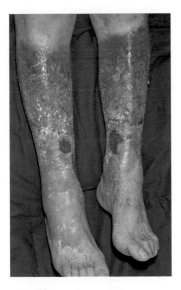

Fig. 2.42 Ulceration caused by varicose veins.

Varicose veins undoubtedly cause aching and seem also to predispose to nocturnal cramps, but aching legs are very common in patients who do not have varicose veins. In patients who have been referred for the treatment of varicose veins, their symptoms are in fact commonly due to arthritis, arterial disease, musculoskeletal pain and many other conditions. Alternative explanations for the patient's symptoms should be carefully considered, as treating the veins will confer no benefit if the symptoms are the result of something else. Typically, a patient with symptomatic varicose veins will report aching felt broadly over the distribution of the varicosities, which is exacerbated by prolonged standing and relieved by putting the legs up.

**Past medical history** A history suggestive of previous DVT (pain with swelling of the leg) should be sought, although two-thirds of DVTs are believed to be asymptomatic and a negative response does not exclude the diagnosis. A previous DVT suggests that the deep venous system may be damaged. It is also a major risk factor for a further DVT in a patient who may be being considered for surgical treatment. Details of other past or concurrent medical conditions should similarly be obtained, as a basis for deciding whether or not to offer surgery.

## General observations

The patient's general state of health should be noted. Advanced age, severe immobility, obesity, dyspnoea and other debilitating conditions may all, to a greater or lesser extent, be contraindications to treatment or may affect choice of treatment.

**Look** at the extent and distribution of the varicose veins. This is best done with the patient standing. The distribution is, however, an unreliable guide to which system is affected. In particular, varicosities confined to the posteromedial aspect of the calf may fill either via the long or the short saphenous system. Varicose veins in the thigh are nonetheless likely to be associated with saphenofemoral incompetence and reflux in the long saphenous vein, while varicosities on the back of the calf suggest short saphenopopliteal reflux.

**Look** at the condition of the skin. Pigmentation alone is harmless, but the presence of varicose eczema (**Fig. 2.41**) is indicative of moderate or severe chronic venous insufficiency.

The key to successful treatment of varicose veins is to identify the sites of superficial venous reflux and then to abolish the reflux, normalising venous function. Older textbooks describe physical methods (Trendelenburg test and tourniquet test) for identifying sites of reflux, but such tests are now obsolete. Sites of reflux are accurately and precisely identified using duplex ultrasound scanning. Any patient in whom invasive treatment for varicose veins is being contemplated should undergo duplex scanning as a basis for planning treatment.

## Care of the patient with varicose veins

Patients whose varicose veins are purely a cosmetic problem do not require treatment. Treatment is in fact not mandatory even in patients who have symptoms and superficial venous reflux, but is warranted if the patient considers the symptoms severe enough to want to undergo it. Compression stockings may be effective treatment for aching and heaviness, but only as long as the stockings are worn. Definitive treatment demands abolition of the superficial venous reflux, combined with removal of the varicosities themselves. In the past this was usually done by tying and stripping the refluxing venous trunk(s). Nowadays, endovascular procedures are generally preferred (endovenous laser ablation, radiofrequency ablation, foam sclerotherapy and others).

## Assessment of chronic venous insufficiency

### Taking the history

Some patients present to vascular clinics not with aching varicose veins but with more advanced symptoms and signs of chronic venous insufficiency, principally leg swelling, chronic inflammation of the skin and subcutaneous tissues (varicose eczema) or leg ulceration. In this group of patients, about a third prove to have superficial venous reflux alone, a third have deep venous reflux alone, and a third have both. Eighty per cent of leg ulcers are due to chronic venous insufficiency, and most of the remainder are due to arterial disease (ischaemia).

A history of a previous DVT should be sought, because two-thirds of DVTs are believed to occur without symptoms, and a negative response does not rule out the condition. An arterial history should also be taken (see page 75). The patient's past medical history in general, co-morbidities, current medication, social circumstances and functional level should also be documented.

## Physical examination

**Look** for evidence of varicose eczema (**Fig. 2.41**) and leg ulceration. Varicose eczema is characterised by thickening of the soft tissues in the gaiter area (the narrowest part of the calf, just above the ankle), erythema, skin staining and hyperkeratosis. Venous leg ulcers (**Fig. 2.42**) are typically irregular in outline, have a red, granular base, are situated in the gaiter area medially or laterally and are surrounded by an area of varicose eczema. Look for ulceration or gangrene on the foot (which is suggestive of arterial disease: venous ulcers do not generally extend below the ankle).

**Feel** and compare the temperature of the feet and feel the peripheral pulses (see page 76).

Patients with varicose eczema and/or leg ulceration require a full arterial assessment, including measurement of ankle blood pressure using a pocket Doppler machine. Duplex ultrasound scanning of the superficial and deep venous systems is also required to determine whether the patient has superficial venous reflux, deep venous reflux, or both.

# Chapter 3
## The respiratory system

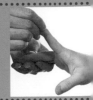

Respiratory diseases often lead to hospital admission, and patients with chronic obstructive pulmonary disease (COPD) may require repeated admissions for infective exacerbations. Carcinoma of the bronchus is the most common cause of cancer death in men, and its prevalence in women has increased in recent years. In the UK, the increasing incidence of pulmonary tuberculosis appears to have halted since 2010. Nevertheless, 10.5 cases still occur per 100,000 population, and the incidence remains 15 times higher in those born outside the UK. There is a greater public awareness of asthma than there was previously, with surveys indicating that over 4 million adults and more than 1 million children are currently receiving treatment for asthma in the UK. Public concern about industrial pollution has led to industry adopting greater safeguards but, nevertheless, occupational lung disease remains an important clinical problem. Smoking remains the single most important cause of respiratory disease despite greater awareness of the dangers of cigarette smoking and health warnings placed in advertisements and on cigarette packets. A total of 15.8% of the adult population were smokers in 2016, with a higher proportion in men than in women. There has been a 6.5% decline in smoking prevalence in the 18–24-year-old group since 2010.

Examination of the nose has been included in this section, as common illnesses affecting the respiratory tract often present with 'upper respiratory tract', or 'coryzal', symptoms. This is the case with the common cold.

## THE NOSE

### Applied anatomy and physiology

The nose comprises the external nose and the two nasal cavities (**Fig. 3.1**). The external nose is given its pyramidal shape by the nasal septum, which articulates with the frontal bone. The nasal cavities form the first part of the respiratory passage and extend from the anterior nares or nostrils to the nasopharynx. The nares are lined with respiratory epithelium, with some olfactory epithelium. The cavities are separated by a midline septum, formed from septal cartilage. The lateral wall of the nose has a large surface area due to the presence of three bony projections – the nasal conchae.

The nose receives its nerve supply from the maxillary nerve in the anterior ethmoidal branch of the ophthalmic nerve; the upper part of the nasal cavity is supplied by the olfactory nerve. Lymphatic drainage is to the submandibular nodes and retropharyngeal nodes. The nose is associated with the paranasal air sinuses: the frontal, ethmoidal, sphenoidal and maxillary sinuses.

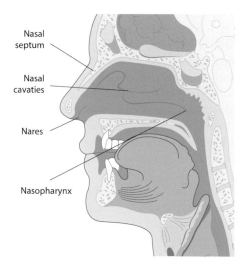

Nasal septum

Nasal cavaties

Nares

Nasopharynx

Fig. 3.1 Anatomy of the nose.

## Assessment and diagnosis

### Taking the history

Patients present with symptoms of nasal obstruction or a change in their sense of smell. Any assessment of the patient begins by observation during history taking.

#### The presenting complaint

**Nasal obstruction** This is one of the most common nasal symptoms, most frequently resulting from the common cold. Patients present with a short history of nasal obstruction and discharge. Other causes of nasal obstruction include polyps and allergic rhinitis.

**Nasal discharge** This may be watery, mucoid, mucopurulent or bloodstained. It is important to ask for details. Sneezing is commonly associated with both nasal obstruction and nasal discharge.

**Sense of smell** The sense of smell is often reduced in inflammatory disorders of the nose; however, both loss of and alteration to the sense of smell can also be caused by a cranial nerve lesion affecting the first cranial nerve.

**Physical aspects** Finally, it is important to ask about any deformity of the nose. Nasal symptoms can be caused by deviation of the nasal septum as a result of previous trauma. The nasal septum can also be affected by Wegener's granulomatosis, syphilis and leprosy.

### Examination of the nose

Look for the shape of the nose and the presence of any deformity or scars. Check the nasal cavities with a nasal speculum. In a child, it is sufficient to look with a pen light. Inspection of the nasopharynx is possible, but only with the use of a postnasal mirror.

## THE LUNGS

## Applied anatomy and physiology

The respiratory tract includes the nose, nasopharynx and larynx, extending down into the alveoli to include the blood supply.

An understanding of the arrangement of the lobes of the lungs is important for a clinical assessment, and this is illustrated in **Fig. 3.2**. The right lung is divided into three lobes – upper, middle and lower – while the left lung is divided into two lobes – the upper and lower, with the lingula (an incomplete left middle lobe) dividing the two.

Examination of the front of the chest is largely that of the upper lobes, whereas examination of the back is largely of the lower lobes. It should be noted, however, that right middle lobe disease will only be detected by careful examination of the front of the chest and axillary area – signs of a right middle lobe pneumonia are often missed.

The muscular effort of inspiration overcomes the elastic resistance of the lungs and chest wall and the non-elastic resistance, which is predominantly found in the airways. In healthy individuals, the large central airways contribute most resistance, with less from small airways due to the larger combined cross-sectional area. In disease, resistance of either kind will greatly increase and call into action the accessory muscles of inspiration (sternomastoid and scaleni) or expiration (abdominals).

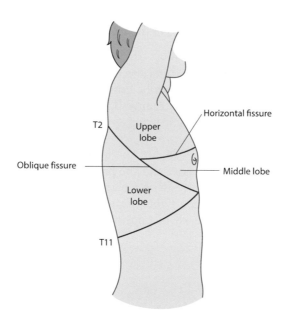

Fig. 3.2 The arrangement of the lobes of the lung, and their surface markings.

## Table 3.1 Disorders causing an alteration in respiratory resistance

| Elastic resistance – increased | Non-elastic resistance (airway resistance) |
|---|---|
| • Pulmonary fibrosis | • Asthma |
| • Pulmonary oedema | • Emphysema |
| • Kyphoscoliosis | • Chronic bronchitis |
| • Ankylosing spondylitis | |
| | |
| Elastic resistance – decreased | |
| • Emphysema | |

Examples of altered respiratory resistance are listed in *Table 3.1*. Gas exchange in the lungs will be efficient only if ventilation is distributed evenly to all parts of the lungs, and if this is matched by uniform distribution of blood flow. Furthermore, this also requires effective diffusion of carbon dioxide and oxygen along the terminal airways and across the alveolar wall.

If the area available for gas exchange is reduced, or if the effective area is decreased by maldistribution of ventilation and perfusion, the overall ability of the lung to transfer gases will also diminish. Such a reduction may not be physiologically significant at rest, but may limit the amount of oxygen that can be taken up during exercise.

## Assessment and diagnosis of respiratory disease

The assessment of a patient with respiratory disease follows the guidelines for general history taking. Some of the questions asked may overlap with those used for assessing the cardiovascular system.

### Taking the history

The six cardinal symptoms of respiratory disease are cough, sputum, haemoptysis, chest pain, dyspnoea and wheeze. These are all unpleasant symptoms that may make the patient tired or too distressed to answer questions easily. Ensure that the patient is sitting up, and do not remove an oxygen mask, if the patient has one, while you are speaking to them; the patient will feel more comfortable this way. As for the cardiovascular system, remember to start your history with an open question.

## The presenting complaint

**Cough** Cough is the forced expulsion of air through a closed glottis. The tracheobronchial tree is richly supplied with mucosal cough receptors, the fibres from which are carried in the vagus nerve. Irritation of these receptors anywhere from the pharynx to the periphery of the lung may initiate coughing. Cough may be caused by infection, inflammation, tumour or foreign body – the full history will help you decide the cause. Cough may be the only symptom in asthma, so ask:

'Does your cough occur after exercise or at night?' as this may suggest cough due to bronchospasm.

Many smokers regard coughing as normal, so you should enquire about a change in its character, as this may be important:

'I understand that you have had a cough for many years. Has it changed recently?'

Patients can often localise a cough to either above or below the larynx. A postnasal drip from rhinitis is an example of the former, which may be associated with a chronically blocked nose. Laryngitis is usually associated with both a cough and a hoarse voice, whereas the appearance of a hoarse voice alone should raise the suspicion of a recurrent laryngeal nerve palsy due to carcinoma of the bronchus.

Try to separate these symptoms in your questioning. The cough in tracheitis is often dry and extremely painful behind the trachea, and is associated with pain on coughing. Cough is also associated with lobar pneumonia and lung collapse due to bronchial obstruction – the two conditions may be accompanied by pleurisy, making the cough distressingly painful over the lungs.

One of the most common causes of coughing is chronic bronchitis, which leads to a chronic or recurrent increase in the volume of mucus secretion that is expectorated. An accepted clinical definition for chronic bronchitis is 'a chronic, or recurrent cough, with sputum on most days for at least 3 months of the year for 2 consecutive years'. It is worth targeting your questions to establish whether this is the case:

'How long have you had this cough? Do you cough every day? Do you bring up sputum or phlegm – what colour is it?'

Ask the patient whether they have coughed up any blood (haemoptysis). Carcinoma of the bronchus is frequently associated with haemoptysis, which may also be seen in pulmonary tuberculosis.

'Have you ever noticed blood in your phlegm?'

Frank haemoptysis is when pure blood is expectorated with the sputum. It is essential to confirm that the blood is coming from the lungs and not the nose or mouth, or is being vomited. The volume and duration of haemoptysis must be noted.

Bronchiectasis is characterised by a cough productive of copious sputum, which is often purulent and very offensive. Other less common causes of cough are the inhalation of foreign bodies (the patient is generally unwell and pyrexial) and parenchymal lung disease (e.g. fibrosing alveolitis). Examples of different types of cough are shown in *Table 3.2*. The common causes of haemoptysis are shown in *Table 3.3*.

**Sputum** It is important to ask all patients with a cough whether they produce sputum or 'phlegm' – this is excessive bronchial secretion, and may be a manifestation of inflammation and infection. You should

## Table 3.2 Different types of cough

| Type of cough | Cause |
| --- | --- |
| Paroxysmal | Chronic bronchitis, asthma, pulmonary vasculitis |
| Copious volume | Bronchiectasis |
| Painful | Pneumonia with pleurisy |
| 'Bovine' (sounding like a cow) | Recurrent laryngeal palsy |
| Associated stridor | Whooping cough or partial laryngeal/tracheal obstruction |

## Table 3.3 Common causes of haemoptysis

- Bronchial carcinoma
- Pulmonary tuberculosis
- Pulmonary embolism and infarction
- Infection involving bronchiectasis
- Pulmonary oedema
- Anticoagulation
- Upper respiratory tract infection (acute bronchitis)
- No cause found

also ask how often they cough up sputum, and whether it is difficult to bring up. You should question about the volume of sputum, its colour, its consistency and its smell:

'How much phlegm do you cough up each day – would it fill an egg cup or a tea cup?'

'What is it like – is it runny or thick?'

'What does it smell like?'

### BOX 3.1 CHARACTERISTICS OF PHLEGM

- **Colour** – sputum is generally described as being either white or grey in colour, the latter particularly in cigarette smokers. In infection, the colour will often change to yellow (due to the presence of leucocytes) or green (as a result of enzymatic action by verdoperoxidase). Sticky and 'rusty' sputum are characteristic of lobar pneumonia, whereas pink, frothy sputum suggests pulmonary oedema.
- **Consistency** – highly viscous sputum with plugs is characteristic of asthma. Viscous sputum is also occasionally associated with viral respiratory infections.
- **Odour** – offensive sputum is seen in association with a lung abscess or bronchiectasis.

**Chest pain (see also Chapter 2)** The most common type of pain coming from the respiratory system is pleural pain due to the rich nerve supply of the parietal pleura (the lungs have no such nerve supply). The pain is described as localised and stabbing in nature, and is made worse by any manoeuvre that apposes the pleural surfaces, such as deep breathing, coughing or sneezing. A similar pain is sometimes seen in association with a pneumothorax.

Pain in the shoulder tip suggests irritation of the diaphragmatic pleura, whereas a dull, 'boring' pain may represent rib erosion by carcinoma of the bronchus. Pain localised to the anterior chest may be accompanied by tenderness on palpation of the costochondral junction as a result of costochondritis.

The questions to ask include:

'Does it hurt when you breathe?'

'What is the pain like?'

'Is it there all the time?'

**Breathlessness** Most types of lung disease will cause dyspnoea or the subjective awareness that an increased amount of effort is required for breathing. It is important to determine the degree of shortness of breath and the resulting functional disability (i.e. how much activity the individual can undertake). Patients will often complain of 'tightness' in the chest, which may result either from angina or lung disease. Ask the patient to distinguish whether they mean pain associated with exercise or breathlessness, but remember that the latter may accompany angina.

Breathlessness may result from the following, either individually or as a combination:

- Altered ventilatory drive to the lungs.
- Impaired ventilation of the lungs.
- Altered gas exchange (or diffusion).
- Changes in perfusion of the lungs.

Examples of such causes are listed in *Table 3.4*. You should question a patient about the duration of the dyspnoea and its variability. Acute dyspnoea may result from a pulmonary embolism, pneumothorax or

## Table 3.4 Causes of breathlessness

Alterations in ventilatory drive
- Hyperventilation syndrome
- Obesity–hypoventilatory syndrome
- Hypothalamic lesions
- Metabolic acidosis

Alterations in ventilatory capacity
- Neuromuscular disease
- Mechanical problems
  - Kyphoscoliosis
  - Ankylosing spondylitis
  - Pleural effusion

Altered gas exchange (ventilation and/or diffusion)
- Chronic bronchitis and emphysema
- Asthma
- Bronchiectasis
- Fibrosing alveolitis
- Pneumonia
- Pneumothorax
- Lung collapse
- Pulmonary oedema

Altered blood supply (perfusion)
- Pulmonary embolism or lung infarction
- Anaemia

acute asthma (*Table 3.5*), while progressive dyspnoea over a period of years suggests chronic airways limitation – particularly in cigarette smokers. Questions about daily activities are helpful to determine more clearly how long the dyspnoea has been present – you should ask the patient how far they can walk on good days, and when they last

## Table 3.5 Conditions associated with increased effort of breathing

- COPD
- Asthma
- Pneumonia
- Pneumothorax
- Pulmonary embolism
- Congestive cardiac failure

visited the shops if they are currently housebound. Remember always to gauge a patient's exercise capacity. In many instances, a spouse or partner may give more reliable answers.

To clarify the variability of the dyspnoea, ask:

'Does your breathlessness come and go?'

This is highly suggestive of asthma, particularly if the patient can describe precipitating or aggravating factors.

**Wheeze** Most patients understand the term 'wheeze', which is a common complaint in patients with diffuse airways obstruction such as chronic bronchitis, emphysema or asthma. Wheezing in patients with chronic bronchitis or emphysema may result from further narrowing of the airways by an intercurrent infection, whereas wheezing in asthmatic individuals may be induced by exposure to an inhaled allergen. A unilateral wheeze should raise concerns about localised bronchial narrowing, by either a tumour or a foreign body.

### Other important points from the history

You should ask the patient about their weight. Weight loss may be associated with carcinoma of the bronchus, pulmonary tuberculosis or, on occasions, chronic airflow limitation. Sleep apnoea syndrome, which is common in obese patients –particularly those with a large neck circumference – may present with sleep disturbance and rest-lessness at night, loud snoring and daytime somnolence. The patient may not complain of these factors, but they may come to light when questioning a patient's partner, or from their reporting:

'Does your partner complain that you snore? Have they ever noticed that you have stopped breathing for a period during the night?'

It is important to ask about this problem as chronic nocturnal hypoxia can cause pulmonary hypertension and heart failure.

## Past medical history

It is essential to take an accurate history of any previous chest complaints, injuries or operations. A previous history of tuberculosis is important, and you should enquire about the length of treatment and/or operative intervention (such as thoracoplasty and phrenic nerve crush, which were commonly performed treatments for pulmonary tuberculosis before the introduction of streptomycin in 1947). A history of childhood asthma, pneumonia or whooping cough is sometimes relevant to the later development of chest symptoms in an adult. Chest injuries and previous pneumonia may explain changes seen on a chest X-ray.

## Personal and social history

Passive smoking (i.e. inhaling someone else's smoke at home or in the workplace) is recognised as a risk for lung disease. Household pets are occasionally associated with chest symptoms, in particular asthma in allergic individuals. Progressive dyspnoea in a person who keeps birds (e.g. pigeons, budgerigars or parrots) may suggest allergic alveolitis, while pneumonia in someone who keeps a parrot or related species raises the possibility of psittacosis.

A detailed occupational history is essential – you should ask the patient whether their work provokes the symptoms, and whether these impair their work. Industrial exposure to noxious gases or particles may be a cause of lung disease – for example, pneumoconiosis in coal miners. You should also enquire about past employment – asbestosis or mesothelioma may not present until many years after exposure. Finally, a question about possible environmental exposure is helpful – remember that the relatives of those who worked in contact with asbestos are also at risk.

## Family history and treatment history

There is a strong inherited component to asthma, and you should enquire about a history of atopy, asthma or eczema in the family. Moreover, you should question, if relevant, about recent tuberculosis in the family. The treatment history should question about the past and present use of bronchodilator inhalers, and how useful they may or may not be. You should also enquire whether any drugs, such as aspirin, non-steroidal anti-inflammatory agents or beta-blockers, have precipitated an asthmatic attack or wheezing in the past. Remember also the possible dangers of steroid therapy in patients with a previous history of tuberculosis.

## Examination of the patient

The patient with respiratory system disease may be short of breath, so it is important to keep this in mind, and not keep asking them to sit forward and back again. Examine everything you can from the front first; then ask the patient to sit forward and repeat the process from behind.

In addition, breathlessness makes people feel tired and anxious. Make sure to remember this – and be patient.

 VIDEO 3.1 **The respiratory examination**

https://www.crcpress.com/cw/kopelman

### BOX 3.2 SOCIAL HISTORY

A detailed social history must be taken, which includes a smoking history. You should substantiate whether the non-smoker has previously smoked and, if so, when they gave up – many patients 'give up' on admission to hospital. Examples of the questions to ask include:

'Do you smoke?'

'When did you start?'

'How many cigarettes do you smoke in an average day?' (Note: record this as pack–years)

'When did you give up?'

'How many were you smoking when you gave up?'

> ## BOX 3.3  CHECKLIST FOR RESPIRATORY HISTORY TAKING
>
> - General approach, introduce yourself, establish rapport, make eye contact.
> - Assess the present complaint and its history (duration of breathlessness, exercise tolerance). Do not forget to ask about cigarette smoking.
> - Ask about past medical history, particularly in relation to childhood chest complaints, and previous hospital attendance.
> - Ask about alcohol intake/treatment and medication use.
> - Ask about social history (e.g. how many stairs, heating in the home, pets, industrial exposure). You may include the smoking history here.
> - Ask about family history – does anyone have asthma or other chronic respiratory illness?
> - Systematic enquiry.
>
> **Listen to the answers!**

## General observations

Observe the general shape of the chest, looking for asymmetry and deformities such as depressed sternum, pigeon chest or kyphoscoliosis (a hunch back). Observe the chest during both normal and deep breathing, and check that the two sides move equally. Diminished movement on one side suggests a lesion on that side. Note whether the thoracic cage expands normally, or if it is fixed and the respiratory movements are predominantly diaphragmatic. Observe the respiratory rate: a normal rate is approximately 12 cycles per minute.

As with the cardiovascular system, it is customary to begin with inspection of the hands, with the patient lying in bed with the chest at a 45° angle. Look for finger clubbing (see **Fig. 2.1**), which is described as an increase in the curvature of the nails in both directions, with loss of the nail angle. This is caused by an increase in the soft tissues of the nail bed and fingertip. It is sometimes subtle and difficult to detect. In these cases, it is worthwhile looking for the diamond sign shown in **Fig. 3.3**. In a healthy individual, when the finger nails are opposed,

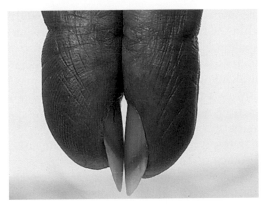

Fig. 3.3 The diamond sign: in normal individuals, a diamond shape can be seen between the nail folds. This disappears if the patient's fingers are clubbed.

a small, diamond-shaped gap can been seen between the base of the nails. In clubbing, this gap is not visible due to loss of the angle of the nail. Long lists of causes of clubbing are available, which will not be duplicated here, but remember the more common intrapulmonary ones: bronchial carcinoma, chronic chest sepsis and fibrosing alveolitis.

Also look for the signs of carbon dioxide retention – a bounding pulse and warm hands with dilated peripheral veins. Look for a flapping tremor by asking the patient to hold their hands out – the flapping tremor is an irregular twitching movement of the hands. The patient with a high level of carbon dioxide may also be peripherally cyanosed.

After your examination of the patient's hands, make sure to look at their face. Is the patient centrally cyanosed (i.e. is there blueness of the mouth and tongue)? Are they breathing out through pursed lips? This is a technique developed by people with chronic airflow limitation to keep their airways open to the end of the respiratory cycle and increase their oxygenation. Look at the patient's neck to assess whether they are using the accessory muscles of respiration.

When the work required to achieve normal ventilation is increased, there will be a larger than normal fall in intrathoracic pressure on inspiration, and this will lead to use of the accessory muscles. Scalenus anterior is the first accessory muscle to be brought into use, followed by the sternomastoids – the latter can be seen contracting. When there is a considerable increase in respiratory work, there will be a large fall of pressure within the chest on inspiration, and recession or indrawing of the intercostal muscles is then easily visible. The use of these accessory muscles increases the negative intrathoracic pressure on inspiration, thereby drawing more air into the lungs. This may be associated in severe cases with a tracheal tug. In expiration, abdominal muscle contraction creates a more positive intrathoracic pressure, helping to push the air out of the lungs.

An increase in respiratory work may result from either an increase in airways resistance or an increase in lung stiffness (see *Table 3.1*). The pattern of abnormal intrathoracic pressure changes varies according to the cause of the increased work, and this may be discernible at the bedside. When there is increased airways resistance (e.g. asthma), expiration is impeded and the respiratory phase of breathing is prolonged. This can be demonstrated by asking a patient to breath out as fast as they can. By contrast, when there is an increase in lung stiffness (e.g. fibrosing alveolitis, **Fig. 3.4**), expiration is aided by elastic recoil, and the chest/lungs are often seen to deflate unusually quickly.

Check to see whether the costal margins expand laterally during a deep inspiration. The ribs usually move upward and outward when the chest inflates (like a bucket handle). Failure to expand, or actual

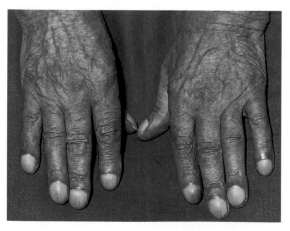

Fig. 3.4 Clubbing and peripheral cyanosis in fibrosing alveolitis.

indrawing of the lowest ribs, suggests a flattened diaphragm and a lung volume larger than normal.

When you examined the cardiovascular system, you will have already noted whether the jugular venous pressure (JVP) is raised. The patient with severe respiratory disease may have associated right heart failure with elevated JVP and swollen ankles.

Finally, look for enlarged lymph nodes in the anterior and posterior triangles of the neck (**Fig. 3.5**), as lymphatic drainage from the lungs is first to the hilum and then up the paratracheal chain to the supraclavicular and cervical nodes. The chest wall lymphatics drain into the axillae and may produce lymphadenopathy; a carcinoma of the bronchus may metastasise here. These lymph nodes are most easily examined from behind by placing your fingertips first in the supraclavicular fossae and then working up the root of the neck on either side of the sternomastoid muscle to the jugulodigastric node at the angle of the jaw, and then the submandibular nodes.

To examine the axillary nodes, support the patient's arm a little away from the chest wall (use your left hand to examine the right axilla, and right hand to examine the left axilla). Palpate anteriorly, posteriorly, medially, laterally and in the apex of the axilla (**Fig. 3.6**). (A more detailed technique is discussed in Chapter 7.) Abnormal lymph nodes (lymphadenopathy) are larger than you expect.

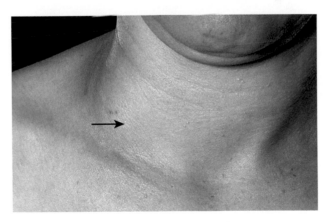

Fig. 3.5 Lymphadenopathy. Note the blurring of the sternomastoid border on the right (arrow).

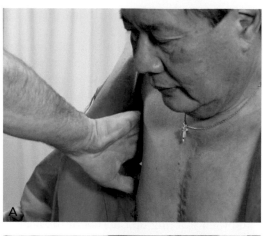

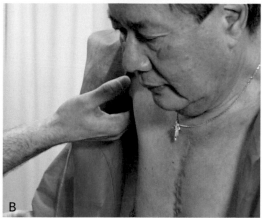

Fig. 3.6A, B Palpation of axillary lymphadenopathy.

They may be enlarged asymmetrically, and may feel hard and fixed in the case of metastases.

Examination of the chest itself follows the sequence inspection, palpation, percussion, auscultation.

## Inspection of the chest

You should now inspect the patient's chest. This is best done with the patient sitting relaxed and bare-chested in front of you.

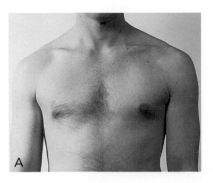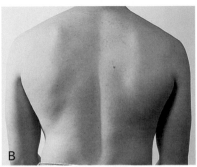

Fig. 3.7A, B Inspect the chest from the front and from the back.

Respiratory disease often results in alteration of the normal chest shape. You should compare the two sides of the chest from the front and back to look for any obvious asymmetry (**Fig. 3.7**). In addition, inspect the patient from the side, to assess the antero-posterior diameter and whether the patient has a kyphosis; kypho-scoliosis is progressive forward and lateral curvature. These result in an increased antero-posterior curvature of the spine, which will increase the diameter of the chest from front to back. If this becomes severe, it may mechanically depress one lung over the other and cause decreased lung expansion on one side.

There is a wide variation in chest shape among healthy individuals, and the only way to become familiar with the normal range is to examine a large number of patients. The normal antero-posterior diameter of the chest should be less than the lateral diameter. The chest wall may be held in hyperinflation and 'remodelled' – a barrel chest – as a result of chronic airflow limitation. This improves the elastic recoil of the lungs, but at the expense of raised lung volumes. Apical fibrosis and scarring may result in flattening of the chest at one or both apices.

It is also important to look again at the movement of the chest wall. To do this, ask the patient to take a few deep breaths in and out. The ribs should move upwards and outwards with inspiration, and this movement should be symmetrical (**Fig. 3.8**). In chronic airflow lim-itation, there is little movement as the ribs are already fixed in the expanded position, while in asymmetrical scarring after tuberculosis, movement is greater on one side than another. As the patient breathes,

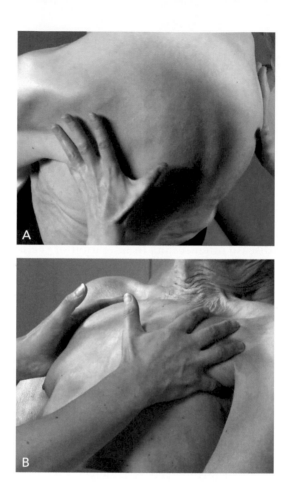

Fig. 3.8A, B Assessment of chest expansion.

listen for stridor, a harsh noise made by respiratory obstruction in the upper respiratory tract. Make sure you check for any scars on the chest that are indicative of previous surgery or trauma.

The rest of the examination of the chest needs to be performed on the front and back. So as not to tire the patient, it is sensible to complete the examination of the front *before* asking them to sit forward. The rest of the examination will include chest expansion, percussion and auscultation.

**Palpation and assessment of chest expansion** Look at the position of the trachea between the heads of the two sternomastoid muscles, and observe for a tug or downwards pulling movement of the skin over the trachea, which you may see in respiratory distress. Next, gently palpate the trachea: using your right hand, place the tips of your index and middle finger to either side of the trachea, and gently feel in the sulcus on either side to gain an impression of the direction the trachea is running and whether it is deviated to the right or left (**Fig. 3.9**). Deviation may be caused by masses in the neck, but can also be due to mediastinal shift. If this is suspected, it can be confirmed by palpating the apex beat, to see whether this is also deviated to the right or left.

To examine chest expansion, place your flat hands around the patient's chest, just below the nipple line (or the breasts in women), with your thumbs stretched out towards the midline and slightly off the skin, and ask the patient to breathe in deeply. Watch your thumbs move apart, and check that they move an equal amount. This procedure should be repeated at the back of the chest.

**Percussion** In percussion and auscultation of the chest, the aim is to compare one side with the other. It is essential to percuss or auscultate systematically to ensure you do not miss any areas. An example of such a system is illustrated in **Figs 3.10** and **3.11**.

To percuss, the non-dominant hand should be placed flat against the chest wall, and the back of the middle finger is then tapped lightly

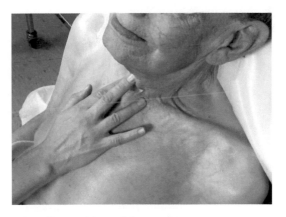

Fig. 3.9 Assessing the position of the trachea.

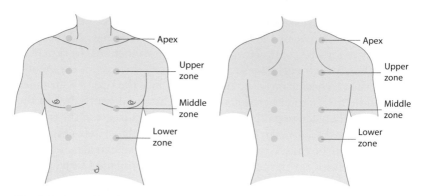

Fig. 3.10 Areas for chest examination (anterior).

Fig. 3.11 Areas for chest examination (posterior).

by the middle finger of the other hand. It is important to tap with your finger tip perpendicular to the middle finger (keep this nail short, otherwise it digs into your other finger). Keep your wrist relaxed, and ensure that most of the movement comes from here, not your elbow.

It is important to start at the apices, by percussing over the clavicles. This can be done by percussing directly onto the bone. Next, compare one side with the other side in the upper, middle and lower zones. It is important to percuss in the axilla as well as the front and back of the chest; abnormalities of the right middle lobe or lingula may only be apparent here.

The percussion note is a measure of the resonance of the chest wall. As the lungs are usually filled with air (hollow), the percussion note is usually resonant. If the intrathoracic space is filled by collapsed or consolidated lung, the percussion note will be dull (as solid material conducts sound less well than air – **Fig. 3.12**). If the space is filled with fluid – as in a pleural effusion – the percussion note will be 'stony' dull (**Fig. 3.13**), as fluid conducts vibration very poorly. If the intrathoracic cavity is filled by air, as in a pneumothorax, the percussion note will be hyper-resonant (**Fig. 3.14**). Hyper-resonance can also occur in association with overinflated lungs as found in patients with emphysema. An illustration of the relationship of some clinical conditions and their percussion notes is shown in *Table 3.6*. Although percussion has a low sensitivity diagnostically, it does have a high specificity.

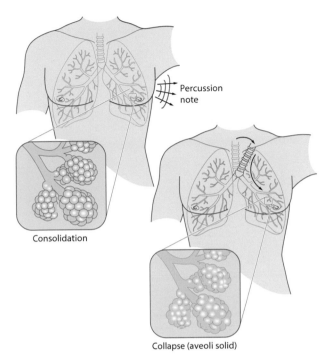

Consolidation

Percussion note

Collapse (aveoli solid)

Fig. 3.12 In consolidation, the percussion note is 'dull'.

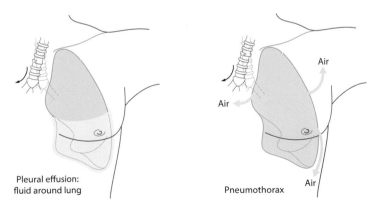

Pleural effusion: fluid around lung

Pneumothorax

Air

Air

Air

Fig. 3.13 In a pleural effusion, the percussion note is 'stony dull'.

Fig. 3.14 In pneumothorax, the percussion note is increased.

## Table 3.6 Conditions affecting conduction of sound through the chest wall

| Problem | Chest wall | Trachea position | Percussion note | Vocal resonance – tactile fremitus | Breath sounds |
|---|---|---|---|---|---|
| Consolidation | Normal | Central | Dull | May be increased over area of consolidation | Bronchial breathing |
| Collapse (larger airways) | Reduced | Deviated towards lesion | Dull | Absent | Absent |
| Pleural effusion | Reduced | Central or deviated away from lesion | Stony dull | Absent | May be bronchial breathing above the fluid + aegophony |
| Pneumothorax (large) | Reduced | Central or deviated away from lesion | Hyper-resonant | Absent | Absent |

**Auscultation** As with percussion, in auscultation it is important to listen over an area on one side, and then compare this directly with the other side (**Figs 3.10** and **3.11**). The diaphragm of the stethoscope should be used for this. Ask the patient to breathe in, and then to breathe right out through an open mouth. Listen over the apices of both lungs first, and then over the upper, middle and lower zones, followed by the axillae. Repeat the auscultation when examining the patient's chest. While listening, it is important to concentrate on the breath sounds themselves, and to listen for added sounds. Normal breath sounds are termed 'vesicular' in nature.

**Sounds** These are produced by the movement of air in and out of healthy lung tissue and airways. They are heard over all normal lung tissue, with no clear pause between inspiration and expiration, and come from the region immediately below the stethoscope. They relate to the flow of air through different airways, and the filtering properties of the surrounding tissues, air, fluid or matter in between the airways and the stethoscope. The differing characteristics of the lungs (e.g. normal versus abnormal tissue; fluid versus solid matter) alter the transmission of these sounds. Bronchial sounds are much

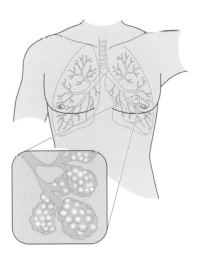

Fig. 3.15 The percussion note is dull, with reduced sounds, as the air passages are occluded in collapse.

more harsh, with a clear pause between inspiration and expiration and a prolonged expiratory phase. They are dominated by the glottic hiss, which is transmitted from the larynx and can usually be heard over the trachea and large airways. In health, they are not heard elsewhere, except in expiration.

Healthy lung tissue and alveolar air usually surround the bronchi and bronchioles, acting as a low-frequency filter or 'muffler'. This allows the transmission of low-frequency sounds but filters out higher frequencies. Consolidation, pulmonary oedema and pleural fluid are better at transmitting higher frequencies. This altered transmission is the cause of different pathological breath sounds and other respiratory signs such as vocal resonance. If the lung tissue becomes solid due to consolidation, there is increased conduction of this bronchial-quality sound to the chest wall, with a reduction in the normal vesicular breathing as air entry is reduced or absent. This is called bronchial breathing and is best heard over the area affected by the consolidation. In consolidation, the alveoli are full of inflammatory exudate but the air passages remain open; this differentiates consolidation from collapse, in which the air passages are occluded (see *Table 3.5*) and bronchial breathing is not heard.

**Vocal resonance** This refers to the character of the patient's voice heard with the stethoscope over the lung fields. Different frequencies of voice sounds are transmitted to the chest wall, and these frequencies are increased, decreased or altered in different disease states (see *Table 3.5*). This can be assessed clinically by asking the patient to say 'ninety-nine' or 'one, one, one', while listening to the chest.

The spoken voice sounds hollow through a stethoscope placed over healthy lung, as low-pitched sounds are transmitted better than high-pitched sounds.

Altered vocal resonance is best heard over areas of consolidation, and is best described as an increase in clarity of the words heard (with an almost booming nature) through the chest wall. This sign is called bronchophony, and is due to the increased sound-conducting properties of solid tissue over air. If vocal resonance is present, it may be easier to hear as 'whispering pectoriloquy'. The whispered voice is conducted very clearly, as it consists largely of high-frequency noises – almost like being in a whispering gallery.

When there is a pleural effusion, the spoken voice heard through the stethoscope is high-pitched, with a nasal quality known as aegophony: this occurs because the improved transmission of high frequencies is accompanied by impaired transmission of the lower frequencies. ('Aegophony' means goat-voice, because of its bleating quality.)

**Tactile vocal fremitus** Vibration of the chest wall is also assessed by palpation. This can be done at this stage, although it is sometimes easier to put into context at the end of the examination of the chest. This test for the transmission of low-frequency vibrations is closely related to auscultation findings, as an increase in tactile vocal fremitus (vibration) is associated with an increase in sound conduction through the chest wall. Place the flat of your hand on the patient's chest, and ask the patient to say 'ninety-nine'. Compare one side with the other over the front and back of the chest in the areas illustrated in **Figs 3.10** and **3.11**. The degree of vibration over each lung should be compared. It is of interest that vocal resonance and tactile vocal fremitus have a sensitivity of over 80% when assessing the presence of a pleural effusion.

**Added sounds** Crackles and wheezes are the most common added sounds you are likely to encounter. Crackles are produced by air bubbles bursting through fluid in the alveoli. They are described as fine or coarse. The noise of fine crackles can be reproduced by rolling your hair between your finger and thumb just in front of your ear. These noises are usually heard at the end of inspiration. Fine crackles are heard in pulmonary oedema, as well as in early bronchopneumonias, where they tend to be basal, and pulmonary fibrosis, where they may be more widespread.

Coarse crackles have a harsh, clicking sound, and are heard in infection and bronchiectasis.

A wheeze comprises continual high-pitched 'musical' sounds heard at the end of inspiration or at the start of expiration.

Airway narrowing allows airflow-induced oscillation of the airway walls, producing acoustic waves. As the airway lumen becomes smaller, the airflow velocity increases, resulting in vibration of the airway wall and the tonal sound. A wheeze on normal quiet expiration or inspiration is most probably pathological. The longer and more high-pitched the wheeze, the more severe the obstruction. It is important to remember that the presence of a wheeze implies that the patient has enough air movement to produce one. Beware the wheezing patient who suddenly becomes silent, as this may mean that air movement is so low that a wheeze cannot be produced.

A few basal crackles may be heard in the healthy upright subject breathing quietly, and this probably results from airways closing in the dependent lung during shallow breathing – this is an effect of gravity. Characteristically, these crackles clear on coughing.

**Pleural rub**   A pleural rub is a creaking sound caused by the inflamed pleural surfaces rubbing against each other. Characteristically, it sounds like creaking leather or, occasionally, walking on dry snow, and is usually located over an area of pleuritic pain. It is heard in both inspiration and expiration, and can be confused with the noise made when listening to the chest through clothing – hence always examine the bare chest. Common causes are pleurisy, lung cancer, pneumonia and pulmonary embolism.

### BOX 3.4  CARING FOR THE PATIENT WITH RESPIRATORY SYSTEM DISEASE

- Appreciate their anxiety.
- Ensure bed rest is in a sitting and not a lying position.
- Make sure oxygen is always available – only 24% oxygen unless otherwise requested.
- Monitor the peak expiratory flow rate (PEFR).
- Regularly check the respiratory rate.
- Cardiac monitoring may be necessary.
- Weigh the patient daily (if there is coexistent heart failure).

## Illustrated physical signs

**Peripheral cyanosis** with dilated veins is a feature of the carbon dioxide retention characteristic of COPD (**Fig. 3.16**). A **kyphoscoliosis** (**Fig. 3.17**) often predisposes a patient to respiratory disease. **Tuberculosis** produces X-ray signs as shown in **Fig. 3.18**. A flattened upper chest can be caused by fibrosis from previous **apical tuberculosis** (**Fig. 3.19**); the patient in the figure also has angulation due to spinal involvement. The appearance of **bronchial carcinoma** is

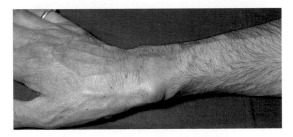

Fig. 3.16 Peripheral cyanosis with dilated peripheral veins, found in carbon dioxide retention.

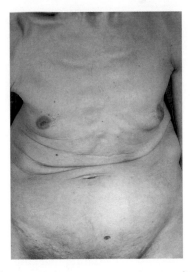

Fig. 3.17 Kyphoscoliosis predisposes to respiratory disease.

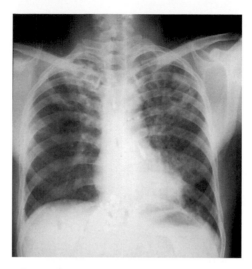

Fig. 3.18 Tuberculosis. Cavitation is seen in the upper lobes.

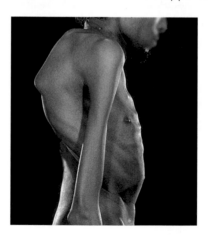

Fig. 3.19 Apical tuberculosis. A flattened apex due to previous tuberculosis, with angulation due to spinal involvement.

shown in **Fig. 3.20**. In a patient with **lobar pneumonia**, there is often coexistent oral herpes simplex infection (**Figs 3.21** and **3.22**). With a **collapsed lung** (pneumothorax), no lung markings can be seen on the X-ray (**Fig. 3.23**).

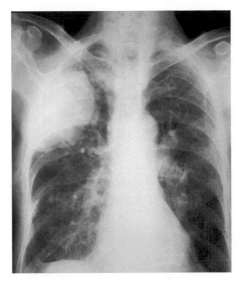

Fig. 3.20 Bronchial carcinoma. A large opacity is shown in the left upper zone.

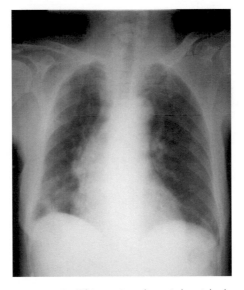

Fig. 3.21 Lobar pneumonia. This patient has right-sided consolidation.

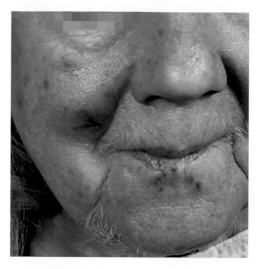

Fig. 3.22 Herpes simplex infection is common in patients with lobar pneumonia.

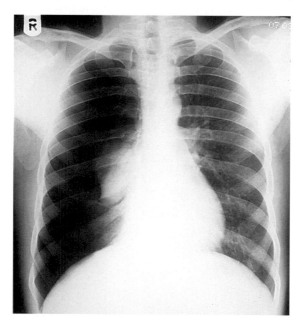

Fig. 3.23 Right-sided pneumothorax with complete absence of lung markings.

## Therapeutic and interventional skills

Peak expiratory flow rate measurement

Either a Wright's peak flow meter or a smaller portable version is needed to measure the PEFR. Ensure that you use a clean disposable mouth-piece for each patient. Ask the patient to take a large breath in through the mouth, then seal their lips around the tube and breathe out as quickly and forcefully as possible into the meter (as if blowing out birthday cake candles). The patient should repeat this three times. This shifts the arrow in the gauge, and the highest recorded value is noted. It is often appropriate to do this before and after treatment with an inhaled bronchodilator, for example salbutamol. The normal PEFR is related to the patient's height – a usual value for a 1.83 m (6 ft) male is around 500–600 L/min.

### BOX 3.5 FINDINGS IN A NORMAL RESPIRATORY SYSTEM EXAMINATION

- Observation – chest wall and respiratory movements are equal and symmetrical.
- Chest expansion – equal and symmetrical.
- Trachea – central.
- Percussion note – resonant.
- Auscultation – breath sounds vesicular, with no added sounds.
- Tactile vocal fremitus – present and equal on both sides.

### BOX 3.6 ARTERIAL BLOOD GAS ESTIMATION

Arterial blood gases are used in the assessment of breathlessness. The results obtained provide vital clues to the underlying cause and the severity of the condition.

 VIDEO 3.2 ABG sampling with a local anaesthetic

https://www.crcpress.com/cw/kopelman

## Inhaler use

If a bronchodilator and steroid inhaler are to be used, the bronchodilator must be used first in order to open the bronchioles and thus maximise the delivery of the steroid. It is helpful to explain the procedure to the patient first, and then instruct them step by step while they follow your instructions:

- Shake the inhaler vigorously; ask the patient to breathe in and then right out.
- Put the inhaler into their mouth and ask them to inhale deeply.
- At the beginning of the inspiration, tell them to press the plunger of the inhaler. This administers the active ingredient in a spray form, which is carried into the lungs with inspiration.
- Tell the patient to hold their breath for 10 seconds and then breathe out.
- Repeat after a pause if two puffs are required.

If the patient is unable to use an inhaler, a spacer device can be used (**Fig. 3.24**). This allows dispersal of the drug into a much larger volume of air. The inhaler is attached at one end, and the patient breathes in and out through the other. A one-way valve ensures delivery of the drug while the patient is breathing in. The other alternative is a Rotahaler. With this technique, the patient breathes

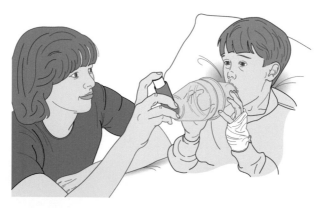

Fig. 3.24 Spacer device being used in conjunction with an inhaler.

in, and the drug delivery system is triggered by the rate of flow of inspired air.

## Key laboratory tests

**Arterial blood gas interpretation** The arterial blood gas measurements indicate the oxygenation and degree of acidosis or alkalosis of the arterial blood.

Respiratory acidosis is caused by hypoventilation. The pH is low, $PaCO_2$ is high and the plasma bicarbonate normal or raised. This may be compensated for if it is long-standing, giving a normal pH and a raised bicarbonate.

---

### BOX 3.7  ARTERIAL BLOOD GAS MEASUREMENT

Values vary from laboratory to laboratory, but a general range of normal values of arterial blood is:

| | |
|---|---|
| $PaO_2$ | 12–13.5 kPa (85–95 mmHg) |
| $PaCO_2$ | 4.5–6.0 kPa (35–45 mmHg) |
| pH | 7.35–7.45 |
| Plasma bicarbonate ($HCO_3$) | 20–30 mmol/L |
| Standard base excess (SBE) | ± 2 mmol/L |
| % $O_2$ saturation | 95–100% |

---

Respiratory alkalosis is caused by hyperventilation. The pH is high, the $PaCO_2$ is low and the plasma bicarbonate is normal or low.

The following illustrations depict the key features of common respiratory conditions: emphysema (**Fig. 3.25**), primary carcinoma of the bronchus (**Fig. 3.26**), asthma (**Fig. 3.27**), pulmonary fibrosis (**Fig. 3.28**), COPD (**Fig. 3.29**) and pulmonary tuberculosis (**Fig. 3.30**).

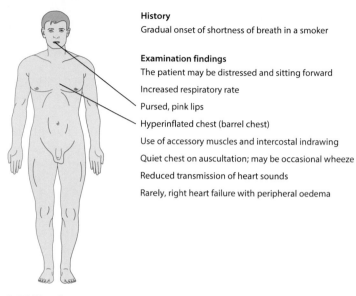

**History**
Gradual onset of shortness of breath in a smoker

**Examination findings**
The patient may be distressed and sitting forward

Increased respiratory rate

Pursed, pink lips

Hyperinflated chest (barrel chest)

Use of accessory muscles and intercostal indrawing

Quiet chest on auscultation; may be occasional wheeze

Reduced transmission of heart sounds

Rarely, right heart failure with peripheral oedema

Fig. 3.25 Emphysema.

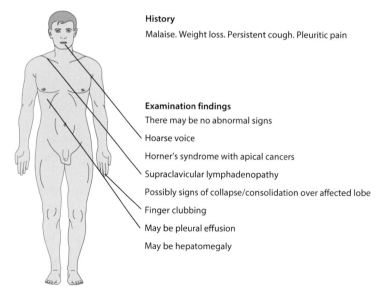

**History**
Malaise. Weight loss. Persistent cough. Pleuritic pain

**Examination findings**
There may be no abnormal signs

Hoarse voice

Horner's syndrome with apical cancers

Supraclavicular lymphadenopathy

Possibly signs of collapse/consolidation over affected lobe

Finger clubbing

May be pleural effusion

May be hepatomegaly

Fig. 3.26 Primary carcinoma of the bronchus.

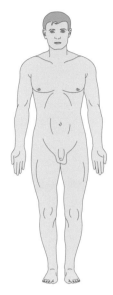

**History**

Intermittent episodes of shortness of breath.

Cough (particularly a troublesome night cough)

**Examination findings**

May be normal between attacks

During attack, the patient may be sitting forward and distressed

During attack, acute dyspnoea with hyperinflated chest

Wheeze throughout chest on auscultation

Fig. 3.27 Asthma.

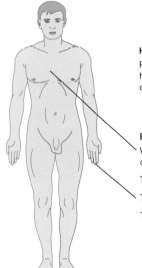

**History**

Progressive shortness of breath. There may be a past history of industrial exposure or associated connective tissue disease

**Examination findings**

Widespread 'showers' of fine crackles that do not clear on coughing

The patient is breathless at rest

There may be finger clubbing

The patient may be cyanosed

Fig. 3.28 Pulmonary fibrosis.

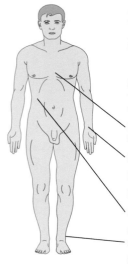

**History**

There is a history of productive cough for at least 2 months in any 2 consecutive years. The patient has repeated chest infections

**Examination findings**

The patient may be distressed and sitting forward, with increased respiratory rate. Barrel chest, blue lips

Use of accessory muscles of respiration, with intercostal indrawing

Bounding pulse and coarse tremor of fingers

Prolonged expiratory phase and expiratory wheezes

Possibly coarse crepitations

Downward displacement of liver

May be associated signs of right heart failure and peripheral oedema. Reduced heart sound transmissions

Severe $CO_2$ retention leads to mental confusion, drowsiness, coma and papilloedema

Fig. 3.29 COPD.

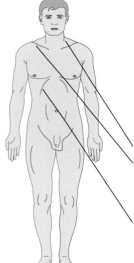

**History**

Persistent cough, possibly haemoptysis

Fever and night sweats

Associated weight loss

Contact with tuberculosis

**Examination findings**

May be unremarkable

Possibly cervical and supraclavicular lymphadenopathy

If there is upper lobe involvement, the percussion note is dull over the clavicle and there is bronchial breathing on auscultation

Elsewhere, possibly localised area of consolidation

May present with pleural effusion

Fig. 3.30 Pulmonary tuberculosis.

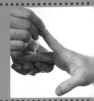

Clinical examination textbooks often split the abdominal examination into systems, separating the gastrointestinal and urinary tracts. Here, however, the approach adopted is the examination of the abdomen and all of its contents to reflect standard bedside practice and the integrated approach that is assessed in clinical examinations.

## Applied anatomy and physiology of the gut

The basic anatomy of the gut is shown in **Fig. 4.1**. The gastrointestinal tract is responsible for the ingestion of food, the absorption of nutrients from food and the excretion of unabsorbed waste products. This process is controlled by the autonomic nervous system, together with hormones including gastrin, secretin and cholecystokinin. The parasympathetic nervous system controls the contraction of smooth muscle and the secretion of digestive hormones. These are secreted in response to stretching of the gut, and to the presence of food in the upper gastrointestinal tract.

The **musculature** of the alimentary tract is composed of smooth muscle from the mid-oesophagus to the external anal sphincter. Smooth muscle has an innate tone that permits sustained and sometimes powerful contraction over long periods of time. On the other hand, the muscle may respond to more gradual stretching by a decrease in tension and an increase in length. Smooth muscle activity is influenced by both neural and humoral components. The sympathetic nervous system has very little influence, while the parasympathetic system has

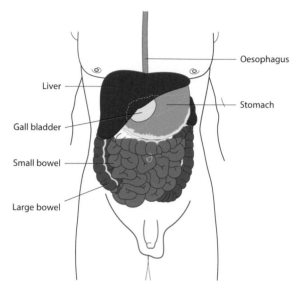

Fig. 4.1 The basic anatomy of the gut.

a profound influence. Humoral influences on smooth muscle include those of neurohumoral transmitters (e.g. 5-hydroxytrytamine and prostaglandins), gastrointestinal hormones (e.g. glucagon) and drugs.

**Gastric peristalsis** occurs at a constant rate of three to four waves per minute. The pylorus, in contrast to the oesophageal sphincter, is not usually in a state of contraction, but at the end of each peristaltic wave it contracts, together with the terminal antrum. Gastric emptying is proportional to the volume in the stomach, with about 1–3% of the gastric contents being emptied each minute. The rate of emptying is delayed by the presence of fat in the duodenum, a low pH or a hypertonic solution. This ensures that the duodenum is not overwhelmed by excessive amounts of hypertonic fluid, and that the intestinal contents are isotonic when they enter the jejunum. The body of the stomach secretes a juice whose main constituents are hydrochloric acid, pepsin and intrinsic factor. Gastric secretion is secreted in three phases – cephalic (neural), gastric (hormonal) and intestinal (hormonal).

The most common movements of the **small intestine** are non-propulsive segmenting contractions whose main function is to mix the intestinal contents. Peristaltic waves propel food along the lumen. The rate of passage through the duodenum is rapid, while the rate of transit in the ileum may be slow. The ileocaecal valve may further delay the passage of the contents in the ileum, facilitating the absorption of water and some nutrients. The exocrine pancreas secretes an aqueous juice with a high bicarbonate concentration, as well as enzymic fluid containing the major proteolytic enzymes of digestion (trypsin, chymotrypsin and carboxypeptidase), amylase and lipase. This secretion is controlled both by neural and hormonal mechanisms (secretin and cholecystokinin).

In the **large bowel**, most contractions are non-propulsive and serve to delay rather than promote transit. This accounts for the paradox that in diarrhoea, intraluminal pressure records show decreased activity, and in constipation increased activity. After receiving the food residues, the caecum exhibits mixing activity and then slowly contracts so that food residues reach the transverse colon over 6–10 hours. Once to three times each day, mass movements occur and propel the contents into the descending and sigmoid colon. Continence is maintained by two sphincters. The internal sphincter reflects the activity of the circular muscle of the intestine; it is usually in tonic contraction. The external sphincter also shows continuous resting activity. Both the external and puborectalis muscle are inhibited on defecation and micturition.

Although no glandular secretion occurs in the small and large intestines, there is a rapid exchange of water and electrolytes across parts of the **mucosa**. Water moves in response to osmotic gradients, a hypertonic solution being rapidly diluted by the movement of water from blood to lumen, and a hypotonic solution being rapidly concentrated by the absorption of water. Sodium is actively absorbed in both the small and large intestine, while potassium is absorbed by the small intestine but secreted by the large intestine. In normal circumstances, albumin leaks into the gut lumen in various secretions such as saliva, gastric juice, succus entericus and bile. The exuded albumin is digested and the nitrogen subsequently absorbed as amino acids. This intestinal loss accounts for approximately 10% of the total albumin catabolism in the normal subject.

## Applied anatomy and physiology of the urinary tract

Normal kidneys lie in the retroperitoneum at the level of vertebrae T11–L3/L4 (see **Fig. 4.11**), are 10–12 cm in length from pole to pole and move with respiration. Congenital abnormalities include pelvic kidneys and horseshoe kidney in which the lower poles are fused. The ureters carry urine to the bladder and have a nerve supply from the L1 and L2 nerve roots. There is usually a single ureter for each kidney, but duplex collecting systems can be found as a congenital anomaly that predisposes to vesico-ureteric reflux. The bladder lies in the pelvis, posterior to the pubic symphysis, and anterior to the rectum in males and the vagina in females. In the healthy state, the bladder can relax to accommodate 500–1000 ml of urine. The bladder outlet is via the urethra, a muscular tube that joins the bladder at the trigone and has its external opening at the urinary meatus. Continence is maintained by an internal sphincter, under autonomic control, within the bladder neck and an external sphincter, under voluntary control, formed by the skeletal muscle of the pelvic floor. The detrusor muscle in the bladder wall relaxes to accommodate increasing volumes of urine, and contracts to ensure bladder emptying on micturition. Sympathetic innervation promotes relaxation of the detrusor muscle to facilitate retention of urine, and parasympathetic innervation promotes contraction of the detrusor muscle to allow micturition. In males, the upper urethra runs through the prostate gland and is prone to obstruction by prostatic hypertrophy in elderly individuals. The male urethra is longer than the female, which contributes to the lower incidence of urinary tract infections.

The excretory function of the kidney regulates water and electrolyte secretion to maintain blood volume, blood pressure and plasma electrolyte composition. A fall in perfusion pressure of the kidney results in homeostatic activation of the renin–angiotensin–aldosterone system, resulting in peripheral vasoconstriction, thirst and sodium retention as measures to raise systemic blood pressure. Renal artery stenosis can mimic hypotension and lead to maladaptive, renin-driven systemic hypertension. Water secretion is regulated by sensing of the tonicity of plasma in the hypothalamus and by baroreceptors. An increase in tonicity of the plasma leads to a release of vasopressin from the posterior pituitary; this stimulates insertion of the protein aquaporin into the walls of the collecting ducts in the distal nephron, leading to water reabsorption. The most common electrolyte disturbances in individuals with chronic kidney disease are hyperkalaemia and metabolic acidosis. Uraemia (known as azotaemia in the USA) is the term applied to the physiological abnormalities that arise due to failure of excretion of a variety of metabolic waste products by the kidney.

The kidney is also an endocrine organ. The 1-hydroxyl group of active vitamin D is added in the kidney, so disorders of calcium and phosphate homeostasis are a common problem in chronic kidney disease. Erythropoietin, which drives erythrocyte production in the bone marrow, is produced by fibroblasts in the renal medulla in response to hypoxia.

## Assessment and diagnosis

### Taking the history

A clear history of abdominal symptoms is important, because it will often discriminate between organic and non-organic (functional) disease. Patients are often vague about their symptoms, and they may be embarrassed when discussing their bowel habit with the doctor. It is important for practitioners to present themselves as sympathetic and caring individuals, and it may be helpful to reassure the patient of the confidentiality of the consultation. It is also important to be very clear what the patient means by their symptoms. This is done using a combination of open questions to encourage the patient to describe the symptoms in their own words, and considerable reiteration and checking by the doctor to make sure they have understood the message. The direction of the interview may also have to be guided, as patients may try to avoid embarrassing or intimate discussions. This can be done using closed and focused questions.

#### The presenting complaint – gastrointestinal system

Any of the symptoms listed in *Table 4.1* may need to be explored with the patient.

## Table 4.1 Symptoms of gastrointestinal disease

| | |
|---|---|
| *Dysphagia* | Difficulty in swallowing |
| *Heartburn* | Retrosternal burning sensation |
| *Indigestion, dyspepsia* | Both are commonly used, but non-specific, terms |
| *Wind* | Describes flatulence, belching or passing of flatus |
| *Nausea* | A feeling of impending vomiting |
| *Retching* | Involuntary spasms with a desire to vomit |
| *Vomiting* | Propulsive regurgitation of stomach contents |
| *Diarrhoea* | Passing increased amounts of loose stool |
| *Constipation* | Difficult passage of hard stool |
| *Pain* | See text |
| *Anorexia* | Loss of appetite |
| *Colic* | Abdominal pain that waxes and wanes |
| *Melaena* | Black stool (altered blood) |
| *Tenesmus* | A painful urge to defecate |

**Dysphagia** The patient may complain that food sticks in their throat, or lower down on swallowing. You should establish where the food sticks, whether it is a consistent site and whether it is more obvious with solids or liquids. Ask the patient to point to the area where they find the food sticks:

'Tell me about the sensation you have of food sticking in your throat.'

'Where does it seem to stick?'

'Is it worse with drinks or solid food?'

'Is swallowing painful?' – odynophagia.

**Heartburn** The patient complains of a burning sensation that occurs in the chest and may extend up into the throat. It is often positional, worse on lying down, and therefore also worse at night. It can be exacerbated by bending over, for example when doing up shoe laces. It is important to ensure that it is not related to exercise, as the symptoms of angina pectoris and heartburn can be difficult to differentiate:

'Describe the burning sensation. Where is it?'

'Does it go anywhere else? Is it related to food intake?'

**Indigestion and dyspepsia** These are vague terms that are widely interpreted by patients. If the patient uses such terms, it is important to establish, by closer questioning, exactly what they mean:

'Describe your indigestion to me. What is it like? When does it come on?'

**Wind** This term is usually used to describe belching or the passing of flatus. It can also be used to describe colicky (intermittent, but intense) abdominal pain. If the patient complains of wind, ask whether it tends to be passed downwards or upwards, and whether it relieves pain or other symptoms:

'Do you feel better after burping or passing wind?'

**Nausea, retching and vomiting** These symptoms tend to, but not always, occur together. It is important to enquire about the frequency of the symptoms and whether they are related to pain. If vomiting is related to pain, does it bring relief? Ask about the approximate amount of vomitus and relate it to common things such as a tea cup, bowl or bucket. What colour is it, and does it have any traces of blood in it? Altered blood from the stomach appears as dark brown flecks and is called 'coffee grounds'. However, vomit often looks brown in the absence of bleeding, and this can be overinterpreted.

'Does the vomit taste sour, and does it contain foods? If so, how long ago were they eaten?'

Vomit containing undigested food suggests a possible delay in gastric emptying, which may accompany pyloric stenosis.

**Diarrhoea** Establish the normal bowel habit, and then ask about any change. Ask how many times the patient goes to the toilet to open their bowels, and compare this with their normal habit. Also ask about the volume and consistency of the stool:

'Is it formed, unformed or watery?'

'Does it smell?'

'Does bulky pale stool float, and is it difficult to flush away?' – steatorrhoea.

'Is there blood and/or mucus associated with the stool? If so, is it mixed in or on top of the stool?'

'Is there pain on, or before, defecation, and is it relieved by defecation?'

Blood mixed into the stool suggests a possible neoplasm or chronic inflammatory bowel disease – blood on the lavatory paper, or on the surface of stool, is more suggestive of haemorrhoids. Both require further investigation.

**Constipation** Patients occasionally misunderstand the term constipation, so it is important to clarify what they mean. Generally, a patient is regarded as constipated if they experience an infrequent passage of small, hard stools that are difficult to pass. There is usually a wide variation in bowel habit, and not everybody opens their bowels every day. Remember to ask about the consistency as well as the frequency of motions:

'Are they difficult to pass?'

'Do they feel small and hard?'

**Pain** The causes of abdominal pain are legion, so keep an open mind about the source of the problem (*Table 4.2*). For example, ischaemic cardiac pain and pleuritic pain can both be referred to the abdomen. Ask about the site of the pain:

'Is it localised or diffuse?'

'Does it radiate?'

'How long has it been there?'

## Table 4.2 Examples of different kinds of abdominal pain

| | |
|---|---|
| *Gnawing pain* | Peptic ulceration |
| *Colicky pain* | Associated with spasm of gall bladder or hollow viscus. Loin-to-groin pain with ureteric colic |
| *Suprapubic pain* | Associated with urinary tract infection |
| *Severe constant boring pain* | Malignancy (e.g. cancer of the pancreas) |

'Has it changed in character during this time?'

'Is it present all the time, or does it come and go?'

'Does it come in spasms, or is it continuous in nature?'

Ask if there is any relationship to eating (i.e. is the pain worse when the patient is hungry or full). Does anything relieve or exacerbate the pain, such as the passing of flatus, or defecation? Painful defecation is suggestive of an anal fissure. Ask for any associated features of the pain such as jaundice or fever. Renal stones cause colicky loin pain, and with ureteric stones the pain classically radiates to the groin. Colicky right upper quadrant pain suggests gall bladder inflammation.

**Anorexia** True anorexia is associated with weight loss, so it is sensible to enquire about both symptoms together. It is also important to decide whether the patient has lost their appetite or is afraid to eat because of pain or other symptoms. You should assess other symptoms as anorexia can be a symptom of diseases outside the gastrointestinal tract:

'How is your appetite? If you were really hungry and I gave you a plate of your favourite food, would you be able to eat it?'

Patients with anorexia nervosa may deny hunger – make sure you ask about weight if the patient looks excessively thin:

'How would you describe your weight?'

'What is your ideal weight?'

The presenting complaint – urinary tract
Symptoms of the urinary tract can be grouped on a functional basis.

**Obstructive**
- Hesitancy – an involuntary delay in starting the urine flow at micturition.
- Poor stream – a reduced urine flow rate. This can be a difficult concept to discuss clearly with the patient. For male patients, you could ask how far away from the toilet pan or urinal they could stand and whether this has changed over time.
- Terminal dribbling – rather than an abrupt cessation of urine flow at the end of micturition.

**Irritative**
- Dysuria – typically described as a burning pain on micturition, and most often due to urinary tract infection.
- Frequency – establish whether this is a frequent voiding of small amounts of urine or of normal volumes, to differentiate problems with bladder capacity or irritation from polyuria.
- Nocturia – may be due to mobilisation of peripheral oedema at night causing polyuria, reduced bladder capacity or bladder irritation.
- Strangury – a painful desire to pass urine with either an empty or completely obstructed bladder.

**Change in appearance of the urine**
- Visible haematuria – as a relatively small amount of blood can stain urine red and may indicate bleeding from anywhere in the urinary tract. Association with a respiratory tract infection is sometimes a feature of IgA nephropathy (synpharyngitic haematuria).
- Brown urine – due to myoglobin release in rhabdomyolysis.
- Passage of stones or 'gravel'.
- Frothy urine – due to proteinuria.

**Change in urine volume**
- Oliguria – an abnormally small daily urine output.
- Polyuria – which must be distinguished from urinary frequency.

**Uraemia** The symptoms of uraemia tend to be non-specific but include fatigue, pruritis, anorexia, nausea, vomiting and dyseugia (a metallic taste in the mouth). Uraemic encephalopathy is uncommon, and delirium in a uraemic patient usually has an alternative cause.

## Past medical history

The patient may have a past history that includes surgery to the gastrointestinal or urinary tract. It is also important to enquire whether the patient has ever been jaundiced and, if so, what the nature of the jaundice was: patients may have suffered from hepatitis in the past and be unaware of the significance.

## Personal and social history

It is essential to enquire how much alcohol a patient drinks. Patients often underestimate this, particularly if they consider that they may have a problem with alcohol. It is important to start cautiously with the questions:

'Do you drink alcohol?'

'How much alcohol might you drink in a week?'

'Is this on social occasions, or are you at home?'

'How much alcohol might you drink at home per day?'

'Is that every day?'

If the patient drinks alcohol most days, enquire how long a bottle of spirits lasts or how many bottles of wine are drunk each week. The unit system used to calculate alcohol intake is illustrated in **Fig. 4.2**.

It is important to make no assumptions about the use of recreational drugs, and enquiry about recreational drug use should be routine. A patient who has used recreational drugs may have been exposed to blood-borne viruses, so it is important to ask if they have ever taken any other substances (which may affect the liver). It may be worthwhile at this point explaining to the patient that you are asking this purely for health reasons, as some of these drugs can affect the liver.

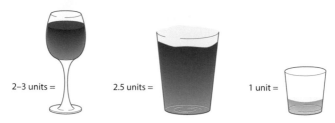

Fig. 4.2 The unit system is used to calculate alcohol intake. In this, 1 unit is 10 ml of ethanol. With increases in alcohol content (now typically 12–14%) and changes in the traditional glass size, one glass of wine (175–250 ml) now contains 2–3 units of alcohol, 1 pint (500 ml) of beer at 5% contains 2.5 units, and 1 measure of spirits (25 ml at 40%) contains 1 unit.

## Family history

In the family history, it is important to know whether any close relatives have suffered from the same symptoms. A history of excessive alcohol consumption also often runs in families. Autosomal dominant polycystic kidney disease is the most common inherited renal disorder, and may be associated with a family history of stroke or sudden death due to a ruptured berry aneurysm.

## Drug history

It is also worth enquiring about drugs, particularly those which may affect the liver, for example methotrexate in the treatment of rheumatoid arthritis or psoriasis. The patient's prescribed medications, and those bought over the counter, need to be noted with particular care if the patient has gastrointestinal problems. Some medications may be a cause of duodenal ulceration (non-steroidal anti-inflammatory drugs, e.g. ibuprofen), diarrhoea (antibiotics) or constipation (opiate-based analgesics). Some drugs (e.g. aminoglycosides) are directly nephrotoxic, while others (drugs blocking the renin–angiotensin system and non-steroidal anti-inflammatory drugs) render the kidney more susceptible to ischaemia with haemodynamic compromise. Chinese herbal remedies containing aristolochic acid are particularly nephrotoxic.

## BOX 4.1 CHECKLIST FOR ABDOMINAL HISTORY TAKING

- General approach:
  - Introduce yourself.
  - Establish rapport.
  - Remember eye contact.
- Assess the presenting complaint (e.g. abdominal pain) and its history:
  - Do not forget to ask about any history of jaundice.
  - Enquire about diet.
- Ask about past medical history (particularly related to gastrointestinal/urinary tract disease, operations and episodes of jaundice).
- Enquire about smoking, drinking and drugs (include in this anything about recreational drugs).
- Enquire about the social history.
- Ask about the family history (any history of peptic ulcer disease).
- Systematic enquiry.

**Listen to the answers!**

## Examination

For the abdominal examination, patients should ideally be exposed from the xiphisternum to the pubis, but, to preserve dignity, do not leave the patient exposed for too long. Ascertain whether they are comfortable when lying flat with one pillow. This is the best way to assess the abdomen, but it is not always practical for some patients. Begin examining the system with the patient sitting up, and only lie them flat when you examine the abdomen itself.

Remember that it may be regarded as threatening if you stand over the patient, and also that it is more comfortable and effective for the clinician to examine the patient at an appropriate height. Either raise the bed to a comfortable working height or sit or kneel by the bedside. If you have cold hands, warm them before starting.

> ▶ VIDEO 4.1 The abdominal examination
> ......................................................
> https://www.crcpress.com/cw/kopelman

## General observations

Melaena indicating significant upper gastrointestinal bleeding has a distinctive offensive sweet smell that, once encountered, is never forgotten. Register the presence of uraemic or hepatic foetor ('bad breath'). Look at the patient's hands, and then the neck, face, mouth and upper back. During the initial assessment, look for any trace of jaundice in the skin and sclerae (**Fig. 4.3**). There may be a lemon-yellow tinge to the skin with uraemia. Pale conjunctivae may indicate anaemia.

**The hands and nails** Look for signs of liver disease. These include liver palms, which is reddening of the peripheral area of the palms due to the peripheral vasodilatation caused by oestrogen excess. Liver palms may be present in liver disease with reduced metabolism of oestrogen in the liver. They may also be found in thyrotoxicosis, in pregnancy and in users of oral contraceptives.

*Dupuytren's contracture* This is a flexion deformity, usually of the fourth and fifth fingers (**Fig. 4.4**). Although there are several other causes for this condition, it may be found in liver disease and alcohol excess.

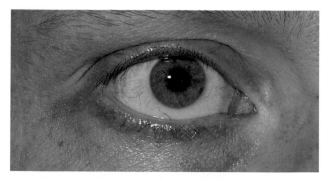

Fig. 4.3 Jaundice, seen as yellowing of the sclera.

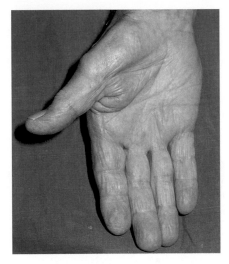

Fig. 4.4 Dupuytren's contracture. Note the tethering of the palmar skin of the ring finger.

*Leuconychia* This is a whitening of the nail bed caused by the hypoproteinaemia associated with liver disease.

*Koilonychia* This refers to the so-called spoon-shaped nails that are associated with iron deficiency.

*Finger clubbing* An increase in curvature of the nail bed in both directions with loss of the nail angle is typically associated with chronic inflammatory conditions, including inflammatory bowel disease and cirrhosis.

*Half and half nails (Lindsay's nails)* The distal nail bed is reddish brown with proximal pallor associated with chronic kidney disease.

**Spider naevi** These are small red vascular malformations associated with oestrogen excess. They are easily identified because they fill from a central arteriole, and can be blanched from the middle. They are found in the distribution of the superior vena cava. A healthy adult may have up to five (see **Figs 4.17** and **4.18**). Remember to look on the scalp.

**Lymph nodes** Examination of the cervical and axillary lymph nodes is described in Chapter 3 (see **Fig. 3.6**, page 108). Virchow's node or Troisier's sign is a hard enlarged left supraclavicular node that is most commonly associated with gastric cancer.

## Assessing the patient's nutritional status

It is always important to assess the nutritional status of a patient during the general examination. Doctors frequently fall into the trap of concentrating on specific symptoms without considering a patient's particular body habitus – signs of weight loss associated with a malignancy may be overlooked because the doctor is focusing on abdominal pain, or the significance of obesity is not immediately recognised in the hypertensive patient. The following are simple clinical measures that can be easily undertaken to assess a patient's overall nutritional status. It is not suggested that all of these are applied on every occasion, although they are indicated in patients with cachexia or extreme obesity.

**Physical appearance** Does the patient look extraordinarily thin or considerably overweight? Many patients have always been underweight, while others will only confirm recent weight loss if asked directly. Remember that denial is sometimes associated with anorexia nervosa. Similarly, a recent increase in weight or long-standing obesity is also of clinical significance – an explanation for the former needs to be found, while the latter is often associated with important complications such as diabetes, osteoarthritis, hypertension and sleep apnoea. It is helpful to note your subjective impression of the patient's body habitus in the patient's case record.

**Body weight and height** Whenever possible, every patient should be weighed on accurate scales, and their height measured using a stadiometer. Changes in weight following treatment are essential measures of success or failure of certain therapies, for example weight reduction in patients with cardiac failure after commencing diuretic treatment, or weight gain following a prescription for supplemental feeds. The body mass index (BMI: weight in kilograms divided by the height in metres squared [$Kg/M^2$]) is a

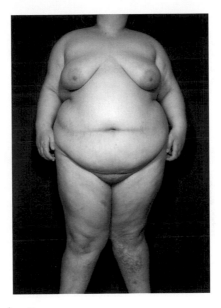

Fig. 4.5 Morbid obesity.

useful estimate of body fatness – the acceptable range is between 19 and 25; a BMI of 25–30 is regarded as overweight and a BMI 30 or greater is defined as obesity. A BMI over 39 is indicative of extreme or 'morbid' obesity and suggests the likelihood of serious associated complications (**Fig. 4.5**).

**Regional fat distribution** Epidemiological studies have confirmed that the distribution of fat within the body is also important in determining increased risk from coronary heart disease, stroke, diabetes mellitus and hyperlipidaemia. Such an increased risk is seen in both men and women who are moderately overweight but in whom fat is deposited predominantly in the upper half of the body (upper body, truncal or 'apple-shaped' obesity). In contrast, this is not found in overweight individuals whose fatness is largely in the lower half of the body (lower body, gynoid or 'pear-shaped' obesity). A simple way of assessing body fat distribution in an overweight patient is by measuring the waist circumference – there is no point in using this measure in a person who has a BMI within the acceptable range. The waist circumference is taken at the point midway between the lower border of the rib cage and the upper margin of the iliac crest.

The gender-specific waist circumference levels in **Box 4.2** denote enhanced relative risk.

### BOX 4.2 WAIST CIRCUMFERENCE LEVELS

| Gender | Increased risk | Substantial risk |
|--------|----------------|------------------|
| Male | >94 cm (~37 inches) | >102 cm (~40 inches) |
| Female | >80 cm (~32 inches) | >88 cm (~35 inches) |

**Skinfold thickness** The measurement of skinfold thickness using skinfold calipers (usually Harpenden calipers) is an additional practical method for estimating body fatness at the bedside. The established system is to measure the skinfold thickness at four sites:

- **Triceps** thickness is measured halfway between the acromial and olecranon processes. A fold of skin and subcutaneous tissue is pinched between your thumb and forefinger. This grip is maintained with your left hand, while the calipers are applied to the skin tuck using your right hand.
- **Biceps** skinfold thickness is measured in the same place as the triceps, but at the front of the arm with the hand supinated.
- **Subscapular** thickness is measured at a 45° angle to the vertical at the lower edge of the left scapula.
- **Suprailiac** thickness is measured in the horizontal plane, just above the iliac crest in the mid-axillary line on the left side.

Tables are available for calculating skinfold percentage fat from the sum of these four skinfolds. These measures of nutritional status should be clearly recorded in the patient's notes; it will be appropriate for measurements to be repeated at intervals after treatment has been commenced.

## Mouth and tongue

Inspect the inside of the mouth, looking particularly at the teeth and gums. Note any obvious caries or periodontal decay and, if the patient has lost many teeth, confirm that the dentures are satisfactory. Look for evidence of oral ulceration, which may be associated with inflammatory bowel disease. White plaques on the oral mucosa or tongue may be due to candidiasis, indicating immunodeficiency or a complication of therapeutic immunosuppression. Look at the tonsils and pharynx using a light and tongue depressor if necessary. Examine the tongue, looking for smoothness (atrophy) of the papillae or soreness. Vitamin $B_{12}$ deficiency leads to uniform atrophy of papillae over the whole tongue, which is often sore and inflamed. Other vitamin deficiency states, including iron, nicotinic acid, pyridoxine and folic acid, may also cause flattening and loss of papillae. Furring of the tongue occurs in a number of acute infections and internal disorders, but is of little help with diagnosis. Macroglossia with dental indentations is a feature of amyloidosis.

Inflammation and soreness of the corners of the mouth (angular stomatitis) is seen in various deficiency states, including lack of iron, riboflavin and nicotinic acid. Most commonly, however, it results from loss of teeth or poorly fitting dentures. Telangiectases on the lips are characteristic of hereditary haemorrhagic telangiectasia, a cause of gastrointestinal bleeding.

Once your quick assessment of the peripheral signs is complete, proceed to examination of the abdomen. Follow the scheme: inspection, palpation, percussion, auscultation.

## Inspection

Inspect the abdomen from the end of the bed, as well as from the side. Begin by looking for distension, which may be caused by masses, dilated bowel, ascites (fluid within the abdominal cavity) or enlarged organs. Take note of any visible scars or dilated subcutaneous veins. Look for signs of obvious weight loss, for example loose, wrinkled skin. Occasionally, dilated veins are seen radiating in all directions from the umbilicus; their appearance, which is described as a caput medusae, indicates elevation of the portal venous pressure (portal hypertension) and results from the formation of portal–systemic anastomosis via the veins in the round ligament.

Peristalsis is not usually visible except in very thin subjects. Peristaltic waves can occasionally be seen in chronic pyloric stenosis or intestinal obstruction.

## Palpation

This is done from the patient's right side with the right hand predominating (even if you are left-handed), with either the bed raised to an appropriate height or the examiner kneeling or sitting next to the patient with their arm horizontal.

Ask if the patient has any tender areas, so you can initially avoid these. Start by palpating gently in the four quadrants shown in **Fig. 4.6**. The approximate location of the organs beneath the skin are shown in **Fig. 4.7**. This gentle palpation should be very systematic (**Fig. 4.8**), allowing the examiner to take note of any obvious tender areas or masses. It is important to look at the patient's face throughout to ensure that you are not causing pain. Generalised peritonitis is obvious at this stage because it causes exquisite tenderness and a rigid abdomen.

**The liver** The normal liver extends from approximately the fifth intercostal space on the right of the midline to the costal margin. It may just be palpable in the normal individual. Occasionally, it becomes palpable because it has been pushed down from above

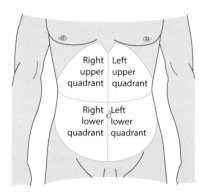

Fig. 4.6 The quadrants of the abdomen.

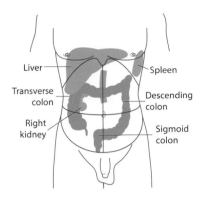

Fig. 4.7 Approximate location of organs beneath the skin in the abdomen related to the quadrants.

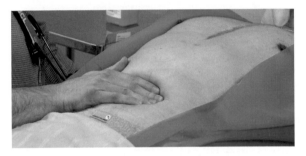

Fig. 4.8 Begin with gentle palpation.

but is still of normal size – for example, if the patient has chronic airflow limitation. This can be checked by percussing out the upper border. To feel the liver, use the flat of the hand with either the side of the index finger or the fingertips parallel to the costal margin. Ask the patient to take deep breaths in and out, and coordinate this with a gentle upward movement of the palpating fingertips as the respiratory effort pushes the liver down. If the liver is enlarged, it is worth beginning the palpation in the right iliac fossa and gradually moving the palpating hand up, coordinating this with respiration.

If a liver is felt, the examiner must describe its consistency. The edge may be smooth or irregular (the latter suggesting metastases or secondary deposits), and the texture soft, firm, hard or nodular. You should also estimate (in centimetres) the amount of palpable liver below the costal margin. A pulsatile liver suggests tricuspid regurgitation. Determination of the precise position of the lower edge of the liver by palpation and percussion can be challenging, particularly in obese individuals. The scratch test, where the diaphragm of the stethoscope is placed over the xiphisternum with gentle scratching of the skin vertically across the costal margin in the mid-clavicular line, results in a change in the intensity of sound transmitted on crossing the lower border of the liver.

Occasionally, the gall bladder is felt when looking for the liver. The gall bladder is a smooth round organ, arising just below the costal margin. Inflammation of the gall bladder, for example in acute cholecystitis, results in tenderness in deep palpation in the right upper quadrant on deep inspiration – Murphy's sign.

**The spleen** The normal spleen is not palpable. It lies behind the ninth rib in the left hypochondrium. It may become palpable as it enlarges; this is usually in the direction of the umbilicus. It is best palpated using the fingertips, coordinating their action with the patient's respiration (**Fig. 4.9**). If the spleen is not palpable with the patient lying flat, ask them to roll towards the examiner and advance your palpating fingers towards, and then under, the left costal margin (**Fig. 4.10**). The left hand can be placed behind the costal margin to bring the spleen forward. Palpation of the splenic notch confirms the findings of an enlarged spleen. While the

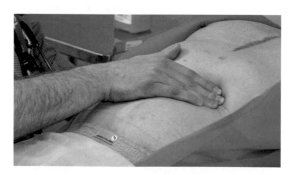

Fig. 4.9 Palpating a patient's abdomen for an enlarged spleen.

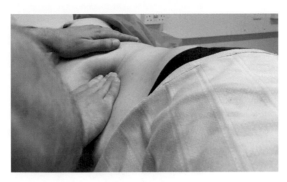

Fig. 4.10 Asking the patient to roll on their side to face you may assist in palpating an enlarged spleen.

patient is in this position, percuss along the line of the seventh rib to ascertain the area of splenic dullness, thereby confirming the palpation findings.

**The kidneys (Fig. 4.11)** Palpation of the kidneys is part of the abdominal examination. In the normal individual, the lower pole of the right kidney may be felt in very thin individuals as it is pushed down by the liver. The kidneys move by up to 4–5cm with respiration.

Examination of the kidneys is performed using both hands. To feel the left kidney, the left hand is placed behind the patient's loin, and the organ pushed forward from the back, onto the palpating right hand (**Fig. 4.12**). This procedure is done in reverse to feel the right kidney. The most characteristic thing about the kidney on palpation is its mobility, in a downwards direction beneath the palpating hand.

The findings are confirmed by percussion as the kidneys are surrounded by perinephric fat with bowel-containing gas above it, and this is resonant to percussion. The palpable left kidney is usually abnormal, except in very thin individuals. Both kidneys are situated posteriorly, and more medially than you may expect. If palpable, and enlarged, they may be ballotable. This means that a renal mass can be pushed between an anterior and a posterior palpating hand. In general, a palpable kidney is either polycystic or contains a large tumour. Massive bilateral polycystic kidneys can be mistaken for hepatosplenomegaly.

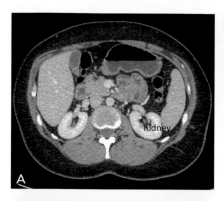

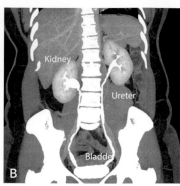

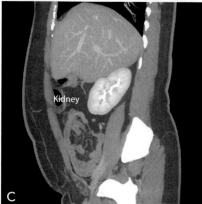

Fig. 4.11A–C Computed tomography scan images of the urinary tract. Axial (A), coronal (B) and sagittal (C) images indicating the position of the kidneys, ureters and bladder. Intravenous contrast, which has been renally excreted, demonstrates the collecting systems in (B). (Courtesy of Dr Uday Patel, Consultant Radiologist, St George's University Hospitals NHS Foundation Trust, London, UK.)

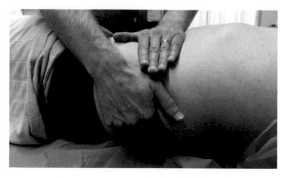

Fig. 4.12 Palpation of the kidneys.

**The bladder** When this is distended, it is felt as a smooth, round swelling extending upward from the pubis. The patient may experience discomfort on pressure over the area, and the swelling is typically dull to percussion. An enlarged uterus or an ovarian cyst may give rise to a swelling that is difficult to distinguish from the bladder on palpation. The distinction can be made, however, if the bladder is emptied either naturally or by means of a urinary catheter.

**Ascites** Ascites is caused by free fluid in the abdominal cavity. It causes abdominal distension, which is often more prominent in the flanks. There are two commonly used methods of detection: percussion, and the detection of a fluid thrill. Percussion for ascites depends on eliciting shifting dullness. This is done by percussing the abdomen from the midline towards the flanks, until the note becomes dull. Keep the hand in the same position and ask the patient to roll towards you; then continue to percuss in that position. If the area where the dullness was confirmed has become resonant, this suggests free fluid in the abdominal cavity. To elicit a fluid thrill, ask an assistant (or the patient) to place their hand longitudinally along the midline. Then flick the flank beneath the area of dullness with the other hand on the opposite side, as if at the other end of a diameter of a circle (**Fig. 4.13**). If there is a fluid thrill, it will be felt shortly after the flick, as a flutter.

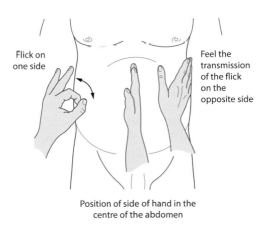

Flick on one side

Feel the transmission of the flick on the opposite side

Position of side of hand in the centre of the abdomen

Fig. 4.13 Eliciting a fluid thrill.

## Auscultation

Auscultation of the normal abdomen reveals peristaltic sounds that are gurgling and bubbling in character. When the intestine is mechanically obstructed, high-pitched tinkling sounds are heard, usually in association with colicky pain. In intestinal paralysis (paralytic ileus), sounds are usually absent.

When there are large amounts of fluid and gas in the stomach (or occasionally in the intestines), a splashing noise is heard when the abdomen is gently shaken. This sign is called a succussion splash; it may be normally heard if the patient has recently been eating or drinking, but is characteristically prominent in patients with delayed gastric emptying, – for example in pyloric stenosis. Vascular sounds are sometimes heard. When there is partial obstruction of the abdominal arteries, systolic murmurs may be produced and heard over the aorta, iliac arteries or renal arteries. The latter (which are rare) may be heard in the renal angle posteriorly and not, as is often taught, by auscultating anteriorly when there is bowel in the way.

Examination of the abdomen is not complete without examination of the external genitalia, inguinal lymph nodes and hernial orifices (see Chapter 8), followed by a rectal examination.

## Rectal examination

Patients are often understandably embarrassed by this part of the examination so it is essential to put them at their ease. Reassure the patient that although the examination may be uncomfortable and unpleasant, it should not be painful. Ask the patient to lower their pants to the knees, lie on their left side, and draw their knees up into the chest. Meanwhile, put a glove on your right hand. With your left hand, lift the right buttock to inspect the anus: note any sores, lesions (such as warts or haemorrhoids), fissures or fistulae. Place the gloved and lubricated index finger of the right hand over the anus and apply gentle pressure. The finger will be gradually admitted to the anal canal, from the front gradually backwards advancing it into the rectum. The rectal mucosa can then be felt posteriorly. The examining finger is then rotated through 360°, and the mucosa felt anteriorly and laterally. Anteriorly in the male, an indentation may be felt, caused by the prostate gland. In a similar position in the female lies the cervix – a small, rounded swelling. There may be polyps (soft and attached to the rectal mucosa) or tumours (hard and irregular), and it is important to learn the difference between these pathologies and the feel of normal or constipated stool. On removing the examining finger, inspect the glove for the presence of melaena, blood or mucus.

## Illustrated physical signs

The following photographs illustrate physical signs that you may see in patients with significant liver disease.

**Ascites (Fig. 4.14)**: this patient has tense, severe ascites. Severe tense swelling of the abdomen is a feature of chronic liver disease.

**Hepatomegaly (Fig. 4.15)**: the large liver of this patient is indicated in the photograph. Patients with liver disease often also exhibit **spider naevi (Fig. 4.16)**.

*Table 4.3* summarises the findings in a normal abdominal examination, and *Table 4.4* the care of the patient with gastrointestinal disease.

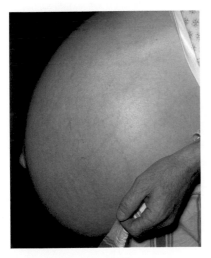

Fig. 4.14 Ascites. Note the tense abdominal distension.

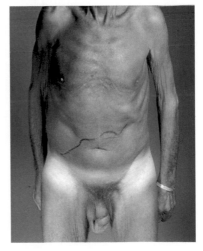

Fig. 4.15 Hepatomegaly. The position of the liver is indicated.

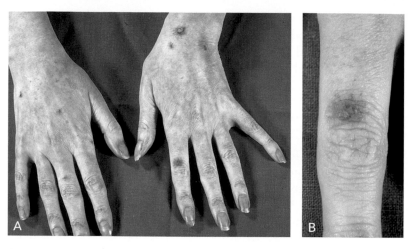

Fig. 4.16A, B Spider naevi in a patient with liver disease.

## Table 4.3 Findings in a normal abdominal examination

- Start by assessing the patient's hands, but do not take too long. Also look for cervical and axillary adenopathy, and signs of abdominal disease in the face
- Expose the patient from the xiphisternum to the pubis
- Ask the patient to identify tender areas, and palpate superficially over the whole abdomen
- Use deep palpation looking for the liver, spleen and kidneys
- Percuss over the palpated areas
- Look for hernias and lymph nodes
- Auscultate over the aorta and renal arteries
- Mention a rectal examination

## Therapeutic and technical skills

### Key laboratory tests

**Liver blood tests** Liver damage is measured by an assessment of hepatic enzymes – alkaline phosphatase (ALP), aspartate aminotransferase (AST) or alanine aminotransferase (ALT) and

## Table 4.4 Care of patients with gastrointestinal disease

- Ensure that adults are able to feed themselves
- Ensure that patients are able to use a commode and/or a bedpan
- Keep stool/vomit charts as necessary: observation of colour, consistency, amount and odour of stool
- Assess patients' dietary needs

gamma-glutamyl transferase ($\gamma$GT) – together with albumin, bilirubin and total serum protein. Bilirubin, AST and ALP are all moderately elevated in hepatocellular jaundice. The ALP is highly elevated in obstructive jaundice – often out of all proportion to the other two enzymes. In this situation, there is usually a corresponding increase in $\gamma$GT. $\gamma$GT is more specifically elevated in alcoholic liver disease – and suggests the presence of excessive alcohol intake, particularly if the other enzymes are normal or mildly raised. Albumin is a measure of hepatic synthetic function, and is a useful marker of the severity of hepatic impairment. Albumin is characteristically reduced in chronic liver disease, whereas the total serum protein level is usually increased.

**Clotting** Clotting is measured by estimating the prothrombin time (PT, or international normalised ratio [INR]), activated partial thromboplastin time (aPTT) and thrombin time (TT). The PT provides an estimate of the performance of the extrinsic and common coagulation pathways. The aPTT is prolonged in abnormalities of either the intrinsic or common pathways. The TT measures the transformation of prothrombin to thrombin; it is prolonged by fibrinogen deficiency. Deficiency of protein C, protein S and anti-thrombin III should be sought in patients with a hypercoagulable state.

**Hepatitis serology** The serological markers of hepatitis B are important in assessing the relative infection risk of carriers. In a patient incubating hepatitis B, or with an acute attack, there are positive tests for HbsAg (surface antigen) and HbeAg (a marker of high infectivity). The patient may also have the antibodies anti-Hbc, immunoglobulin (Ig) G and IgM. In the carrier state, HbsAg is positive. HbeAg is either positive or negative, depending on whether the patient is highly (positive HbeAg) or not very highly (negative HbeAg) infectious. In the convalescence phase of an acute attack, the HbsAg and HbeAg are negative, but anti-Hbs and anti-Hbi antibodies become positive. After successful vaccination, the patient is positive for anti-Hbs only. The presence of viraemia should be confirmed by quantifying hepatitis B viral DNA in the blood. Evidence of previous hepatitis C virus infection is indicated by serology with quantification of viral RNA in the blood and genotyping to guide therapy.

## Urinalysis and microscopy

In a patient with suspected renal disease, a mid-stream specimen of urine should be analysed at the first opportunity: even though the patient is currently passing urine, they may not be in a few hours time. Inspect the urine. Red urine may indicate haematuria or treatment with rifampicin. Less intense haematuria gives the urine a smokey appearance. Myoglobin in urine in rhabdomyolysis turns urine dark brown. A turbid appearance is most commonly due to pyuria caused by urinary tract infection. Infection is most unlikely in the presence of crystal-clear urine. Widely available test strips identify the following substances in urine

**Protein** This is actually a test for albumin with a threshold for a positive result of 3 g/L and does not detect globular proteins (myoglobin or Ig light chains in myeloma). Proteinuria may either indicate urinary tract infection or glomerular damage.

**Blood** This is actually a test for haemoglobin detecting intact or lysed erythrocytes, and cross-reacts with myoglobin, which is present in urine if there is rhabdomyolysis. Urinary tract infection is the most common cause of haematuria, but it may indicate bleeding from anywhere in the urinary tract from the glomerulus to the urethra due to inflammation, stones or neoplasm. Identification of dysmorphic erythrocytes and erythrocyte casts on urine microscopy suggests a diagnosis of glomerulonephritis.

**pH** Normal urine is acidic. Alkaline urine may indicate renal tubular acidosis, urinary infection with urease-producing organisms or diuretic treatment.

**Nitrite and leucocytes** Nitrite is produced by some but not all bacteria that cause urinary tract infections. Leucocyturia is a cardinal feature of urinary tract infection. A positive test for nitrite in the absence of leucocyturia is likely to be due to a contaminated specimen.

## Tests of renal function

Creatinine, which is generated in skeletal muscle and excreted in urine, is the endogenous biomarker that is used most widely to estimate glomerular filtration rate (GFR). Equations to predict estimated GFR (eGFR) use serum creatinine with factors that estimate body muscle mass. The MDRD (Modification of Diet in Renal Disease) equation is only precise for GFRs up to 60 ml/min, but the more recently introduced CKD-EPI (Chronic Kidney Disease Epidemiology Collaboration) equation can be used across the full range of GFRs.

## Quantification of proteinuria

Spot early morning urine specimens can be used to measure the ratio of creatinine to either albumin, which is more sensitive for screening, or total protein, which corrects for urine concentration. An albumin:creatinine ratio of 30 mg/mmol or a protein:creatinine ratio of 50 mg/mmol equates roughly to 0.5 g protein excretion per 24 hours.

The following figures demonstrate the features required to make a diagnosis of common gastrointestinal and genitourinary diseases: peptic ulceration (**Fig. 4.17**), large bowel carcinoma (**Fig. 4.18**), inflammatory bowel disease (**Fig. 4.19**), chronic liver disease (**Fig. 4.20**), chronic renal failure (**Fig. 4.21**) and urinary tract infection (**Fig. 4.22**).

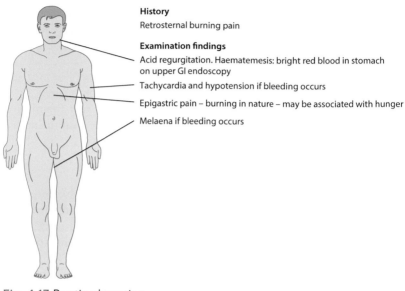

**History**
Retrosternal burning pain

**Examination findings**
Acid regurgitation. Haematemesis: bright red blood in stomach on upper GI endoscopy
Tachycardia and hypotension if bleeding occurs
Epigastric pain – burning in nature – may be associated with hunger
Melaena if bleeding occurs

Fig. 4.17 Peptic ulceration.

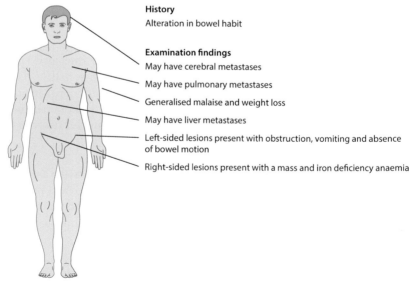

**History**
Alteration in bowel habit

**Examination findings**
May have cerebral metastases
May have pulmonary metastases
Generalised malaise and weight loss
May have liver metastases
Left-sided lesions present with obstruction, vomiting and absence of bowel motion
Right-sided lesions present with a mass and iron deficiency anaemia

Fig. 4.18 Large bowel carcinoma.

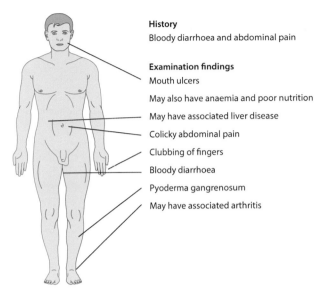

**History**
Bloody diarrhoea and abdominal pain

**Examination findings**
Mouth ulcers

May also have anaemia and poor nutrition

May have associated liver disease

Colicky abdominal pain

Clubbing of fingers

Bloody diarrhoea

Pyoderma gangrenosum

May have associated arthritis

Fig. 4.19 Inflammatory bowel disease.

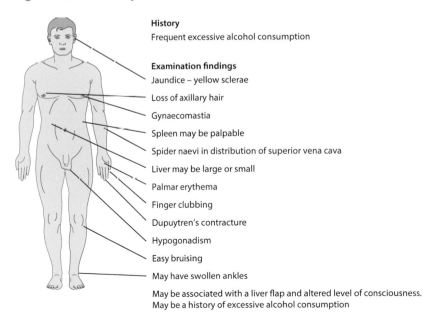

**History**
Frequent excessive alcohol consumption

**Examination findings**
Jaundice – yellow sclerae

Loss of axillary hair

Gynaecomastia

Spleen may be palpable

Spider naevi in distribution of superior vena cava

Liver may be large or small

Palmar erythema

Finger clubbing

Dupuytren's contracture

Hypogonadism

Easy bruising

May have swollen ankles

May be associated with a liver flap and altered level of consciousness.
May be a history of excessive alcohol consumption

Fig. 4.20 Chronic liver disease.

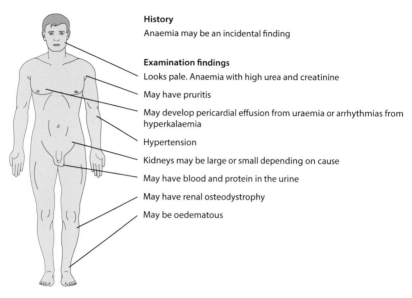

**History**
Anaemia may be an incidental finding

**Examination findings**
Looks pale. Anaemia with high urea and creatinine

May have pruritis

May develop pericardial effusion from uraemia or arrhythmias from hyperkalaemia

Hypertension

Kidneys may be large or small depending on cause

May have blood and protein in the urine

May have renal osteodystrophy

May be oedematous

Fig. 4.21 Chronic kidney disease.

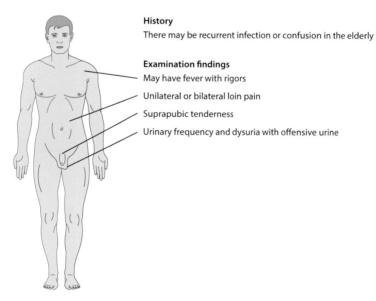

**History**
There may be recurrent infection or confusion in the elderly

**Examination findings**
May have fever with rigors

Unilateral or bilateral loin pain

Suprapubic tenderness

Urinary frequency and dysuria with offensive urine

Fig. 4.22 Urinary tract infection.

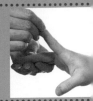

Locomotor disorders are one of the most common causes of pain and disability, both in hospital and within the community. Almost everyone has had some time off work with back pain during their career or has suffered a similar minor locomotor problem. Examination of the locomotor system is quite difficult, particularly as it is somewhat diverse – the high prevalence of rheumatic conditions in the general population is not reflected by the quality of rheumatological examination in practice. Conditions affecting the locomotor system are diverse, and range from very minor soft tissue conditions such as tennis elbow to very severe, life-threatening connective tissue diseases such as systemic lupus erythematosus (SLE). This requires history taking and examination to be extremely flexible, allowing for a quick 'spot' diagnosis, or time and understanding to be given where necessary to patients with more complex problems.

## Applied anatomy and physiology of the joints

The locomotor system is made up of muscles and joints. The two basic structures of joints that permit mobility are cartilage and fibrous tissue. **Cartilaginous joints** are those in which a wide range of movement is required. The anatomy of the synovial joint is shown in **Fig. 5.1**.

In a **fibrous joint**, there is less mobility, and therefore the joint is simpler in structure and associated with fewer medical problems.

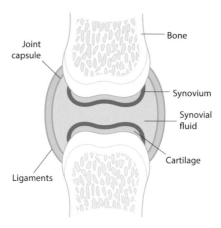

Fig. 5.1 The anatomy of a synovial joint.

In a **synovial joint**, the bony ends are covered by hyaline cartilage and surrounded by a capsule. The inside of the capsule is covered by a synovial membrane, which has secretory and absorptive tissue. The synovial membrane produces synovial fluid by ultrafiltration.

In addition to joints, there are several other fluid-filled sacs within the body known as bursae. These can also become inflamed and symptomatic.

The joints are moved by the actions of muscles, which are attached to bone by tendons. The two main causes of arthritis or joint disease are degenerative change and inflammatory change:

- **Degenerative** change is seen in patients with osteoarthritis in whom the cartilage layers have become thinned and fibrillated and thus degenerate, giving rise to symptoms.
- **Inflammatory** joint disease occurs in patients in whom there is synovitis, or inflammation of the synovium, causing joint inflammation and thus secondary damage to the joint.

Tendons, ligaments and fascial structures are attached to the periosteum by a specialised structure, the enthesis, and this can become inflamed, causing an enthesitis, for example plantar fasciitis.

## Assessment and diagnosis of joint disease

Assessment of a patient with disease of the musculoskeletal system involves an assessment of not only the history of their symptoms, but also the degree of disability and handicap.

## Taking the history

The cardinal symptoms of joint disease are pain, stiffness, swelling, deformity, disability and systemic illness (*Table 5.1*). It is often the history and the pattern of joint involvement that lead to the diagnosis of a rheumatic condition. For example, a symmetrical polyarthritis that is inflammatory and mainly affects small joints is likely to be rheumatoid arthritis.

### The presenting complaint

**Pain** Pain is the most common reason for a rheumatological consultation, but it is often quite a vague symptom and requires specific questioning. The degree of pain does not relate directly to the severity of the condition. Although open questions are essential to start the consultation, a question such as 'Where is the pain?' may get a vague answer. Thus, it is important to use focused and closed questions, and also to ask the patient to point not only to the general area of the pain, but also to the place where the pain is at its maximum intensity:

'Where do you get the pain?'

'Does it go anywhere else?'

'Show me the worst spot.'

'Does it go down your arms or legs?'

## Table 5.1  Important areas of enquiry

| | |
|---|---|
| • Pain | • Deformity |
| • Stiffness | • Disability |
| • Swelling | • Systemic illness |

**BOX 5.1 LOCOMOTOR HISTORY TAKING**

A locomotor history allows the doctor to answer the four following questions and thus make a diagnosis:

- Is the patient's problem caused by a symmetrical or an asymmetrical arthritis?
- Is it a monoarthritis, or does it affect several joints – a polyarthritis?
- Is it an inflammatory or a non-inflammatory arthritis?
- Does it affect large joints or small joints?

As some locomotor system problems, such as a prolapsed intervertebral disc, may cause nerve root irritation, the pain may be in a dermatomal distribution and quite distant from the original problem. Rheumatological pain is also referred; for example, shoulder pain is felt in the upper arm, and hip pain is felt in the knee. It is important also to enquire whether the pain is associated with other symptoms of locomotor problems, such as stiffness and swelling.

Locomotor pain is often related to movement, and it is important to enquire whether the pain gets better with rest or improves with increased activity. Pain that gets better with activity or as the day progresses is more likely to be due to inflammation. Pain that gets worse during the day is likely to be due to degenerative change:

'When is the pain at its worst?'

'Does it get better or worse during the day?'

Most locomotor system pain is better at night; however, pain from severe arthritis and also malignant disease keeps the patient awake. Night pain is likely to suggest a more significant problem, such as a hip that needs replacing or a disease with a poorer prognosis. Some locomotor system pain is caused by fairly specific abnormalities, such as tennis elbow. In these patients, the pain is very specific and is localised to one particular spot. The patient can often show the exact spot:

'Can you find the exact spot?'

Some patients have many non-specific aches and pains that may have a non-organic cause. This is often called arthralgia. It is important to exclude organic causes before reassuring the patient that nothing is seriously amiss.

**Stiffness** Patients with locomotor system problems often complain of stiffness. This is an inability to get the joints moving again after a period of rest. In inflammatory conditions, this stiffness is much worse in the mornings and gradually wears off over a period of 1 or 2 hours. The length of time that the stiffness lasts is related to the severity of the inflammation. Patients with degenerative change also have stiffness, but the stiffness is related to inactivity, and tends to come on when sitting down for a period of 10 minutes or longer. It is sometimes called gelling.

The stiffness usually takes less than half an hour to resolve, but is worse as the day progresses:

'Do you feel stiff?'

'When?'

'How long does it take you to get going when you get up in the morning?'

**Swelling** In patients with joint pain and stiffness, it is important to enquire about local swelling. Swelling may be symmetrical or asymmetrical, depending on the kind of arthritis, and is of three kinds (*Table 5.2*):

- **Synovial swelling** – this feels soft and 'boggy', and is associated with heat and local inflammation. It is often symmetrical and is associated with inflammatory conditions.
- **Bony swelling** – this is associated with degenerative conditions and causes joint deformity, but little associated heat and redness. It has often been present for longer than soft tissue swelling.
- **Fluctuant swelling** – this is caused by fluid and may feel hot, but is not compressible. It is important to ask the patient whether

### Table 5.2 Examples of different kinds of joint swelling

| | |
|---|---|
| Synovitis | 'Boggy', symmetrical swelling that feels hot |
| Osteoarthritis | Hard, bony swelling that generally feels cool |
| Fluid | Soft, fluctuant swelling that feels hot |

the swollen joint is hot and red, and whether the swelling is there permanently or whether it comes and goes.

- Ask: 'Do your joints swell? Which joints are affected? Do they feel hot to the touch? Do they go red?'

**Deformity** Deformity is often the end result of an arthritic process. Ask over what period of time the deformity has been developing, and the association of the deformity with swelling and pain:

'How long has this been going on?'

**Disability** Disability is frequently the result of an arthritic process. In the history, you should estimate how much the patient is able to do and how much the disease interferes with their day-to-day life. The sort of questions you should ask will depend on the patient's daily activity and whether they can carry out their normal job. For example, a tennis elbow or a frozen shoulder may be severely disabling in somebody who needs to use their upper limb (a librarian, a painter or a secretary), while painful feet are a serious disability in a postman. It is a useful exercise to ask the patient to take you through an average day – and enquire how they do things like shopping or cooking – and whether they have help from other people or uses appliances.

**Systemic illness** Connective tissue diseases, which are multisystem diseases, may present with locomotor system problems. It is therefore important to ask patients whether they have noticed fever, weight loss, a tendency to fatigue or lethargy. In addition, there may have been a problem with rashes, particularly the photosensitive rash of SLE.

In general, although locomotor system problems are rarely life-threatening, they may cause significant disability in those who suffer them, and are frequently associated with subclinical symptoms of depression. You should enquire whether the patient has suffered from feelings of depression, excessive tiredness or weepiness. These may be part of a primary problem or they may have developed secondary to the locomotor system problem.

Recent advances in the treatment of inflammatory conditions with biological agents has resulted in an increase in susceptibility to infection. Patients being treated with biological therapy may present with the symptoms of an underlying infection. These symptoms may be subtle, and are often systemic.

## Past medical history

Rheumatological complaints may have a long history, so it is important to establish whether there is any locomotor system problem in the past medical history.

For example, a patient with generalised osteoarthritis may have a problem with one large joint affected by osteoarthritis, and may also have had evidence of cervical spondylosis in the past. The patient may feel that this new pain is part of a different condition. You must establish whether there has been a history of acute injury or damage to a particular joint. This is important in osteoarthritis, where mechanical damage may predispose to the condition; for example, footballers are likely to get osteoarthritis of the knee. In the inflammatory arthritides, it is important to enquire about associated conditions such as iritis. Inflammatory conditions like rheumatoid arthritis wax and wane over a prolonged period. Periods of severe flares of arthritis should be documented, and note taken of alleviating factors.

## Personal and social history

Some occupations predispose to specific problems: for example, dentists may develop osteoarthritis of the neck due to their working position, and dancers may develop osteoarthritis of the feet. Leisure activities can also predispose to osteoarthritis, and you should enquire about particularly violent types of physical exercise.

There are some specific occupational rheumatic diseases that have now become common parlance – for example, housemaid's knee (pre-patellar bursitis), tennis elbow (lateral epicondylitis) and weaver's bottom (ischial bursitis).

## Family history and treatment history

There is an inherited component to inflammatory musculoskeletal diseases such as rheumatoid arthritis and ankylosing spondylitis, so you should enquire about any familial history of inflammatory arthritis. Recent research in twins has suggested that osteoarthritis also runs in families. However, many patients may remember that their grandparents had rheumatism but cannot recall the diagnosis. It may be helpful to ask the patient to describe the abnormalities they remember, as well as to tell you what they think was wrong.

You need to enquire about drugs such as aspirin and non-steroidal anti-inflammatory drugs, not only to assess their efficacy but also to assess their side effects (in particular gastric irritation and gastrointestinal bleeding). Patients with rheumatoid arthritis are particularly prone to this. Remember also that some patients with inflammatory arthritic conditions may be on long-term steroid therapy and have associated side effects. Many patients with inflammatory conditions are now on biological therapies. These medications predispose patients to infection. The criteria for being prescribed a biological therapy include the failure of previous treatments as a result of either inefficacy or side effects. It is important to ask which disease-modifying drugs a patient has taken in the past, and why they were stopped. As inflammatory conditions are lifelong, there is a risk of giving a patient a drug that they have reacted to in the past but have forgotten about.

Finally, it is important not to forget that some connective tissue diseases can be drug-induced. Beware the patient with SLE who has been taking long-term phenothiazines for a psychiatric condition and who has developed the condition as a consequence of the drug intake.

## BOX 5.2 CHECKLIST FOR RHEUMATOLOGICAL HISTORY TAKING

- General approach, establish rapport, make eye contact.
- Assess the patient's complaint, particularly with relation to pain.
- Ask about a past medical history of rheumatic problems.
- Take a detailed drug history of the drugs that may precipitate and be used to treat the condition.
- Ask about the social and occupational history.
- Ask about the family history; remember that several rheumatic problems are inherited.
- Systematic enquiry.

**Listen to the answers!**

## Examination of the patient

Examination of the locomotor system can be complicated, so for the purpose of this book a rheumatological screen will be described, followed by a simple system for examining other joints. The screen is known as the 'GALS' locomotor system screen.

**BOX 5.3 THE 'GALS' LOCOMOTOR SYSTEM SCREEN (VIDEO 5.1)**

G = Look at the **G**ait          L = **L**egs
A = **A**rms                        S = **S**pine

▶ VIDEO 5.1 **The GALS examination**

https://www.crcpress.com/cw/kopelman

## General observations

**Gait** Observe the patient from the front and sides while they are standing in their underwear (**Figs 5.2** and **5.3**), looking for any kind of asymmetry and deformity such as one leg being shorter or longer (**Fig. 5.4**) than the other, or abnormality of the spinal curvature (kyphosis, scoliosis or a loss of lumbar lordosis). Observe the patient walking to make sure that the gait is normal, that they are swinging the

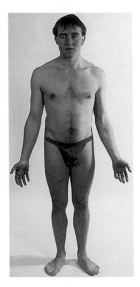

Fig. 5.2 Look at the patient from the front.

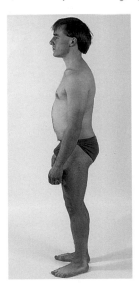

Fig. 5.3 Look at the patient from the side.

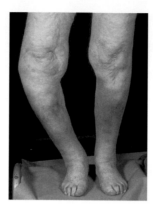

Fig. 5.4 Paget's disease of the tibia (a sabre tibia) and secondary osteoarthritis of the knee.

arms and moving the legs symmetrically. Look out for an antalgic gait, and make sure that both the person's knees are straight. An antalgic gait is an abnormality of gait rhythm in which the patient avoids bearing weight on the painful leg and spends most of the gait cycle on the unaffected limb. This may suggest a problem of the hip, knee, hindfoot, midfoot or forefoot.

## BOX 5.4 EXAMINATION OF THE ARMS (1)

During the general inspection, you should inspect for abnormalities such as swelling or deformity, and look for any skin changes that may be associated with arthritis, for example digital vasculitis in SLE or evidence of peripheral infarcts from Raynaud's phenomenon.

- Ask the patient to show you their hands, palms down, and then turn them over – this is an assessment of the radioulnar joint, which is a common site for rheumatoid arthritis (**Fig. 5.5**). Remember to ask the patient to keep their elbows tucked in; otherwise they may use their shoulders to perform this movement.
- Ask the patient to make a tight fist with each hand (**Fig. 5.6**); this is a position of function of the hands, and you can also assess power grip.

*(Continued)*

> **BOX 5.4 (*Continued*) EXAMINATION OF THE ARMS (1)**
>
> - Ask the patient to place the tip of each finger onto the tip of the thumb in turn (**Fig. 5.7**); this permits an assessment of the dexterity and fine movement of the hand, which is limited in rheumatoid arthritis.

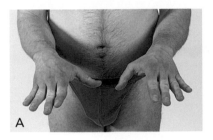 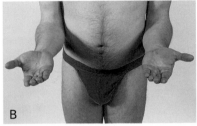

Fig. 5.5A, B  Assessment of radioulnar joint movement.

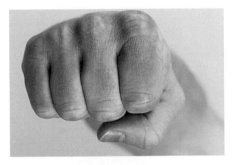

Fig. 5.6  Ask the patient to make a fist.

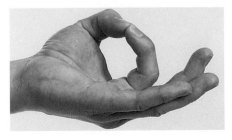

Fig. 5.7  Opposition of the thumb.

**BOX 5.5 EXAMINATION OF THE ARMS (2)**

- Squeeze across from the second to the fifth metacarpals (**Fig. 5.8**); this is an assessment of joint tenderness. Tenderness across the metacarpophalangeal joints is a sign of rheumatoid arthritis.
- Next, ask the patient to put their hands behind their head, pressing the shoulders right back; this is an assessment of abduction and external rotation of the shoulder with flexion of the elbow (**Fig. 5.9**). It is a measurement of shoulder and elbow movement as well as of function; it is not possible to put on a tie or comb your hair unless you can do this manoeuvre.

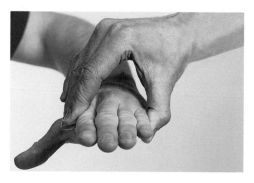

Fig. 5.8 Assessment of metacarpophalangeal tenderness.

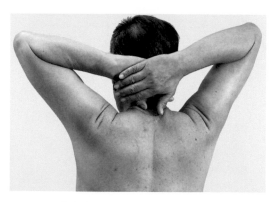

Fig. 5.9 Assessment of abduction and external rotation of the shoulders.

## BOX 5.6 EXAMINATION OF THE LEGS

- Ask the patient to lie back on the couch and flex the hip and knee while holding the knee. Ensure normal knee flexion, feel for crepitus and also test hip flexion.
- Then passively and internally rotate the hip with the knee and hip still flexed (**Fig. 5.10**); this is a measurement of knee movement and internal rotation of the hip.
- Ask the patient to flex, extend, invert and evert the ankle in order to assess tibiotalar (affected by osteoarthritis) and subtalar (affected by inflammatory arthritis) movements (**Figs 5.11** and **5.12**).
- Squeeze the metatarsals, looking for rheumatoid arthritis in the same way as for the metacarpals.

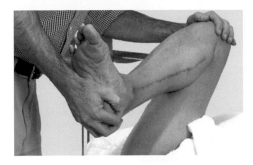

Fig. 5.10 Assessment of knee flexion and hip internal rotation.

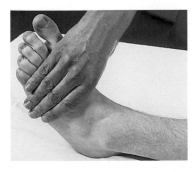

Fig. 5.11 Assessment of tibiotalar movement.

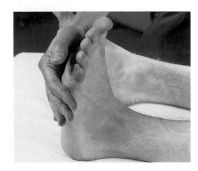

Fig. 5.12 Assessment of subtalar movement.

## BOX 5.7 EXAMINATION OF THE SPINE

- Ask the patient to stand up and to put their ear onto each shoulder in turn; this is an assessment of lateral flexion of the neck (**Fig. 5.13**), which is lost with either osteoarthritis or rheumatoid arthritis affecting the neck.
- Put two fingers over adjacent spinous processes in the lumbar region and then ask the patient to bend over and touch their toes; your fingers should move apart. This is a modification of Schober's test, which is designed to pick up a lack of movement associated with ankylosing spondylitis (**Fig. 5.14**).

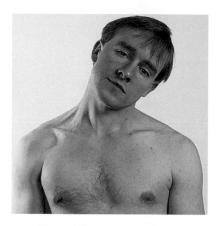

Fig. 5.13 Assessment of lateral flexion of the neck.

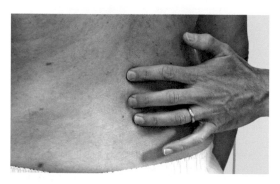

Fig. 5.14 A modification of Schober's test for spinal movement.

## Regional joint examination

**Low back pain** The lumbar spine should be examined with the patient standing, supine and prone:

- With the patient standing, assess the curvature of the spine. Scoliosis may be due to muscle spasm in acute sciatica or may be postural in leg length inequality. Loss of the normal lordosis is a sign of inflammatory spinal disease, such as ankylosing spondylitis.
- Palpate the erector spinae muscles to assess spasm.
- Perform a modified Schober's test (see **Box 5.7** and **Fig. 5.14**).
- Ask the patient to lean over to each side in turn and run their hand down the side of the leg to the knee; this assesses lateral flexion.
- Then ask the patient to lean over backwards to assess extension. If extension is painful, facet joint disease (usually degenerative) may be present.

With the patient supine on the couch, assess straight leg raising:

- Lift the leg by placing your hand underneath the ankle and passively flex the hip, keeping the knee extended. When the limit is reached, perform the sciatic stretch test by passively dorsiflexing the ankle. The test assesses irritation of the low lumbar and upper sacral nerve roots. The result is positive if the patient complains of sensory disturbance (pains, pins and needles, or numbness) anywhere below the knee.
- Now ask the patient to turn over. Remove the pillow from the head of the couch and place it under their pelvis and abdomen. This slightly flexes the lumbar spine and is a comfortable position for the patient. Palpate down the spinous processes in turn and along the erector spinae muscles, looking for tenderness.
- Then perform the femoral stretch test. This is the counterpart of the sciatic stretch test and assesses irritation in the upper lumbar nerve roots, which contribute to the femoral nerve. Passively flex the person's knee and, holding the foot, gently extend the hip. If this provokes spasm of the quadriceps and the patient complains of sensory disturbance over the front of the thigh, the test is positive.

**Hip pain**  Hip joint disease produces pain in the groin that may radiate down the anterior thigh to the knee. Pain over the lateral pelvis and thigh is more likely to be due to trochanteric bursitis, and pain in the buttock may be due to ischial bursitis, sacroiliitis or lumbar spine disease.

- To assess the hip joints, ask the patient to lie supine on the couch. Look for flexion deformity at the hip. The hip joints are deep and cannot be directly palpated. Assess flexion at the hip with the knee flexed to relax the hamstrings.
- Then assess internal and external rotation in flexion. Internal rotation is frequently restricted early in hip disease. Place the hip in the neutral position, extend the knee and abduct and adduct the hip in turn. Extension is assessed either by hanging the leg over the side of the couch or with the patient in the prone position.

**Knee pain**  Ensure the patient is sitting propped up on the couch with the knees extended and the legs relaxed. Look for flexion deformity and for valgus and varus deformities.

- Look at the quadriceps muscles, which may be wasted in significant knee disease.
- Look for swelling. A large effusion will cause obvious suprapatellar swelling. Depress the patella with your fingertips; when the pressure is released, it will bounce up (the 'patella tap') if a large effusion is present.
- A small effusion may be detected by the 'bulge' test. To perform this test, empty the hollow next to the medial aspect of the patella by stroking it firmly, and then push with the flat of your hand against the lateral aspect of the knee. If the medial hollow becomes filled in by a bulge, an effusion is present (the normal knee contains only 1–2 ml of fluid, and this is insufficient to cause a bulge). Palpate the popliteal fossa for swelling, which is most often due to a Baker's cyst caused by posterior leakage of a large effusion in the direction of the calf (see **Fig. 5.22**). This can be confused with a deep vein thrombosis.
- Flex and extend the knee to its fullest extent in either direction, with your hand placed on the knee to feel for crepitus. Look for hyperextension, which is a feature of hypermobility syndrome and is commonly associated with mechanical knee pain.

- Assess stability of the knee by attempting to distract the knee first medially and then laterally while holding the knee in a few degrees of flexion. If there is abnormal movement, the collateral ligaments are lax.

**Shoulder pain**  The shoulder is a complex structure and shoulder pain may have many causes. Pain from the glenohumeral joint (the shoulder joint proper) radiates to the front and side of the upper arm. Pain over the top of the shoulder suggests acromioclavicular joint disease, and this may be confirmed by point tenderness over the joint and pain on forced extension of the shoulder.

- With the patient sitting and facing you, observe the shoulders for asymmetry and swelling. Effusions point anteriorly.
- Palpate the capsule over the anterior humeral head and the supra-spinatus tendon over the lateral upper humerus for tenderness.
- Assess flexion, extension, abduction, adduction and internal and external rotation, both actively and passively.

In glenohumeral joint disease, such as adhesive capsulitis and rheu-matoid arthritis (degenerative disease of this joint is not common), pas-sive and active movements will be equally restricted. In contrast, disease of the rotator cuff, such as calcific tendinitis or degenerative rupture, causes restricted active movements, but passive movements remain full. Painful arc syndrome is a feature of rotator cuff disease affecting the supraspinatus component. It is detected by asking the patient to hold their arms up above the head, close to the ears, with the palms turned outwards (that is, with the shoulders internally rotated) and then asking them to lower the arms slowly sideways. Increased pain, due to com-pression of the inflamed tendon between the acromion and the rotating humeral head, occurs at some point within the arc of movement.

**Pain in the hand and wrist**  The hand is examined in some detail in the GALS screen (see **Box 5.5** and **Video 5.1**). The following should be noted in addition.

When examining the hands, stand in front of the patient and exam-ine both hands at the same time, comparing the two sides. When you ask the patient to hold out their hands, make sure that the hands are held free of the knees, with the fingers spread. Unless this is done, you will miss minor degrees of flexion deformity of the fingers and the dropped fingers characteristic of extensor tendon rupture. Pain in the fingers may be due to osteoarthritis; look for bony swellings on the distal interphalangeal joints (Heberden's nodes) and on the proximal interphalangeal joints (Bouchard's nodes). Pronounced soft tissue swelling of these joints indicates inflammatory arthritis. Severe inflammatory arthritides, such as rheumatoid or psoriatic arthritis, with marked bone loss may lead to 'telescoping' of the fingers, with redundancy of the soft tissues, and to flail joints, which have lost all integrity. A combination of fixed joints (due to bony ankylosis) and flail joints is a feature of psoriatic arthritis.

Examination of the hand is not complete without an assessment of function. Hand the patient a pen and ask them to write, ask the patient to do up and undo buttons, and to hold a cup and bring it to their lips.

Should you find specific abnormalities in the locomotor system using this system, you should then do a regional joint examination remembering the mnemonic 'look, feel, move':

- **Look** for swelling and deformity.
- **Feel** to see whether the swelling is hot and symmetrical.
- Then **move** the joint.

Do not worry if you cannot remember the range of movement of all joints as you may compare this either on the patient – who may have a normal joint on the other side – or with your own joints.

## Recording a normal locomotor system examination

Examination findings are recorded as shown in *Table 5.3*.

### Table 5.3 Recording a normal locomotor system examination

| GALS | | Appearance | Movement |
|---|---|:---:|:---:|
| **G** | Gait | ✓ | ✓ |
| **A** | Arms | ✓ | ✓ |
| **L** | Legs | ✓ | ✓ |
| **S** | Spine | ✓ | ✓ |

## Illustrated physical signs

The following photographs illustrate some common locomotor system abnormalities.

**Rheumatoid hands (Fig. 5.15)**: note the symmetrical small joint polyarthritis with ulnar deviation and swan-neck deformities.

**Osteoarthritis of the hands (Fig. 5.16)**: note the squaring of the hand caused by first carpometacarpal and distal interphalangeal joint involvement.

**Gout of the great toe (Fig. 5.17)**: this photograph is characteristic of acute gout. **Scleroderma** causes characteristic skin thickening **(Fig. 5.18)**, while **SLE** causes a photosensitive rash in a characteristic butterfly distribution **(Fig. 5.19)**.

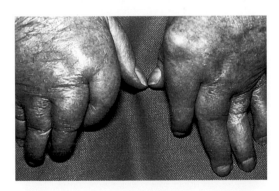

Fig. 5.15 Rheumatoid hands with swelling and swan-neck deformities.

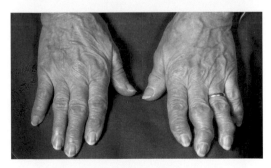

Fig. 5.16 Osteoarthritis of the hands with squaring at the first carpometacarpal joint, and Heberden's nodes.

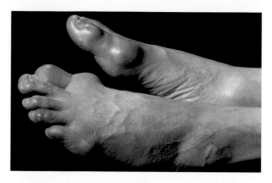

Fig. 5.17 Gout of the great toe. Note the erythema and swelling.

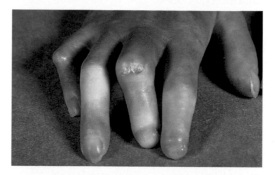

Fig. 5.18 Scleroderma of the hands. Note the tight, shiny skin.

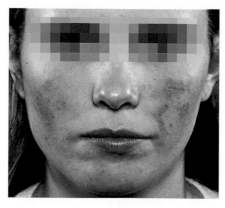

Fig. 5.19 The photosensitive rash of SLE.

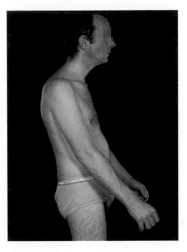

Fig. 5.20 Ankylosing spondylitis.

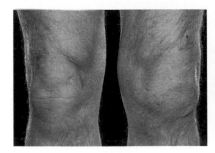

Fig. 5.21 Baker's cyst (front view). Note the swollen left knee.

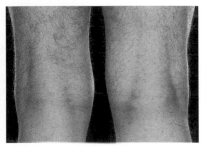

Fig. 5.22 Baker's cyst (back view). The joint has ruptured into the calf. A popliteal cyst results from fluid from the joint.

**Ankylosing spondylitis** causes characteristic changes in posture (**Fig. 5.20**), and **arthritis** of the knee (**Fig. 5.21**) may rupture into the calf (**Fig. 5.22**).

## Therapeutic and interventional skills

### Key laboratory tests

**Erythrocyte sedimentation rate (ESR)** The ESR is a non-specific test of inflammation and is often raised in inflammatory locomotor system disease. You need to be a little cautious about its interpretation, as intercurrent infections can also cause the level to be elevated.

**Rheumatoid factor** This is positive in the majority of patients with rheumatoid arthritis. However, rheumatoid disease can be present with a negative rheumatoid factor. This emphasises that rheumatoid arthritis is a clinical diagnosis.

**Anti-CCP (cyclic citrullinated peptide)** This test is positive in patients with rheumatoid arthritis. It is more specific, but slightly less sensitive, than the rheumatoid factor test. If the anti-CCP test is positive, the patient is highly likely to have rheumatoid arthritis.

**Anti-nuclear antibodies** These antibodies are positive in patients with connective tissue diseases. Patients with SLE may also have a high circulating level of anti-DNA or SM antibodies. Patients with other connective tissue diseases may have high levels of extractable nuclear antigens (ENA). The antibodies are helpful in predicting the pattern of involvement of the disease, and therefore the outcome.

*Table 5.4* outlines the principles underlying the management of patients with locomotor disease.

The following illustrations highlight key features of common rheumatology conditions: rheumatoid arthritis (**Fig. 5.23**), osteoarthritis (**Fig. 5.24**), connective tissue disease (SLE) (**Fig. 5.25**) and gout (**Fig 5.26**).

## Table 5.4  Care of the patient with locomotor disease

- Use physical as well as pharmacological measures to relieve pain
- Encourage movement and muscle strength by using physiotherapy
- Encourage the patient to continue their normal life in spite of their disability
- Refer patients early to occupational therapists for aids and appliances
- Encourage patients to keep as mobile as possible
- Be aware that patients may be depressed

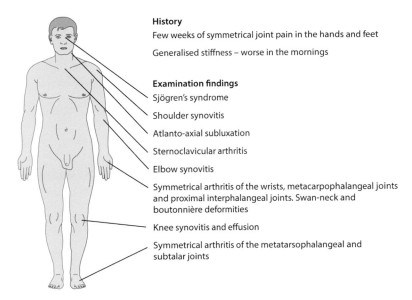

**History**

Few weeks of symmetrical joint pain in the hands and feet

Generalised stiffness – worse in the mornings

**Examination findings**

Sjögren's syndrome

Shoulder synovitis

Atlanto-axial subluxation

Sternoclavicular arthritis

Elbow synovitis

Symmetrical arthritis of the wrists, metacarpophalangeal joints and proximal interphalangeal joints. Swan-neck and boutonnière deformities

Knee synovitis and effusion

Symmetrical arthritis of the metatarsophalangeal and subtalar joints

Fig. 5.23 Rheumatoid arthritis.

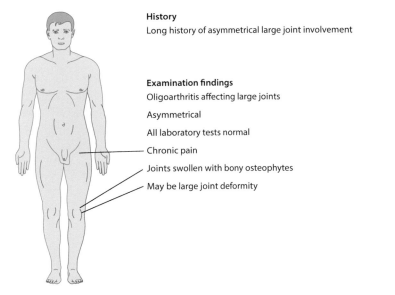

**History**

Long history of asymmetrical large joint involvement

**Examination findings**

Oligoarthritis affecting large joints

Asymmetrical

All laboratory tests normal

Chronic pain

Joints swollen with bony osteophytes

May be large joint deformity

Fig. 5.24 Osteoarthritis.

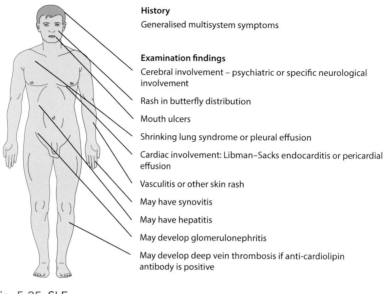

**History**
Generalised multisystem symptoms

**Examination findings**
Cerebral involvement – psychiatric or specific neurological involvement

Rash in butterfly distribution

Mouth ulcers

Shrinking lung syndrome or pleural effusion

Cardiac involvement: Libman–Sacks endocarditis or pericardial effusion

Vasculitis or other skin rash

May have synovitis

May have hepatitis

May develop glomerulonephritis

May develop deep vein thrombosis if anti-cardiolipin antibody is positive

Fig. 5.25  SLE.

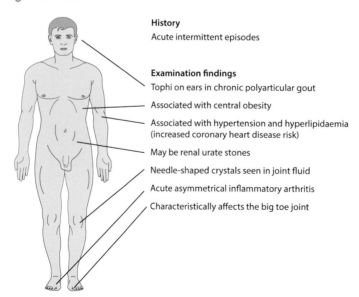

**History**
Acute intermittent episodes

**Examination findings**
Tophi on ears in chronic polyarticular gout

Associated with central obesity

Associated with hypertension and hyperlipidaemia (increased coronary heart disease risk)

May be renal urate stones

Needle-shaped crystals seen in joint fluid

Acute asymmetrical inflammatory arthritis

Characteristically affects the big toe joint

Fig. 5.26  Gout.

# Chapter 6
## The nervous system

Most students and many qualified doctors find the examination of the nervous system somewhat daunting. However, such concerns will prove unfounded provided that you remember a basic outline of neuroanatomy and apply some simple neurophysiological principles.

A fully comprehensive clinical examination of the nervous system may take a considerable time; in practice, this is often unfeasible. You should be able with time (and a little experience) to judge the need for a comprehensive examination after taking a careful history of the patient's symptoms. This is an extremely important prelude to the neurological examination, not only because it may help to determine which aspects of the nervous system require most attention, but also because it provides useful clues to the patient's mental and intellectual state.

## Applied anatomy and physiology

Disorders of the nervous system usually present with a combination of abnormal neurological signs that are often predictable from the history, provided that you are familiar with the anatomy of the nervous system and neuronal pathways.

### The motor system

The motor system (**Fig. 6.1**) is responsible for the action of muscle groups (i.e. the initiation of voluntary and skilled movements).

- The **lower motor neurone** (LMN) consists of anterior horn cells, the efferent (those transmitting impulses away from the spinal cord)

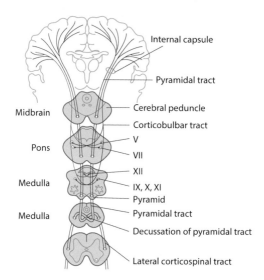

Fig. 6.1 The motor (pyramidal) system and location of nuclei of the lower cranial nerves.

nerve fibres that pass via the anterior spinal nerve root, and peripheral nerves to the muscles.

- The **corticospinal (pyramidal) system** consists of the central pathway that directly links the pyramidal cells of the motor cortex with motor neurones in the brainstem and spinal cord (**Fig. 6.1**).
- The **motor area** of the cortex is located in the anterior aspect of the central sulcus (pre-central gyrus). Localisation of function in the motor cortex with different parts separately represented is shown in **Fig. 6.2**.
- The **corticospinal fibres** descend from the motor cortex into the internal capsule, with fibres for the face located anteriorly and those for the lower limbs posteriorly. They pass through the cerebral peduncles in the midbrain, the pons and the medulla. In the upper part of the medulla, they occupy the pyramids, while, in the lower part, the majority of corticospinal fibres decussate (cross over each other) with those of the opposite side and pass posteriorly into the spinal cord to form the lateral corticospinal tracts.

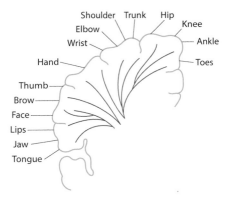

Fig. 6.2 Representation of function in the motor cortex (coronal section).

The corticospinal fibres terminate in the grey matter of the brain-stem motor nuclei or in the anterior horns of the spinal cord. The corticospinal system is concerned with the initiation of voluntary and skilled movements.

• The **extrapyramidal system** consists of those parts of the nervous system, excluding the motor cortex and corticospinal pathways, that are concerned with movement and posture. The system includes the basal ganglia, the subthalamic nuclei, the substantia nigra and other structures in the brainstem. The connections of these extrapyramidal centres are complicated and include fibres from the cerebral cortex and thalamus. The extrapyramidal system is important in the control of posture and in the initiation of movement.

## Coordination

The cerebellum acts as a 'control centre' for coordinated movements. The connections of the cerebellum include links with the skin, muscles, ears (both auditory and vestibular), eyes and viscera. In addition, corticocerebellar pathways provide links with information from the cerebral cortex. The cerebellum uses this information to control the maintenance of postural muscles (particularly those concerned with balance) and to achieve coordination of voluntary movements.

## The sensory system

Afferent fibres convey stimuli to the spinal cord. They enter the spinal cord via the posterior root ganglia and posterior roots. The majority of afferent fibres terminate in the grey matter of the posterior horn, at or near the level at which they enter. The second-order sensory neurone fibres arise from these cells in the posterior horn (**Fig. 6.3**). Sensations of pain and temperature ascend in the lateral spinothalamic tract, with fibres from the lower part of the body being placed laterally and those from the upper part medially. These fibres cross immediately, or within a few segments, to the opposite lateral and anterior columns of the cord, and ascend to the brainstem as the anterior and lateral spinothalamic tracts. Simple touch also follows this route, largely in the anterior spinothalamic tract. The other afferent fibres do not synapse in the grey matter of the posterior horns of the spinal cord, but ascend in the ipsilateral posterior columns (**Fig. 6.4**) (transmitting joint position sense, size, shape, discrimination and vibration sense).

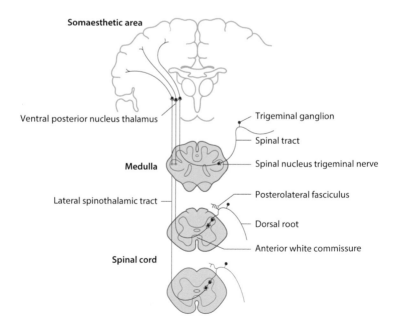

Fig. 6.3 The sensory system (pain and temperature).

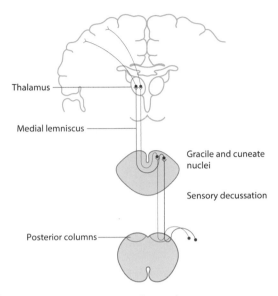

Thalamus

Medial lemniscus

Gracile and cuneate
nuclei

Sensory decussation

Posterior columns

Fig. 6.4 The sensory system – proprioception.

At the upper end of the spinal cord, the posterior column termi-
nates in the gracile and cuneate nuclei. The fibres of the second-order
sensory neurone originate in these nuclei and immediately cross to the
opposite side of the medulla in the sensory decussation.

At the level of the medulla, the spinothalamic fibres touch and
pass laterally, while the posterior columns enter the medial lemniscus. A lesion at the level of the medulla (or above) will involve
all sensory fibres from the opposite half of the body. Higher in the
brainstem, the two sensory pathways are joined by the second-order
sensory fibres from cranial nerve nuclei (**Fig. 6.3**). The fibres of the
medial lemniscus and spinothalamic tract synapse in the thalamus.
The fibres finally ascend through the internal capsule to the cerebral cortex.

## Vascular supply
The brain is supplied by the internal carotid and the vertebral arteries.
The blood supply to the brain is illustrated in **Fig. 6.5**.

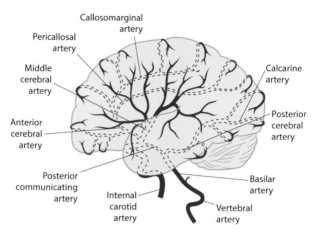

Fig. 6.5 Left lateral view of the principal arteries of the cerebrum.

## Assessment and diagnosis

## Taking the history

### The presenting complaint

If you suspect a disease of the nervous system, it is essential to take a comprehensive history. Included in this history must be the duration of the symptom, its development and its subsequent course, because this provides a clue to the underlying diagnosis. The nature of the condition sometimes makes it difficult to obtain an accurate account from the patient as they may be confused; in such circumstances, it is important to question a relative, a friend or a witness of any event. For example, in multiple sclerosis the episodes of neurological loss occur in relapses and remissions, with slow progression that may occur over several years. Symptoms particularly relevant to the central nervous system (CNS) are shown in *Table 6.1*.

**Headache** Headache is a common presentation in neurological disease. It is also very commonly felt by patients with no neurological pathology. In such cases, there may be psychological reasons that should be explored and discussed with the patient.

## Table 6.1 Symptoms of CNS disease

- Headache
- Visual disturbance
- Unconsciousness, faints or fits
- Problems with speech
- Difficulty in performing simple tasks
- Difficulty with walking
- Bowel and urinary disturbances
- Numbness
- Muscle weakness

## Table 6.2 Examples of different types of headache

- Migraine
- Stress
- Brain tumour
- Cervical spondylosis
- Temporal arteritis
- Referred pain – toothache, jaw, sinus, eyes

Determining the site and distribution of the headache may help in diagnosis: pain may be localised to an extracranial structure or may overlie an intracranial tumour. Remember that headache can arise as a result of disease affecting the teeth, sinuses, eyes, ears or cervical spine (*Table 6.2*). Migrainous headaches may occur at regular intervals or be confined to particular times, while tension headaches are typically associated with stress. Headache due to raised intracranial pressure is commonly aggravated by movement or sudden changes in posture, and may be worse in the morning.

A headache that has been present for years is unlikely to signify progressive disease, while one present over a period of weeks or months suggests the possibility of an expanding intracranial lesion. The following phrases may be helpful in assessing a headache:

'How long have you had this headache?'

'Where do you feel the pain?'

'How bad is it?'

'At what time of day does it affect you?'

'What makes it worse?'

'Does anything make it better?'

**Unconsciousness, fits or faints** Whenever possible, obtain a history and description from someone who knows the patient and/ or has witnessed an attack. What the patient remembers may be of great significance. A seizure is characteristically instantaneous, but is sometimes preceded by a premonitory sensation or aura. The fit can be accompanied by tongue biting and incontinence of urine and/or faeces.

'Do you remember anything about the attack?'

'Did anyone see you fall to the ground?'

'How did they describe it?'

'Did you hurt yourself or wet yourself?'

'Did you bite your tongue?'

**Problems with speech** Problems associated with speech include difficulties of expression, impairment of comprehension and indistinct articulation. These problems may not be voiced by the patient – but you should notice the problem during your history taking. It may not be appropriate to continue the history in these circumstances, so you should consider moving directly to the examination.

**Difficulty in performing simple tasks** Patients will occasionally volunteer problems in accomplishing simple day-to-day tasks – for example, difficulty doing up buttons.

**Difficulty with walking** Patients occasionally complain that they have experienced some difficulty with walking, and find that they 'reel' from side to side.

**Bowel and urinary disturbance** The development of urinary and/or bowel disturbance is important. Incontinence of urine may occur when higher cerebral functions are impaired as a result of organic disease.

It is important to ask about this directly but sensitively, as the patient may be embarrassed and not volunteer the information.

'Have you had any trouble with passing water?'

'Have you unintentionally messed yourself?'

Retention of urine can be associated with spinal cord or conus medullaris disease, while incontinence of faeces may be a feature of nervous system disease, particularly of the spinal cord.

### BOX 6.1  CHECKLIST FOR NEUROLOGICAL HISTORY TAKING

- Introduce yourself.
- Presenting complaint – enquire about headache, blackouts, etc. Assess the time course of the problem.
- Past medical history – enquire about fits and faints.
- Personal and social history – ask about alcohol and recreational drugs.
- Family and treatment history – ask about a history of epilepsy or neurological disease; in a woman, ask about use of the combined oral contraceptive pill
- Systems review (see **Box 6.2**).

**Listen to the answers!**

### BOX 6.2  A SCHEME FOR THE EXAMINATION OF THE NERVOUS SYSTEM

- Assess speech and mental function. If the level of consciousness appears to be impaired, assess this using the Glasgow Coma Scale (*Table 6.3*).
- Test the cranial nerves.
- Test motor function.
- Test the reflexes.
- Test coordination (cerebellar function).
- Test sensory function.
- Examine related structures.
- When appropriate, assess walking gait.

## Table 6.3 Glasgow Coma Scale

| Behaviour | Response | Score |
|---|---|---|
| Eye opening response | Spontaneously | 4 |
| | To speech | 3 |
| | To pain | 2 |
| | No response | 1 |
| Best verbal response | Oriented to time, place and person | 5 |
| | Confused | 4 |
| | Inappropriate words | 3 |
| | Incomprehensible sounds | 2 |
| | No response | 1 |
| Best motor response | Obeys commands | 6 |
| | Moves to localised pain | 5 |
| | Flexion withdrawal from pain | 4 |
| | Abnormal flexion (decorticate) | 3 |
| | Abnormal extension (decerebrate) | 2 |
| | No response | 1 |
| Total score | *Best response* | 15 |
| | *Comatose patient* | 8 or less |
| | *Totally unresponsive* | 3 |

### BOX 6.3 CARE OF THE PATIENT WITH NEUROLOGICAL DISEASE

- Consider the positioning of disabled limbs.
- Regular turning and pressure area care.
- Appropriate communication aids for patients with receptive/expressive speech defects.
- Continuity of nursing care for patients with delirium or dementia.
- Prevention of self-harm in patients prone to fits or seizures.

If the patient's presenting complaint does not suggest neurological disease, a series of routine questions usually suffices to exclude any possibility of disease within the nervous system.

## Systems review

Important areas of enquiry are as follows (these questions can be asked as part of the systems review in patient with no symptoms of neurological disease):

'Has there been any change in your mood, memory or powers of concentration?'

'Have you suffered unduly from headaches?'

'Have you ever had any fits, faints or blackouts?'

'Have you noticed any change in your sense of smell, taste, sight or hearing?'

'Have you noticed any difficulty in talking or swallowing?'

'Have you experienced any numbness, burning or tingling sensations or pins and needles in the face, limbs or trunk?'

'Have you noticed any weakness in either the arms or legs?'

'Have you noticed any unsteadiness or difficulty in walking?'

'Have you had any problems in passing urine or opening your bowels?'

## Examination of the nervous system

### Undertaking an assessment and diagnosis

If the patient's main complaint appears to be unrelated to disease of the nervous system, and the replies to the screening questions are all negative, the examination of the nervous system may be relatively brief. It should include a short assessment of intellectual function, tests of motor function (including tendon reflex responses) and tests of sensory function.

 VIDEO 6.1 The neurological examination

https://www.crcpress.com/cw/kopelman

Examination of the nervous system is complex. A full neurological examination may take some time. It can sometimes be quite difficult for the patient to cooperate, so you may need to take a break and return later. In addition, remember that good communication and avoidance of jargon is crucial. You are asking the patient to perform tricks that may seem very odd.

- You must ask whether the patient is right- or left-handed – the left hemisphere is dominant in right-handed people, while the reverse is usually true for left-handed people. Hand dominance is clinically significant: the side of hand dominance correlates with the side of the dominant cerebral hemisphere and thus has important localising value.
- If the speech appears abnormal, try to identify the type of abnormality.
- It is important that you understand the difference between aphasia and dysarthria and are able to distinguish, wherever possible, the different types of aphasia (see below).

**Aphasia** This is a disturbance of the ability to use language, while dysarthria represents a difficulty in articulation of the spoken word (*Table 6.4*).

You should test for expressive aphasia by asking the patient to name certain objects – a comb, the teeth of the comb, a watch, the strap of the watch, a glass, the rim of the glass. Ask:

'What is this?'

'Is this part of it?'

It is not uncommon for a nervous patient to stumble over one or two of the questions, but consistent failure usually signifies an expressive aphasia. Receptive aphasia (difficulty in understanding) is tested by asking the patient to perform simple tasks, for example:

'Close your eyes and then scratch your nose with your right hand'.

Patients with a posterior superior temporal gyrus lesion will be unable to follow the instructions.

## Table 6.4 Dysfunction of speech

| Condition | Cause |
|---|---|
| **Dysarthria** is a disorder of speech articulation – comprehension and speech content are not affected | Typically seen with cerebellar dysfunction, but may be present in other conditions, including alcohol or drug intoxication |
| **Dysphonia** is a disorder of sound production (phonation) | Dysfunction of the larynx and/or vocal cords |
| **Aphasia** is a disturbance of the ability to use language | |
| **Expressive aphasia** – a disorder of speech fluency (word production). Speech is laboured and short, lacks normal intonation and is grammatically simple and monotonous | Damage to Broca's area (posterior inferior frontal gyrus, dominant hemisphere). Typically a lesion of the superior division of the middle cerebral artery |
| **Receptive aphasia** – a disorder of language comprehension. Speech fluency is typically not affected. Patient's speech is meaningless or strange, and may include inappropriate words/phrases | Damage to Wernicke's area (posterior superior temporal gyrus, dominant hemisphere). Typically a lesion of the inferior division of the middle cerebral artery |
| A **combination** of expressive and receptive aphasia may result from an extensive lesion involving both Broca's and Wernicke's areas | |

The recognition and detection of aphasia is extremely important, even when it is a minor deficit, because it reflects disease in localised areas of the dominant hemisphere (in right-handed people, generally the left). Lesions in the left frontal region predominantly affect articulation and fluency, while lesions in the left parieto-occipital area impair reading and left parietal lesions impair several other associative functions, particularly writing. An assessment of articulation and fluency combined with reading and writing enables the recognition of lesions in front of or behind the central sulcus – those in front largely affect expression and those behind largely affect understanding or reception. Failure of recognition may lead to a mistaken diagnosis of delirium or dementia, which implies a diffuse rather than a localised brain lesion.

**Dysarthria** Dysarthria may be made more apparent by asking the patient to repeat a sentence such as, 'West Register Street'.

Dysarthria may result from peripheral nerve lesions affecting the muscles used in speech or their neuromuscular junctions, or the nerve supply of these muscles. Alternatively, it may be caused by a disruption of the nerve supply of the structures within the brain which control and regulate the peripheral mechanisms.

**Apraxia** This is an inability to perform certain motor acts in the absence of motor or sensory paralysis. Damage to the left parietal cortex or disease involving the connections between the two cerebral hemispheres, through the corpus callosum, may result in a patient suffering apraxia. An example is the patient who is unable to demonstrate the use of a hammer, but is able independently to pick up the hammer. In testing for apraxia, first establish that there is no receptive aphasia and no impairment of power or coordination ability. Then ask the patient to perform a task, for example:

'Show me how you would take your jacket off.'

'Show me how you would tie a shoe lace.'

The patient does not know how to approach the task.

**Gerstmann's syndrome** is a disorder of higher visuospatial function that is typically associated with a lesion in the angular gyrus of the dominant parietal lobe. It results in acalculia (difficulty with arithmetic), agraphia (difficulty with writing) and left/right confusion with finger agnosia (difficulty in identifying each finger).

## Assessment of mental state, personality and intellectual function

(See Chapter 12 for a detailed assessment of the mental state.)

The patient's appearance should be noted – are they unkempt? What is the state of their clothing? Disease of the nervous system may mean that the ability to communicate is less than might be expected from the patient's social status and apparent educational level. However, mental confusion or emotional disturbance will make any assessment difficult. It is important to describe the patient's mental state at the first examination, since future management may depend on an accurate assessment of any changes that have taken place.

Test whether the patient is orientated in time and place by asking their name, age, present location and the date:

'Can you tell me your name? ... Do you know where you are? ... What is the date?'

Remember that patients who have been in hospital for some time may have difficulty with the date. Assess whether the patient appears depressed – sad expression, little mobility of facial expression, general slowness of action, agitation and possibly spontaneous weeping and less eye contact than you may expect.

High spirits or euphoria, which apparently is out of character with the patient's presenting complaint, may be seen in multiple sclerosis, while general immobility and an expressionless face is commonly seen in Parkinson's disease (**Fig. 6.6**).

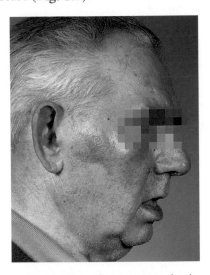

Fig. 6.6 Parkinsonian facies. Note the associated seborrhoea – and lack of expression.

A change in personality, which is usually reported by a close relative, may be early evidence of disease affecting the brain.

You should discover whether there has been a deterioration in mental capacity by testing a patient's concentration, memory and reasoning capacity, to see whether they correspond with an assessment of the patient's level of educational attainment. A test which will help with this evaluation might include 10 simple questions (see **Box 6.4**).

### BOX 6.4 TEN SIMPLE QUESTIONS FOR A MENTAL TEST

| | | |
|---|---|---|
| 1 | Age | How old are you? |
| 2 | Time (hour) | What time is it? |
| 3 | Year | What year is it? |
| 4 | Name of place | Where are we now? |
| 5 | Recognition of two people | Who am I? Who is this person? (nurse) |
| 6 | Date of birth | When were you born? |
| 7 | Date of World War II | When did the Second World War start? |
| 8 | National leader | Who is our Prime Minister/President/Head of State? |
| 9 | Counting backwards | Can you count backwards from 20? |
| 10 | Five-minute recall | Can you try to remember this address? (42 East Street) |

## Examination of the cranial nerves

It is easier to remember the sequence and the abnormalities if you examine the cranial nerves in sequence from I to XII. The following descriptions outline the important features of each test.

### I. Olfactory nerve

You should ask the patient if they have noticed any change in sense of smell, and then ask them to identify and distinguish various smells. It is permissible to use objects found by the bedside such as deodorants, perfumes, strongly smelling fruit or soap. Test each nostril individually and ask the patient to close their eyes – unilateral anosmia suggests a nerve lesion, but bilateral anosmia is usually the result of local nasal disease such as a cold. Ask:

- 'Can you smell this?'
- Do you know what it is?'

## II. Optic nerve

Remember to test each eye separately, and that form and detail of vision are best perceived in the central field.

Test the patient's visual acuity (with the patient wearing glasses if necessary) by asking them to read small print by near vision and large print at a distance. Assess the visual fields by the method of 'confrontation' – sit at the same level as the patient, and try to be absolutely opposite them. Then ask them to cover or close one eye. You should cover or close your opposite eye. The patient should then fix the gaze of their open eye on your open eye while you bring a pin, or your finger, into their (and your) vision from the middle of each of the quadrants of the visual field (**Fig. 6.7A**). Ask the patient to tell you when the advancing object is visible to them, and compare this with when you first see the object. This is repeated for the upper and lower temporal (outer) fields and the upper and lower nasal (inner) fields (**Fig. 6.7B**).

Each eye is tested separately, and then the two together, to check for sensory inattention, which may occur with a parietal stroke. You should now repeat the examination using a red pin instead of your finger to outline the central or macular field – a central area of impaired vision (central scotoma) is recognised by an inability to see the red pin compared with your own vision. This is particularly important, as the area of loss may be enlarged in conditions such as senile macular degeneration and diabetes, which can affect the macular area.

**Use of the ophthalmoscope** The optic fundi must be examined with an ophthalmoscope (**Fig. 6.8**). Ophthalmoscopy is a difficult part of the examination, and one with which students often have problems. It is made much easier if the patient is cooperative. The only way to become adept in ophthalmoscopy is to practise as much as possible. If you do not have perfect vision, you will find it more difficult. Either correct for your refractive problem with the ophthalmoscope lens, or wear glasses or contact lenses.

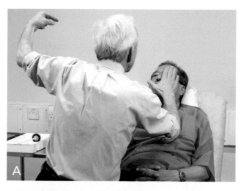

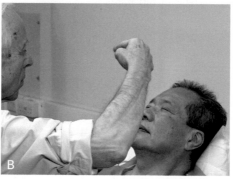

Fig. 6.7A, B Confrontation testing of visual fields. Patient and examiner each close one eye. (A) Assessment of the upper and lower temporal fields. (B) Assessment of the upper and lower nasal fields.

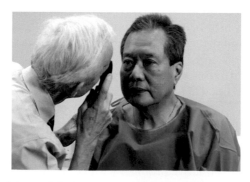

Fig. 6.8 Use of the ophthalmoscope. Use your right eye to look in the patient's right eye.

## BOX 6.5  USING THE OPHTHALMOSCOPE

- Correct for refraction. Ask the patient if they wear glasses, and take your own visual acuity into account. If they and/or you have a significant refractive problem, make sure glasses are worn. Use your right eye for the patient's right eye and vice versa, or you will find you are rubbing noses. Make sure you are sitting comfortably and are opposite the patient.
- Put your non-dominant hand on their shoulder so that you can gauge how close you are. Ask the patient to focus on a distant object, but warn them to keep looking in that direction even if you get in the way.
- Begin by assessing the red reflex. Hold the ophthalmoscope to your own eye and look through it from a distance of about 1 metre. You should see a red light similar to that seen on a photograph when a flash bulb has gone off.
- Set your ophthalmoscope at the highest negative number on the focus dial. This may be red or black, depending on the instrument you are using. Look through the lens from a distance of just less than 1 metre, aiming at the pupil, and gradually bring the ophthalmoscope closer to the patient's eye. You will find that the retina suddenly comes into focus when you are approximately 2–3 cm from the eye. Focus on the anterior structures of the eye before concentrating on the fundus.
- Then focus on the optic disc. This consists of a yellow circle crossed by blood vessels. Note its colour and clarity, and the depth of the physiological cup – swelling with indistinct margins suggests papilloedema; extreme paleness indicates optic atrophy.
- Look at the macula and retinal background structures for any additional abnormalities.

Always introduce yourself and explain what you are going to do and why. Outline how you will perform the examination and ask the patient if they have any questions. Check the controls on the ophthalmoscope and make sure that the batteries are working; it is a good idea to get into the habit of doing this.

You will need to see several retinal photographs before the technique becomes familiar. Look temporally to see the macula, a reddish blob. It is helpful to describe what you see as you go along. Search the 'background' (i.e. not the disc or the macula) for haemorrhages and exudates, and examine the retinal blood vessels, noting their calibre and regularity – arterioles should be about two-thirds the diameter of veins and should be regular in outline. Examples of a healthy optic disc and one in diabetes, hypertension, papilloedema and optic atrophy are shown (**Figs 6.9–6.13**).

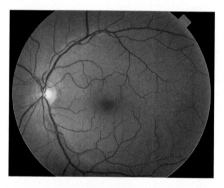

Fig. 6.9 A normal optic disc and retina.

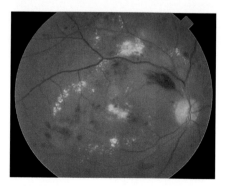

Fig. 6.10 A fundus in a patient with diabetes. Note the dot and blot haemorrhages and exudates.

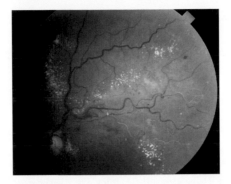

Fig. 6.11 A fundus in a patient with hypertension. Note the increased tortuosity of the vessels.

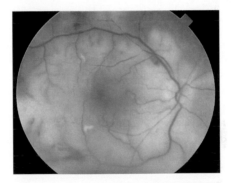

Fig. 6.12 Papilloedema. Note the blurring of the disc margins.

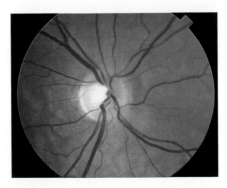

Fig. 6.13 Optic atrophy. Note that the disc is clear and pale.

## III, IV and VI. Oculomotor, trochlear and abducens nerves (eye movement)

The abducens nerve innervates the lateral rectus and the trochlear nerve innervates the superior oblique muscle. All the other external ocular muscles, the sphincter pupillae (muscle of accommodation) and the levator palpebrae are supplied by the oculomotor nerve. A simple way to remember the muscle innervation is $LR_6SO_4$ – Remainder 3: lateral rectus = abducens (cranial nerve no. 6), superior oblique = trochlear (cranial nerve no. 4) and the remainder = oculomotor (cranial nerve no. 3).

The actions of the external muscles are illustrated in **Fig. 6.14**. The superior and inferior recti act as elevators and depressors alone when the eye is abducted; the superior and inferior recti act similarly when the eye is in adduction. Movements of the eyes are usually symmetrical or conjugate – conjugate movements depend on brainstem integration of the IIIrd, IVth and VIth nuclei. Ask the patient to look at your finger and follow its movement with their eyes. Also ask them to tell you if they see double. This suggests a lack of conjugate eye movements, and may occur in nerve palsies. If the patient sees double, it may confirm your suspicions. Move your finger to the patient's right, then up and down, then to their left, and then up and down. As in **Fig. 6.7**, keep your non-dominant hand on the patient's chin to ensure that you

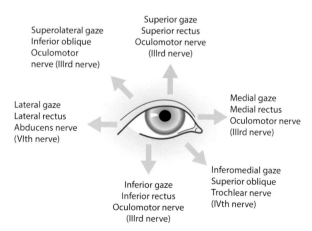

Fig. 6.14 The actions of the external ocular muscles.

are not too far away – an arm's length is sufficient (**Figs 6.15** and **6.16**). If you move your finger too far laterally, you will see one or two beats of physiological nystagmus – this is normal. Obvious nystagmus in one direction (see below) suggests a cerebellar lesion on that side.

You must observe the size, shape and equality of the pupils – note whether the pupils are large or small, and whether they have

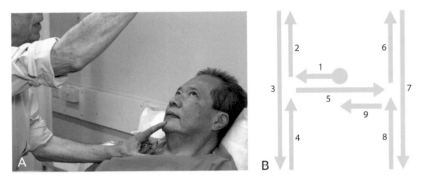

Fig. 6.15A, B Assessment of upward gaze (A). Note the examiner's hand is on the patient's chin to ensure an appropriate distance between doctor and patient. The directions to follow when testing eye movement (B).

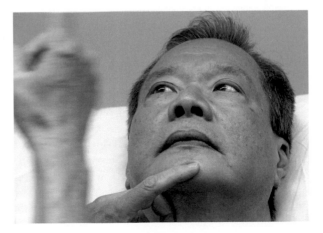

Fig. 6.16 Assessment of lateral gaze. Note that, even in healthy people, looking too far laterally induces nystagmus.

an irregular contour. Test their reaction to a bright light. Ask the patient to look across the room, and then shine a bright light into one eye – both pupils should constrict almost immediately (known as a consensual pupil reaction). You should then test for accommodation, asking the patient to look away at a distant object and then quickly look at your finger, which is held close to their nose – as the eyes converge to accomplish this, the pupils should become smaller. Look for drooping of the eyelid (ptosis). Ptosis with enophthalmos and a small pupil suggests a Horner's syndrome caused by a cervical sympathetic nerve problem.

**Nystagmus** This is the term applied to a disturbance of ocular movement characterised by involuntary, conjugate and often rhythmical oscillations of the eyes. These movements may be horizontal, vertical or rotary. For any given direction of gaze, the movements are usually quicker in one direction than the other – the quicker movement indicates the direction of the nystagmus. The patient should be asked to look straight ahead to see whether the eyes remain steady. They should then look to the extreme right, and then to the left, to see whether any jerking of the eyes is present. This should be followed by the patient looking up and then down to test for vertical nystagmus.

## V. Trigeminal nerve

The trigeminal nerve has motor and sensory functions. You should test sensation to pin-prick and touch over the three divisions of the nerve: ophthalmic (the forehead), maxillary (the cheek) and mandibular (the jaw). Remember to keep near the midline as the upper cervical nerve roots may supply the lateral aspects of the face.

Compare the size of the masseter and temporalis muscle on each side by palpation while the patient's teeth are clenched. Ask the patient to open their mouth: deviation of the jaw to one side suggests weakness of the pterygoids on the same side. Test the jaw jerk by gently tapping your finger placed across the patient's chin with the patella hammer. An abnormally brisk jaw jerk is a sign of bilateral upper motor neurone (UMN) disease; a depressed or absent jaw jerk or bulbar palsy is a sign of an LMN lesion (see below).

Now elicit the corneal reflex – the patient is asked to look straight ahead and the cornea is then lightly touched with a wisp of cotton wool

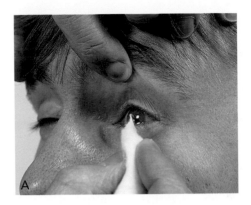

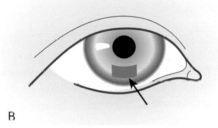

Fig. 6.17A, B Testing for the corneal reflex (A). The shaded area over the iris (arrow) shows where the cornea is touched to elicit a corneal reflex (B).

to elicit a blink (**Fig. 6.17A**). The precise position is shown in **Fig. 6.17B**. You can guarantee that you will touch the cornea if you are over the iris. If your wisp is outside the shaded area in **Fig. 6.17B** you run the risk of touching the sclera, and getting a false-negative response.

## VII. Facial nerve

The facial nerve is almost entirely a motor nerve, supplying all the muscles of the scalp and face except the levator palpebrae superioris. The chorda tympani travels with the facial nerve during part of its course, so taste may also be lost on the anterior two-thirds of the tongue when the proximal part of the nerve is damaged.

You should test movements of the face by asking the patient to wrinkle the forehead, screw up the eyes, show the teeth and whistle.

LMN lesions of the VIIth nerve or its nucleus produce weakness of the whole side of the face (Bell's palsy), whereas a unilateral lesion of the supranuclear pathways (UMN) spares the forehead – the patient is able to frown or wrinkle the brow. To test taste, strong solutions such as sugar, salt or a coffee granule can be applied to the protruding tongue and the patient asked to identify the taste before withdrawing the tongue into the mouth.

## VIII. Auditory nerve

Begin an examination of the VIIIth nerve by an assessment of the external auditory meatus with an auriscope. Check that the batteries work before you begin, and that a clean and appropriately sized speculum is attached to the light. It is sensible to examine both ears, starting with the non-affected side.

Hold on to the pinna of the ear and point it gently upwards and backwards, while stabilising the patient's head with the knuckles of the same hand. Insert the auriscope speculum gently into the external auditory meatus, holding the body of the scope upside down. Look at the external ear and for a foreign body or any sign of inflammation, and then look at the eardrum. It should look pink and shiny. Check for perforation, swelling, redness or a fluid level behind the drum (seen in secretory otitis media).

You should test the hearing initially by whispering, or by applying a ticking wrist watch, to each ear. If there is an impairment, define whether it is due to middle ear disease (conductive deafness) or to a lesion of the nerve (perceptive deafness). Rinne's test is a comparison of the noise heard by a patient from a tuning fork (256 Hz 'C' tuning fork) held close to the ear (air conduction) with the noise heard from a tuning fork placed on the mastoid bone (bone conduction; **Fig. 6.18**). In the normal situation, and in patients with perceptive nerve deafness, air conduction is better than bone conduction, whereas in patients with conductive deafness the reverse is true. Weber's test may also help to distinguish between unilateral conductive and perceptive nerve deafness – a tuning fork placed on the centre of the forehead is usually heard equally well in both ears (**Fig. 6.19**). In conductive deafness it is generally heard loudest in the deaf ear, as the sound is transmitted to the nerve through the bone, while in perceptive deafness it is heard loudest in the healthy ear.

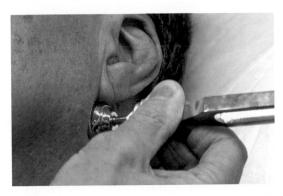

Fig. 6.18 In a healthy patient, air conduction of sound should be greater than bone conduction (Rinne's test).

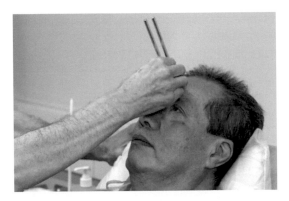

Fig. 6.19 A tuning fork in the centre of the forehead is usually heard equally well in both ears.

## IX and X. Glossopharyngeal and vagus nerves

The glossopharyngeal nerve is sensory from the posterior third of the tongue and the mucous membrane of the pharynx. It contains taste fibres from the posterior third of the tongue. The glossopharyngeal nerve is very rarely damaged alone. The vagus is motor for the soft palate, pharynx and larynx. It is also sensory and motor for the respiratory passages, the heart and – through the parasympathetic ganglia – most of the abdominal viscera.

Damage to the vagus is clinically obvious through its palatine and laryngeal branches.

You should note whether the uvula rises in the midline when the patient says 'Aah' – a unilateral palatal palsy causes drooping of the affected side, and on phonation the palate deviates to the opposite side. To test sensation, touch the tonsillar fossa or posterior pharyngeal wall with a spatula – this will provoke a gag reflex in the normal situation.

## XI. Accessory nerve

Test the power of the sternomastoid and trapezius muscles by asking the patient to shrug their shoulders while you push down on them (a test of trapezius function), and then to push against your hand placed against their jaw (a test of sternomastoid function) (**Fig. 6.20**).

## XII. Hypoglossal nerve

The hypoglossal is purely a motor nerve. Look for wasting or abnormal movements (fasciculation) of the tongue, and then ask the patient to protrude the tongue: a unilateral lesion causes protrusion towards the side of the lesion. The presence of wasting indicates that this is an LMN lesion (nuclear or infranuclear). Tremor of the tongue is common in Parkinson's disease with the tongue either at rest or protruded.

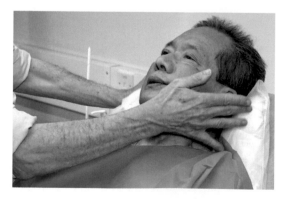

Fig. 6.20 Normal sternomastoid function reflects an intact accessory nerve (XI).

## The motor and sensory systems

First, observe the patient's posture and gait, which may give immediate pointers to nervous system disease – this should be done before the patient climbs on to the examination couch. Possible alterations in gait are summarised in *Table 6.5*.

### Examination of motor function

You should now observe the patient lying on the examination couch. It is important to observe the patient's overall musculature, including muscle groups that are not visible with the patient lying flat. Wasting of muscles is evident from a reduction in bulk and a 'flabby' appearance. Look also for any involuntary (spontaneous) movements of the limbs, or tremor of the fingers. This may be emphasised by lightly flicking the muscles. Fasciculations are caused by spontaneous firing of motor units and are typically a sign of an LMN lesion.

**Muscular tone** Muscle tone is a state of tension found in healthy muscles. An increase in tone is called hypertonia and a decrease

### Table 6.5  Examples of abnormal gait

| Type | Signs | Cause |
|---|---|---|
| Ataxic | Drunken or staggering quality, wide-based stance to accommodate instability | Cerebellar lesions<br>Alcohol and/or drug toxicity<br>Demyelination |
| Bradykinesia | Slowness or poverty of movement, decreased ability to initiate movement | Parkinson's disease<br>Extrapyramidal lesion |
| Spasticity | Stiff, foot-dragging walk caused by long muscle contraction | Cerebral infarction or haemorrhage – middle cerebral artery region<br>Multiple sclerosis<br>Spinal cord injury |

**BOX 6.6 ROMBERG'S TEST**

- This is a simple test to determine whether an ataxic gait (or a patient's unsteadiness) results from a cerebellar or a proprioceptive lesion. The patient is asked to stand with feet together and then to close their eyes and maintain their posture for 60 seconds. Where there is loss of proprioception, the patient immediately loses stability (a positive Romberg's test); this is not the case in a cerebellar lesion.

is hypotonia. Tone is assessed by passively moving the major joints of the arm and legs (elbow, hips and knees); the elbow is extended and then flexed, the arm is turned into pronation and then supination, and the hips and knees are flexed and extended. Hypotonia is easily recognised (it feels 'floppy' and is usually accompanied by profound muscle weakness), but hypertonia may be missed. Spasticity is an initial resistance to attempted stretch of the muscle that increases with applied force until there is a sudden give at a certain tension – the 'clasp-knife' effect. This is caused by a pyramidal or UMN lesion, such as a stroke in the internal capsule, or a spinal cord lesion in the neck. Rigidity is, in contrast, a resistance to passive movement that continues unaltered throughout the range of movement, and so has a plastic or 'lead-pipe' quality. Rigidity is classically seen in extrapyramidal lesions and most particularly Parkinson's disease. Cogwheel rigidity is resistance during passive ranges of movement that intermittently gives way like a lever pulling over a ratchet. It is a sign of extrapyramidal dysfunction and characteristically seen in Parkinson's disease.

**Muscle strength** The strength of individual muscle groups in the arms and legs must always be assessed. The innervation of the muscle groups is shown in *Table 6.6*. Each movement made should be compared with your own strength, or with what you regard as normal power for the patient. It is easiest to make an assessment of power starting from the shoulders and then working down.

A numerical system for grading muscle power is listed in *Table 6.7*: this is based on the Medical Research Council system of classification.

## Table 6.6 Segmentation and innervation of the muscles to joints

| | |
|---|---|
| Abduction of shoulder | C5 |
| Adduction of shoulder | C5 |
| Flexion of elbow | C5 |
| Extension of elbow | C7 |
| Flexion of wrist | C6, C7, C8 |
| Extension of wrist | C6, C7 |
| Finger movements | C8, T1 |
| Flexion of hip | L1, L2, L3 |
| Extension of hip | L5, S1 |
| Adduction of hip | L5, S1 |
| Abduction of hip | L4, L5, S1 |
| Flexion of knee | L4, L5, S1, S2 |
| Extension of knee | L3, L4 |
| Dorsiflexion of foot | L4, L5 |
| Plantar flexion of foot | S1 |
| Inversion of foot | L4 |
| Eversion of ankle | L5, S1 |
| Dorsiflexion of toes | L5 |

## Table 6.7 Grading of muscle power

| Grade | Description |
|---|---|
| 5 | Normal |
| 4 | Weak, but can overcome gravity and resistance |
| 3 | Very weak, but can overcome gravity |
| 2 | Able to move the limb only if supported against gravity |
| 1 | Flicker or trace of contraction |
| 0 | No movement at all |

## BOX 6.7 ASSESSING MUSCLE POWER

First ask the patient to extend both arms straight and the palms facing to the ceiling. Downward arm drift and flexion of the wrist and elbow are sensitive signs of subtle UMN weakness (pronator drift).

- To assess deltoid power, ask the patient to push their abducted arms up, or 'Put your wings up', and demonstrate the movement. Then test their power against yours, by trying to overcome them (**Fig. 6.21**).
- Test the biceps by asking the patient to hold an arm in the position shown in **Fig. 6.22** and then tell them 'Pull me towards you.'
- Assessment of triceps power is made by maintaining the previous position and asking the patient to 'Push me away' (**Fig. 6.22**). Ask the patient to push your hand up (wrist extension) and push it down (wrist flexion) with their hand.
- Power in the small joints of the hand is tested by asking the patient to 'Spread your fingers wide apart' (**Fig. 6.23**), and then to hold their fingers together while you try to separate them.
- In the leg, test the hip flexors, extensors, adductors and abductors by asking the patient to push the thighs 'up', 'down', 'outwards' and 'inwards', as shown in **Fig. 6.24**.

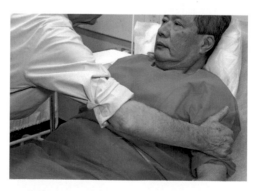

Fig. 6.21 Power: abduction of the shoulder (C5).

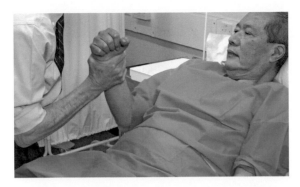

Fig. 6.22 Assessment of biceps and triceps. Elbow flexion (C5) and extension (C7).

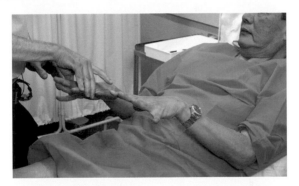

Fig. 6.23 Power in the small joints of the hand (C8, T1).

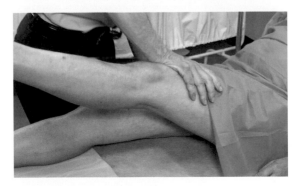

Fig. 6.24 Assessment of hip flexion (L1, L2, L3).

## BOX 6.8 ASSESSING FLEXION

- Knee flexion is tested by holding the leg under the flexed knee with one hand and asking the patient to 'Pull me towards you', and then 'Push me away' (**Fig. 6.25**).
- For dorsiflexion and plantar flexion of the foot, inversion and eversion, ask the patient to 'Cock your foot up towards your head' (**Fig. 6.26**) and 'down', 'out towards me' and 'in'.

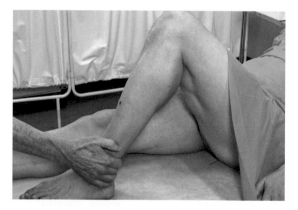

Fig. 6.25 Assessment of knee flexion (L4, L5 S1, S2) and extension (L3, L4).

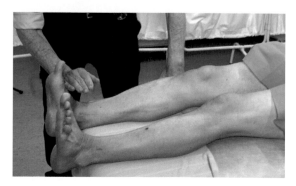

Fig. 6.26 Assessment of dorsiflexion of the foot (L4, L5).

**Tendon reflexes** Testing the reflexes assesses the reflex arc and the supraspinal influences that operate on it. If the tendon of the stretched muscle is gently struck using a reflex hammer, the muscle briefly contracts. This demonstrates the integrity of the afferent and efferent pathways and the excitability of the anterior horn cells in the spinal segment of the stretched muscle.

It is important to become skilled in testing the reflexes. You should always stand on the same side of the bed, elicit the tendon jerks in the same manner and ensure that the patient is relaxed. Swing the patella hammer gently – and allow it to fall under its own weight. Reflex responses are very variable between individuals in the normal situation – some usually have very brisk responses, whereas the response may be depressed in others. Always 'reinforce' if you cannot elicit a reflex. This is done by asking the patient to grit their teeth or clench their hands together while you try to elicit the reflex again. It is a way of distracting the patient and thus reducing the cortical influence on the reflex response.

### BOX 6.9 SYSTEM FOR GRADING THE REFLEX RESPONSE

| | |
|---|---|
| Absent | – |
| Present only with reinforcement | +/– |
| Just present | + |
| Brisk response | ++ |
| Exaggerated response | +++ |

Clonus is a rhythmic, sustained muscular contraction initiated by a brisk stretching force in a muscle group. Clonus results from pronounced hyper-reflexia as a consequence of a UMN lesion. Clonus is most commonly elicited in the ankle by abrupt passive dorsiflexion. The rhythmic contractions are generally sustained until the ankle is released.

The reflexes that are commonly tested are the biceps, triceps, supinator, knee and ankle jerks. Test the biceps by tapping the biceps tendon on the flexor surface of the elbow (**Fig. 6.27**), the triceps by tapping the tendon on the extensor surface of the elbow (**Fig. 6.28**) and the supinator by tapping the radial surface of the wrist (**Fig. 6.29**).

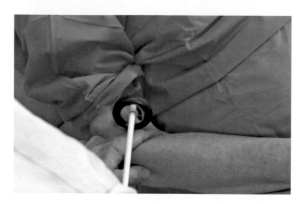

Fig. 6.27 The biceps jerk (C5, C6).

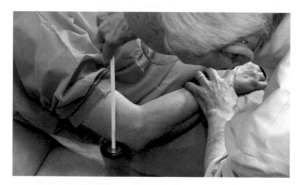

Fig. 6.28 The triceps jerk (C7).

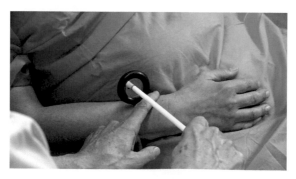

Fig. 6.29 The supinator jerk (C5, C6).

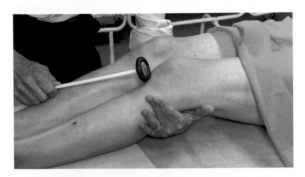

Fig. 6.30 The knee jerk (L4, L5).

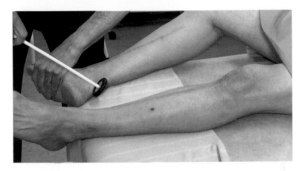

Fig. 6.31 The ankle jerk (L5, S1).

In the leg, the reflexes are the knee jerk (**Fig. 6.30**), which is elicited by tapping the patellar tendon, and the ankle jerk, elicited by dorsi-flexing the foot to stretch the Achilles tendon and tapping the tendon (**Fig. 6.31**). It is easier to elicit if the patient crosses the ankle over the other leg.

Reflexes are reduced or absent in LMN lesions and brisk or exag-gerated in UMN lesions.

**Abdominal reflex** A light stroke applied over each of the four quadrants of the abdomen will, in healthy individuals, elicit a brisk contraction of the underlying muscles. The upper reflexes are subserved by segments T9–T10 and the lower by T11–T12. Particular attention should be paid to the symmetry of the abdominal reflex response, since its absence on one side may be good evidence of a UMN lesion.

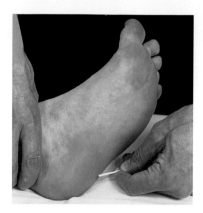

Fig. 6.32 The plantar response.

**Plantar response** The plantar response (**Fig. 6.32**) is elicited by applying firm pressure (usually with your fingernail or a blunt orange stick) along the lateral border of the dorsum of the foot, and observing the metatarsophalangeal joint of the great toe. In normal circumstances, the toe flexes (goes down); with pyramidal and corticospinal (UMN) lesions, the great toe shows an extensor response called the Babinski response (the toes goes up, with an associated fanning of the toes). Results are denoted as follows: flexor plantar response down (↓); extensor response up (↑); and an equivocal response up/down (↑↓).

## Tests of coordination

These are not worth attempting if the patient has significant weakness:

- **Finger-to-nose test:** ask the patient to touch the point of their nose first with the index finger, and then with the other, and then to touch one of your fingers with the same finger. Ask them to repeat this exercise as fast as possible. The patient can keep their eyes open while you change the position of your finger. If this is normal, there is no need to progress to additional tests. If the movement is not fluid, you should ask them to repeat the action of touching their nose with the eyes closed. Additional difficulty suggests an abnormality of joint position sense (**Fig. 6.33**).

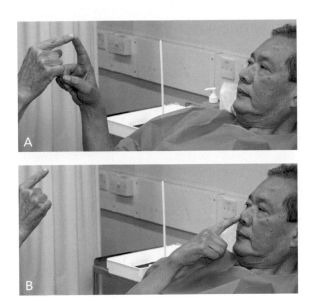

Fig. 6.33A, B The finger-to-nose test.

- **Dysdiadochokinesia:** this is the term used to characterise an inability to perform rapidly repeated movements. It can be tested by asking the patient to pretend to screw a light bulb into a socket. Another useful test is to ask the patient to perform simple repetitive movements, such as drawing a circle with a finger on the back of one, and then the other, hand. Slow, awkward movements indicate dysdiadochokinesia.
- **Heel-to-shin test:** to assess lower limb coordination, ask the patient to slide the heel of one foot in a straight line down the shin of the other leg. In cerebellar ataxia, the heel wavers across the intended target.

## Examination of the sensory system

The assessment of sensory function starts with the history because symptoms of sensory dysfunction sometimes precede any objective abnormality on clinical testing. In addition, the patient's symptoms may direct you to a particular area of the body or to the type of sensory function that requires most attention.

The areas and modalities tested will depend on the type of sensory disturbance suggested by the patient's symptoms and history. However, it is sensible to be thinking whether the pattern fits with a dermatomal distribution or a peripheral neuropathy. The modalities of sensation are light touch, pain, temperature, vibration and proprioception. First, test on a part where you know the sensation is normal to confirm that the patient can feel the stimulus and understands what to do. Then follow a dermatomal pattern (**Fig. 6.34**). If the sensory loss looks as if it is in a glove or stocking distribution, start at the tips of the fingers or toes, and work up until you find a sensory level.

- **Light touch:** this is tested with a wisp of cotton wool applied at a single point with the patient's eyes closed. Do not drag the wool across the skin as this sensation may be transmitted via pain fibres.

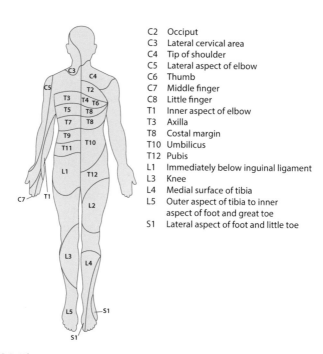

| | |
|---|---|
| C2 | Occiput |
| C3 | Lateral cervical area |
| C4 | Tip of shoulder |
| C5 | Lateral aspect of elbow |
| C6 | Thumb |
| C7 | Middle finger |
| C8 | Little finger |
| T1 | Inner aspect of elbow |
| T3 | Axilla |
| T8 | Costal margin |
| T10 | Umbilicus |
| T12 | Pubis |
| L1 | Immediately below inguinal ligament |
| L3 | Knee |
| L4 | Medial surface of tibia |
| L5 | Outer aspect of tibia to inner aspect of foot and great toe |
| S1 | Lateral aspect of foot and little toe |

Fig. 6.34 The segmental (dermatomal) innervation.

- **Pain:** this is best tested using a broken orange stick or a specially designed 'neurotip' (which creates a sharp point). A needle point should be avoided because it may easily puncture the skin and is a potential source of infection.
- **Vibration sense:** this is commonly reduced or absent in elderly patients; nevertheless, it may be valuable in patients suspected of having a peripheral sensory neuropathy. It is best tested using a 128 Hz 'C' tuning fork, testing both the lower and upper limbs and the trunk.
- **Proprioception:** joint position sense should be tested with the patient's eyes closed. The system for testing joint position sense in the fingers and toes is illustrated in **Figs 6.35** and **6.36**. The digit should be separated from any adjacent digits and the joint being tested moved up and/or down. Ask the patient which way the digit is being moved.

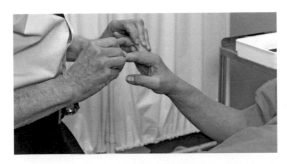

Fig. 6.35 The system for testing joint position sense in the fingers.

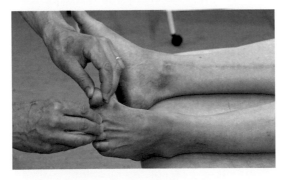

Fig. 6.36 The system for testing joint position sense in the toes.

- **Temperature:** this is rarely tested as a routine. If it is indicated, the simplest way is to fill either a blood sample bottle or a metal tube with either ice or warm water. Follow the scheme of looking for first a dermatomal, and then a peripheral neuropathy, distribution of loss.
- **Weight, shape, size and texture:** coins are useful objects for this test. A coin is placed in the palm of the patient's hand with their eyes closed, and the patient is then asked to describe it. The weight of different coins can be compared by simultaneously placing different ones in each hand.

Summaries of sensory loss and of sensory loss localising lesions are shown in *Tables 6.8* and *6.9.*

## Examination of related structures

The neurological examination is incomplete unless related structures are also examined. These include skeletal structures (skull and spine), extracranial blood vessels and the skin.

- The shape and size of the skull must be observed, and the head palpated to look for bony defects or swellings.
- You should examine the spinal curvature and palpate for local tenderness all the way down the spine. Test spinal movements and measure the extent of straight leg raising. Look for limitation of movement of the cervical spine – this is generally the result of cervical spondylosis, but occasionally the consequence of meningeal irritation.

## Table 6.8  Loss of sensory modality and associated sensory pathway

| Modality | Pathway |
| --- | --- |
| Light touch, vibration and proprioception | Predominantly mediated via dorsal column tract and medial lemniscus pathway |
| Pain and temperature | Mediated by spinothalamic tract |

## Table 6.9 Localisation of signs associated with sensory loss

| Location | Signs |
|---|---|
| Sensory cortex | Contralateral complete hemi-sensory loss |
| Anterior limb, internal capsule | Contralateral hemi-sensory loss over face, arm and leg |
| Thalamus | Most common cause of pure contralateral hemi-sensory loss in the absence of motor findings |
| Brainstem | Crossed motor and sensory deficit. Cranial nerve nuclear dysfunction in region of the lesion causes ipsilateral cranial nerve abnormalities |
| Spinal cord | Ipsilateral loss of light touch, vibration and proprioception, contralateral loss of pain and temperature. Characteristic in complete cord lesions is a sensory level (discrete loss of sensation below a certain dermatomal level) |
| Radiculopathy | Disorders of nerve roots typically cause positive (dysaethesia or burning or paraesthesia, pain) and negative (anaesthesia or numbness) sensory findings |
| Peripheral neuropathy | Complete sensory loss is length dependent and caused by axonal degeneration (e.g. diabetes mellitus or alcohol)<br><br>Compression neuropathy caused by mechanical injury |

- Remember not only to palpate the carotid arteries (one at a time), but also to listen over them for bruits. You should also examine the skin for vascular malformations, neuromas and café-au-lait spots, which may be seen in association with certain neurological diseases.

## Illustrated physical signs

### Physical signs caused by optic nerve lesions (cranial nerve II)

Light from an object on the left side of the body falls on the right half of each retina – the temporal or outer half of each retina is eventually connected to the occipital cortex on the same side, while the nasal or inner half is connected to the occipital cortex on the opposite side by nerve fibres that cross the midline in the optic chiasm (**Fig. 6.37**).

A visual field defect may be due to a lesion affecting the eye or optic nerve, optic chiasm, optic tract between the chiasm and the lateral geniculate bodies, optic radiation or occipital cortex. A diagrammatic outline of the visual pathways is shown in **Fig. 6.37**. Included in the illustration are the common abnormalities you may encounter and the anatomical location of the various lesions.

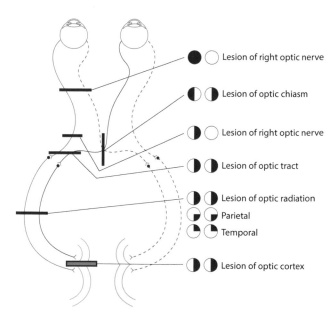

Fig. 6.37 Visual field defects caused by optic nerve lesions.

## Physical signs caused by defects of the IIIrd, IVth and VIth cranial nerves

- Infranuclear (LMN) lesions of the IIIrd, IVth and VIth nerves result in paralysis of individual eye muscles or groups of muscles. Supranuclear (UMN) lesions will result in paralysis of conjugate eye movements of the eyes.
- In infranuclear lesions of the IIIrd nerve (IIIrd nerve palsy), the eye has a complete ptosis (**Fig. 6.38**), and when the eye is open, the gaze is displaced downwards and outwards (**Fig. 6.39**). The pupil is usually dilated and fixed, and there is loss of accommodation. However, the lesion may be only partial, with one or a few of these functions being lost.
- A IVth nerve palsy results in an impaired movement, with the eyeball being rotated outwards when the subject attempts to look down in the mid-position of gaze.
- In a VIth nerve palsy, there is an inability to move the eye outwards, and diplopia occurs when this is attempted.

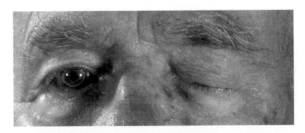

Fig. 6.38 A IIIrd nerve palsy. The patient has a complete ptosis.

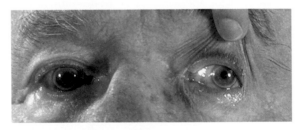

Fig. 6.39 A IIIrd nerve palsy. With the eye open, the gaze is deviated downwards and outwards.

Signs of an infranuclear lesion involving one or more of these three nerves may include:

- Defective movement of the eye.
- The presence of a squint (or strabismus).
- The presence of diplopia.
- Pupillary abnormalities.

---

### BOX 6.10 DIPLOPIA: DETECTING WEAK OCULAR MUSCLES

- The diplopia may consist of images that are side by side (horizontal diplopia), one above the other (vertical diplopia), or both. Pure horizontal diplopia must be due to weakness of a lateral or medial rectus. Vertical diplopia may be due to weakness of any of the other muscles.
- Separation of the images is maximal when the gaze is turned in the direction of action of the weak muscle (e.g. maximal separation on looking to the right indicates weakness of the left medial or right lateral rectus).
- When the gaze is directed so as to cause maximal separation of the images, the abnormal image from the lagging eye is displaced further in the direction of the gaze (e.g. if horizontal diplopia is maximal on looking to the right and the image furthest to the right comes from the right eye (tested by covering each eye separately), the right lateral rectus is weak).

---

**Strabismus** This is an abnormality of ocular movement such that the visual axes do not meet at the point of fixation (**Fig. 6.40**). Paralytic strabismus is due to weakness of one or more of the extraocular muscles. The following clinical features are seen in paralytic strabismus:

- Limitation of movement: a prominent feature is impairment of ocular movement in the direction of action of the muscles affected.
- False orientation of the field of vision: there is erroneous judgement by the patient of the position of the object in that portion of the field of vision towards which the paralysed muscles should

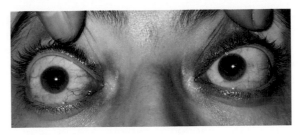

Fig. 6.40 Strabismus. Note the lack of conjugate gaze.

usually move the eye. Patients point wide of an object if they close the unaffected eye.
- Diplopia: patients with paralytic strabismus complain of double vision.

**Box 6.10** contains three rules that may help you detect which of the ocular muscles is weak in a patient with diplopia.

Supranuclear lesions do not produce diplopia, and the ocular axes remain parallel because the supranuclear centres regulate conjugate gaze and do not control individual eye movements. The frontal and occipital cortical ocular motor areas control lateral conjugate gaze to the opposite side, with the result that destructive lesions at these sites cause deviation of the gaze towards the side of the lesion in the brain (but away from any associated weakness in the limbs). The supranuclear centres for vertical gaze are situated in the midbrain, and lesions at this site produce weakness of vertical conjugate gaze.

The pathways that subserve lateral conjugate gaze pass to the brainstem and decussate below the IIIrd nerve nucleus to reach the pontine centres for lateral conjugate gaze, which are close to the vestibular nuclei and direct the gaze towards the same side. A lesion of the pons producing hemiplegia may therefore be associated with fixed deviation of the eyes towards the weak limbs.

The fibres from the pontine centre for lateral gaze are distributed to the ipsilateral VIth nerve nucleus and, via the medial longitudinal bundle, to the portion of the contralateral IIIrd nerve nucleus innervating the medial rectus. A lesion of the medial longitudinal bundle will therefore produce **internuclear ophthalmoplegia**, characterised by selective paralysis of the medial rectus on horizontal gaze, with monocular nystagmus of the contralateral abducting eye.

Internuclear ophthalmoplegia is characterised by impaired adduction of the eye on the abnormal side and horizontal jerk nystagmus in the opposite eye on lateral gaze from the side of the lesion. The remainder of the extraocular movements, including convergence, are normal (see **Box 6.10**).

**Control of pupillary size** The size of the pupil is controlled by two divisions of the autonomic nervous system acting mainly in response to the level of illumination and distance of focus. The iris sphincter muscle makes the pupil smaller (miosis), and is innervated by parasympathetic nerves; the iris dilator muscle makes the pupil larger (mydriasis), and is innervated by sympathetic nerves.

The parasympathetic fibres control both pupillary constriction and contraction of the ciliary muscle, which produces accommodation; these fibres arise from the Edinger–Westphal nucleus. They travel via the IIIrd cranial nerve to the ciliary ganglion in the orbit. Postganglionic fibres are distributed via the ciliary nerves.

A lesion of the parasympathetic nerves produces a dilated pupil that is unreactive to light or accommodation. The pupillary response to light depends on the integrity of the afferent pathways, and is lost when the retina or optic nerve is damaged. A unilateral lesion of the retina or optic nerve results in loss of the pupillary reflex when a light is shone in that eye (direct light reaction), but there will still be a response when the unaffected eye is tested (indirect light reaction).

The sympathetic fibres supplying the eye arise from the eighth cervical and first two thoracic segments of the spinal cord and pass via the carotid plexus to the orbit. The activity of these fibres is controlled by hypothalamic centres from which central sympathetic pathways pass to the spinal cord.

A lesion of the ocular sympathetic pathways produces a constricted pupil that may become smaller in response to a bright light, but will not dilate normally in response to shade.

**Horner's syndrome** This is due to paralysis of the cervical sympathetic chain. It consists of slight drooping of the eye (ptosis), pupillary constriction, absence of pupillary dilatation on shading the eye and absence of sweating on the corresponding half of the face and neck (**Fig. 6.41**). Enophthalmos (apparent indrawing of the eye) is often also present. The pupil of a completely blind eye is dilated

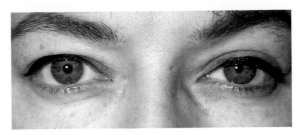

Fig. 6.41 Horner's syndrome. The left pupil is small, and there is ptosis and enophthalmos.

and fails to react to light, but it constricts when light is shone into the opposite normal eye.

Horner's syndrome may be caused by hypothalamic lesions, lateral medullary syndrome or lesions of the second-order sympathetic nerve in the cervical region of the neck. Examples of the latter include an aortic aneurysm and Pancoast tumour.

**Holmes–Adie pupil** This is distinguished by unilateral mydriasis (dilatation) and diminished or absent pupillary light reflex. It is caused by injury to the ciliary ganglion and/or postganglionic fibres. It is most commonly idiopathic or benign.

**Nystagmus** This is most commonly due to disorders of the vestibular system or to lesions involving central pathways concerned with ocular movements, for example vestibulocerebellar connections in the brainstem or the medial longitudinal bundle. It may also on occasion result from weakness in the ocular muscles. Nystagmus may be induced by toxic levels of certain drugs, for example phenytoin. It may also be congenital in origin, where it shows a pendular quality. A few irregular jerks of the eyes may be seen in full lateral deviation in healthy subjects. Optokinetic nystagmus may be observed in healthy subjects when the eyes are repeatedly fixed on a moving stimulus; an example is seen when a person tries to read an advertisement on a station platform as the train departs.

## Physical signs caused by the Vth cranial nerve (trigeminal)

Lesions of the whole trigeminal nerve lead to loss of sensation in the skin and mucous membrane of the face and nasopharynx, and a reduction in salivary, buccal and lacrimal secretions. Taste is spared, but lack of oral secretions may result in subjective changes. A characteristic feature is weakness of the muscles of mastication. Pain in the distribution of the ophthalmic division of the trigeminal nerve may be caused by herpes zoster infection.

## Physical signs caused by the VIIth cranial nerve (facial)

A unilateral LMN lesion causes weakness of all the muscles of facial expression on the same side as the lesion. There is weakness of the frontalis muscle, the eye will not close, and there is a risk of corneal ulceration. The angle of the mouth falls, and dribbling from the corner of the mouth is common. Damage to the facial nerve in the temporal bone (e.g. Bell's palsy, trauma, herpes zoster or middle ear infection) may be associated with undue sensitivity to sounds (hyperacusis) and loss of taste to the anterior two-thirds of the tongue (**Fig. 6.42**).

A UMN lesion causes weakness of the lower part of the face on the opposite side. Upper facial muscles are spared because of the bilateral cortical innervation of neurones supplying the upper face. Wrinkling of the forehead is normal.

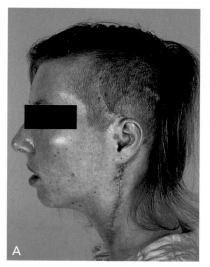 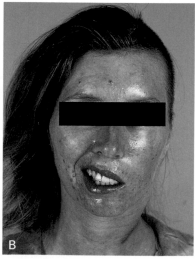

Fig. 6.42A, B A LMN facial palsy (VIIth cranial nerve). Note the involvement of the forehead.

## Physical signs caused by the VIIIth cranial nerve (auditory vestibular)

**Tinnitus** In the case of the VIIIth nerve, abnormal auditory sensations may occur. A patient may complain of 'ringing in the ears' (tinnitus). This symptom is common but only rarely due to neurological disease. Hyperacusis is the term used when even slight sounds are heard with painful intensity; this sometimes occurs with paralysis of the stapedius muscle due to a facial palsy. Patients with sensorineural deafness due to damage of the cochlea may also complain of a similar problem – an example is Ménière's disease.

**Vertigo** Patients often complain of giddiness or dizziness. In true vertigo, external objects seem to move around the patient. Vertigo may occur in disease of the vestibular system, for example of the ear, vestibulococlear nerve, brainstem or temporal lobe.

## Physical signs caused by the IXth–XIIth cranial nerves (glossopharyngeal, accessory, vagus, hypoglossal)

**Bulbar and pseudobulbar palsy** Unilateral damage of the pathways from the cortex to the lower cranial nerve nuclei (the corticobulbar tracts) may produce transient weakness of the many muscles supplied by these nerves. This results in temporary unilateral weakness of the muscles of the jaw, lower parts of the face, palate, pharynx, larynx, neck and tongue. There is a rapid recovery even after extensive lesions because the corticobulbar tract on the other side can generally take over the function. Bilateral damage (which may follow repeated strokes) results in persistent weakness and spasticity of the muscles supplied by the bulbar nuclei. As a result, there is slurring of speech and dysphagia (difficulty in swallowing), the jaw jerk is abnormally brisk and movements of the tongue are reduced in amplitude. In addition, there is loss of voluntary control of emotional expression and the patient may laugh or cry without apparent provocation.

A contrasting situation is bilateral LMN lesions in the same nuclei or cranial nerves, which causes a bulbar palsy. In this case, there is wasting and weakness of the jaw, face, palate, larynx, neck and tongue, with accompanying dysarthria and dysphagia, but a depressed jaw jerk and an absence of emotional lability. In both pseudobulbar and bulbar palsies, it is often necessary to feed patients through a fine-bore nasogastric tube – the poor coordination of the pharyngeal/laryngeal muscles make these patients liable to aspirate food or liquid.

## Abnormalities of the motor system

The ability to walk and to maintain a normal posture of the body when standing are very sensitive tests of the nervous system that are frequently overlooked. These actions require normal sensory, motor and coordination function: a defect of posture or gait may result from a sensory deficit, muscle weakness or cerebellar incoordination. Certain abnormalities of gait are distinctive. In paralysis of the dorsiflexors, the foot may not clear the ground when walking, resulting in foot drop – the knee has to be raised high as the leg is moved forward and the foot is slapped onto the ground. Proximal leg weakness leads to a curious waddling gait. In a hemiparesis (weakness of arm and leg), the affected arm may not swing and the stiff leg is dragged along the floor. Loss of proprioception in the legs produces a high-stepping, broad-based gait with the patient carefully watching the feet and the ground. In cerebellar disease, the rhythmic coordination of the movements that comprise walking are lost, and the patient reels from side to side as if drunk (cerebellar ataxia). Ataxia is made more obvious by asking the patient to walk heel-to-toe along a straight line – cerebellar ataxia, unlike sensory ataxia, cannot be compensated by visual clues.

With regard to the appearance of the muscles, wasting is characteristically seen in LMN lesions, but may also occur as a result of poor nutrition with weight loss, malignancy and injury, leading to disuse as a consequence of immobility of a muscle group. In the latter case, strength may be relatively well preserved in relation to the degree of wasting. Occasionally, muscles appear hypertrophied but are weak on testing (pseudohypertrophy). This situation is found in muscular dystrophy, where the muscles are infiltrated by fat and connective tissue.

Muscle weakness may result from primary muscle weakness, an LMN lesion (motor nerve or anterior horn cell) or a lesion of the UMNs (corticospinal and pyramidal tracts). An LMN weakness from a T1 lesion causing a claw hand is shown in **Fig. 6.43**.

## Therapeutic and technical skills

### Key laboratory tests

Neurology is anatomically based, so the most important investigations involve imaging. Computed tomography and magnetic resonance imaging are essential components of neurological assessment – and are

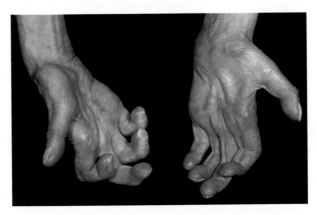

Fig. 6.43 Claw hands from T1 involvement in the spine.

### BOX 6.11 ABNORMAL REFLEX RESPONSES: INVOLUNTARY MOVEMENTS

The following more common abnormalities may occasionally be seen:

- **Tics and habit spasms:** these are twitching or jerking movements often associated with anxiety conditions.
- **Myoclonus:** these are sudden, rapid, irregular jerking movements of a group of muscles. They can occur with lesions at many levels in the nervous system, and do not have any localising value.
- **Tremor:** this refers to regular or irregular distal movements with an oscillatory character. In thyrotoxicosis, tremors are rapid and fine, but in familial disorders they tend to be of a coarser character (benign essential tremor). In intention tremor, a coarse tremor occurs only with voluntary movement; this is best demonstrated by asking the patient to touch your finger and then their own nose (**Fig. 6.33**). A rapid, alternating and rhythmic tremor is present in Parkinson's disease ('pill rolling'), while a flapping tremor (of the outstretched fingers) is seen in association with carbon dioxide retention and hepatic encephalopathy.

*(Continued)*

---

### BOX 6.11 (Continued) ABNORMAL REFLEX RESPONSES: INVOLUNTARY MOVEMENTS

- **Athetosis:** this is writhing movements of a limb. The movements may be unilateral or generalised; the latter are seen with degenerative disease of the basal ganglia.
- **Chorea:** this comprises rapid, jerking and darting movements that may affect the face, tongue and, in particular, distal portions of the arms and legs. Huntington's chorea is an example that occurs in adults and is accompanied by progressive dementia. Senile chorea may be seen in association with widespread cerebral atherosclerosis; chorea is also occasionally seen with systemic lupus erythematosus and may be induced by certain drugs (e.g. phenothiazines).
- **Tetany:** this is recognisable by a characteristic posture of the hand (*main d'accoucheur*) and is caused by hypocalcaemia or profound alkalosis. Inflating a sphygmomanometer cuff above the arterial pressure for 2–3 minutes will produce or augment this sign (Trousseau's sign).
- **LMN lesions:** the tendon reflexes are absent with lesions affecting the afferent pathways, the anterior horn cells or the efferent pathways.
- **UMN lesions:** these occur at all levels above the anterior horn cells – exaggerated reflexes (hyper-reflexia) follow. This may occur with anxiety or thyrotoxicosis, and is therefore only of pathological significance if it is associated with other signs of a UMN lesion.

---

a specialist area. The techniques are best performed in conjunction with a neuroradiologist.

The following figures illustrate features of CNS disease: lateral medullary syndrome (**Fig. 6.44**), cerebral infarction (**Fig. 6.45**), a spinal cord lesion (**Fig. 6.46**), peripheral nerve lesions (**Fig. 6.47**), Parkinson's disease (**Fig. 6.48**), motor neurone disease (**Fig. 6.49**) and brainstem stroke (**Fig. 6.50**).

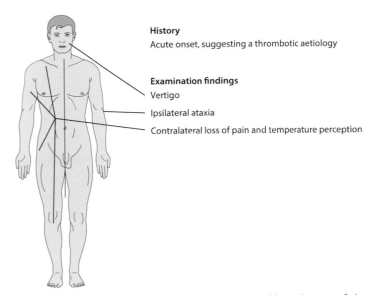

**History**
Acute onset, suggesting a thrombotic aetiology

**Examination findings**
Vertigo

Ipsilateral ataxia

Contralateral loss of pain and temperature perception

Fig. 6.44 The lateral medullary syndrome, caused by a lesion of the posterior inferior cerebellar artery.

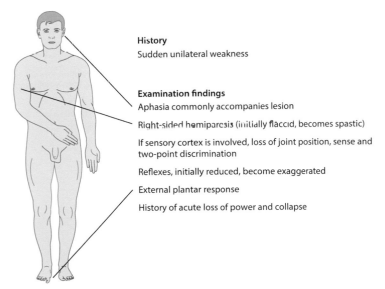

**History**
Sudden unilateral weakness

**Examination findings**
Aphasia commonly accompanies lesion

Right-sided hemiparesis (initially flaccid, becomes spastic)

If sensory cortex is involved, loss of joint position, sense and two-point discrimination

Reflexes, initially reduced, become exaggerated

External plantar response

History of acute loss of power and collapse

Fig. 6.45 Cerebral infarction – middle cerebral artery territory.

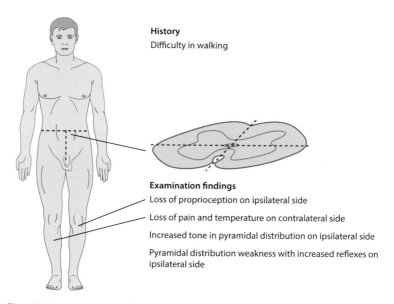

**History**
Difficulty in walking

**Examination findings**
Loss of proprioception on ipsilateral side

Loss of pain and temperature on contralateral side

Increased tone in pyramidal distribution on ipsilateral side

Pyramidal distribution weakness with increased reflexes on ipsilateral side

Fig. 6.46 A spinal cord lesion.

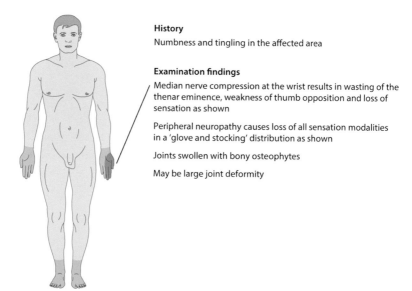

**History**
Numbness and tingling in the affected area

**Examination findings**
Median nerve compression at the wrist results in wasting of the thenar eminence, weakness of thumb opposition and loss of sensation as shown

Peripheral neuropathy causes loss of all sensation modalities in a 'glove and stocking' distribution as shown

Joints swollen with bony osteophytes

May be large joint deformity

Fig. 6.47 Peripheral nerve lesions.

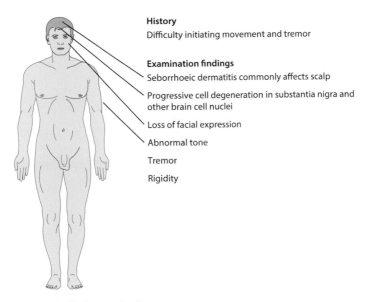

**History**
Difficulty initiating movement and tremor

**Examination findings**
Seborrhoeic dermatitis commonly affects scalp

Progressive cell degeneration in substantia nigra and other brain cell nuclei

Loss of facial expression

Abnormal tone

Tremor

Rigidity

Fig. 6.48 Parkinson's disease.

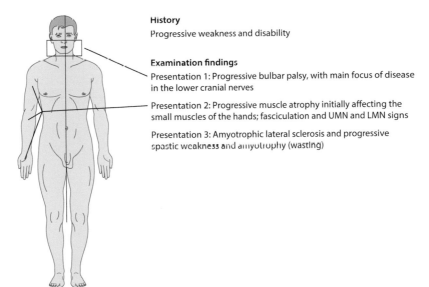

**History**
Progressive weakness and disability

**Examination findings**
Presentation 1: Progressive bulbar palsy, with main focus of disease in the lower cranial nerves

Presentation 2: Progressive muscle atrophy initially affecting the small muscles of the hands; fasciculation and UMN and LMN signs

Presentation 3: Amyotrophic lateral sclerosis and progressive spastic weakness and amyotrophy (wasting)

Fig. 6.49 Motor neurone disease.

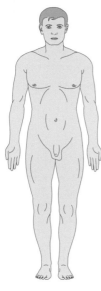

**History**

Sudden collapse with loss of consciousness

**Examination findings**

Deeply unconscious. Pyrexia

Bilateral brisk tendon reflex responses

Bilateral extensor plantar responses

Decerebrate posture

Rigidity

Constricted pupils

Cheyne–Stokes respiration may be present

Fig. 6.50 Brainstem stroke.

## OBSTETRICS AND GYNAECOLOGY

Women's health forms a large part of clinical practice, and includes pre-pregnancy planning, pregnancy, childbirth, disorders of menstruation, pelvic tumours, incontinence, pelvic organ prolapse, contraception and fertility. Much of the time the women are not ill, but the role of healthcare professionals is to identify when something is becoming abnormal, and then to act appropriately. Technological developments are both exciting and diverse, but accurate and sensitive history taking together with gentle examination is the cornerstone of good care and will never let you down. To highlight the need for care, consider the figures for maternal mortality. In 2015 in the UK, maternal mortality was 8.2 per 100,000 live births, with just under 700,000 deliveries a year; by contrast, in Afghanistan, maternal mortality was 1575 mothers per 100,000 live births.

There is a wide range of 'normal' in the physiology and anatomy of structures within the pelvis. Additionally, there are variations in function through the lifetime of a normal woman, including puberty, pregnancy, lactation and the climacteric (menopause), each of which can have a profound effect on systemic signs and symptoms. Never be tramlined in your thinking when assessing a gynaecological history, as so many systemic diseases can present with an alteration in vaginal or uterine function. A good example is recurrent vaginal yeast infections; this is a very common gynaecological problem, but it may be the presenting complaint in women with undiagnosed diabetes mellitus.

## Applied anatomy and physiology

Knowledge of the embryological development of the urogenital system is relevant because there are clinical problems that may present in childhood and early adult life as a direct consequence of congenital anatomical abnormalities.

The ovaries develop from primitive gonads that are common to genetically male or female embryos. Testes are formed in the presence of an XY chromosome; otherwise ovaries develop. The fallopian tubes, uterus, cervix and upper vagina develop by fusion of the dual mesonephric systems. The lower vagina is developed from an invagination of the cloacal pit. When the process of fusion is not complete, two uteruses, two cervixes and a double vagina may be found.

### BOX 7.1 THE MENSTRUAL CYCLE

The menstrual cycle starts on the first day of a period. Shedding of the endometrium normally lasts 5 days, and is associated with a blood loss of 30 ml. Endometrial haemostasis is a complex process and includes fibrinolysis, which prevents clot formation. As a result, a normal period is not associated with blood clotting.

After the period ceases, the follicular phase is associated with the development of a graafian follicle, culminating in ovulation on day 14 of a normal 28-day cycle. The egg is released from a mature follicle, which measures 18–22 mm. Follicles can be clearly seen on ultrasound examination. Release of the egg can be painful, and is referred to as 'Mittelschmerz' (German for 'middle pain'). The time from ovulation to the start of the next period – the luteal phase – is always 14 days, but the length of time from the end of a period to ovulation varies from month to month and from woman to woman. If the egg has been fertilised, the corpus luteum persists and the next period does not start.

The fine balance of the menstrual cycle is easily influenced. Weight loss, for example, reduces hypothalamic function to a point where ovulation stops. For example, few full-time ballet dancers or athletes have a regular menstrual cycle.

## Assessment and diagnosis of obstetric and gynaecological problems

### Taking the history

Many features of the gynaecological history are common to both women who are pregnant and those who are not. The guidelines for general history taking, which were outlined in Chapter 1, still apply. The history must be taken in an unrushed manner, and in an environment that reduces embarrassment. An overview of the gynaecological history will be considered first, and then the specific points about pregnant women will be added.

It helps to be logical and ask in chronological order. Begin by asking how old the woman was when her periods started, and how the cycle changed in the following years. Ask about pregnancies and whether the patient has had children (see below for details). Establish when the patient's last menstrual period (LMP) was. When you ask, 'When was your last menstrual period?', document day 1 of the last period. Ask what form of contraception she is using, if any. Taking a sensitive sexual history is also important.

Establish when she last had screening tests (appropriate for her age) and the results of those tests; these include a cervical smear, human papillomavirus (HPV) test, sexual health screen, mammogram, bone density scan and test for ovarian cancer.

You can ask several questions to gain an idea about the regularity and usual pattern of the menstrual cycle (see **Box 7.2**).

### BOX 7.2 QUESTIONS TO ASK ABOUT THE MENSTRUAL CYCLE

'How old were you when your periods started?'

'How have they changed over the years?'

'Do they always start on the same day of the month?'

'How many days bleeding do you have?'

## The presenting complaint

**Abnormal periods** This is the most frequently seen problem in the gynaecology clinic. It implies a knowledge of what is 'normal', and needless to say there is a huge range of normality. After birth, female babies may have a little vaginal bleeding on day 2, in response to withdrawal of the oestrogen levels that the baby is exposed to *in utero*. Periods most commonly start at the age of 12 years (menarche), although quite normally they may start between 9 and 16 years. Menstruation is preceded by breast development (thelarche).

The normal menstrual cycle involves 2–7 days' bleeding every 23–34 days. It is not normal to bleed in early pregnancy, and menstruation may or may not restart during lactation. The mean age at which a woman has her last period (menopause) is 51 years, and climacteric symptoms (flushing, sweating, etc.) associated with the menopause last for 5 years in 60% of women. After the periods have ceased for 6 months, there should be no vaginal bleeding. If bleeding occurs after this time, it is very important to investigate thoroughly as 'post-menopausal bleeding' may be the first symptom of pelvic malignancy.

When presenting the history, try to describe the bleeding pattern rather than using terms like 'menorrhagia' or 'oligomenorrhoea', even though you need an understanding of these terms. Sample questions may be:

'When you have a period, do you have to use double protection, such as pads and tampons?'

'When you have a period, do you notice clots? How large are they?'

**Menorrhagia** This is the term to describe heavy periods. The normal blood loss during a period is 30 ml, but when the loss exceeds 80 ml, 90% of women will complain of heavy bleeding. The common 'local' causes are fibroids, endometriosis and pelvic infection. The patient will typically have noticed the passage of blood clots up to 3–4 cm in diameter, and she will have noticed flooding such that she needs to use 'super' tampons in conjunction with other methods of protection. Additionally, the period of bleeding may be excessive. Ask about general problems of bleeding elsewhere in the body, including ease of bruising. There are rare conditions, for example von Willebrand's disease, that are associated with heavy periods.

**Amenorrhoea** There are two types:

- **Primary:** if a woman has never had a period at the age of 16, she has primary amenorrhoea.
- **Secondary:** if menstruation has been established and then stops, the problem is described as secondary amenorrhoea.

The most common cause of secondary amenorrhoea is pregnancy, and this should always be considered as a possible diagnosis. The next most common cause is excessive weight loss, sometimes associated with emotional stress, so ask about changes in body weight, deliberate or otherwise.

**Climacteric symptoms** In women with secondary amenorrhoea, ask about the symptoms attributed to falling oestrogen levels at the climacteric. The word 'menopause' refers to the last period. The mean age of menopause is 51 years, and premature menopause is when the last period occurs below the age of 40. Hot flushes, particularly on the face and neck, and also 'night sweats' are characteristic. Patients wake at night, fling off the duvet and go to the window 'while my partner is shivering on the other side of the bed'. Associated with this may be a sensation of dryness in the vagina, short-term memory loss and other symptoms including epigastric pain/reflux, joint pain and alteration in body weight.

**Dysmenorrhoea** When periods have always been associated with pain that is not caused by a specific condition such as endometriosis, the condition is termed 'primary dysmenorrhoea'. In contrast, if painless menstruation has been followed by an increase in pain not due to a specific condition, the condition is described as 'secondary dysmenorrhoea'. Pain is described as central in the pelvis, cramp-like with radiation down the top of the thighs, and is often associated with nausea. Ask whether the pain starts with the onset of bleeding or whether it precedes it by a few days. The importance of this is that endometriosis is a common cause of secondary dysmenorrhoea and is characterised by several days of premenstrual pain.

**Metrorrhagia** This is a condition of irregular and unpredictable periods with a menstrual cycle falling outside the normal 28 (±5) days.

Frequently, irregular periods are the result of systemic hormonal upset. In young women, 'polycystic ovaries' is the most common finding, so ask about excessive hair growth with male distribution, caused by increased circulating androgens.

**Intermenstrual bleeding** Mid-cycle spotting associated with ovulation occurs regularly 14 days before the onset of a period, and is not abnormal. Any other form of bleeding is abnormal, and its cause must be identified.

**Post-coital bleeding** Bleeding after intercourse occurs as a response to inflammation or tumour of the endocervix, ectocervix, vagina or vulva (including the urethra).

**Premenstrual symptoms** Most women are aware of breast tenderness, fluid retention and mood swings before a period. Ask about specific problems including depression, tearfulness, psychiatric disturbances and cyclical systemic symptoms such as migraine headache.

**Vaginal discharge** The normal vagina is liberally coated by mucus from ducts at the introitus (Bartholin's glands) and columnar epithelium on the endocervix. Discharge increases and becomes thinner at the time of ovulation, and is often absent after the menopause. An alteration in vaginal discharge causing an offensive loss, or a loss that itches, is significant. At this point, remember to ask about any infections that the woman's partner may have had.

**Pain** The normal menstrual cycle can be associated with pain at ovulation on day 14 of a 28-day cycle, as well as during the first days of a period. This pain should be helped by simple analgesics. Any other pain should be investigated. You must ask about the relationship of pain to the menstrual cycle, bowel function and urinary function. Ask if the pain is made worse by intercourse (dyspareunia).

It is difficult to make generalisations about different types of pain. As a guideline, pain from the ovaries is felt in the iliac fossae. If an ovary undergoes torsion (an ovary with a cyst may twist on the infundibulopelvic ligament), it may pull on the obturator nerve and cause pain down the medial side of the thigh. In addition, torsion of the ovary can distort the ureter, causing pain in the renal area exactly like that of renal colic. However, rupture or bleeding into an ovarian cyst produces sudden-onset pain.

Pain originating in the uterus is felt centrally. Endometritis, for example, gives low suprapubic pain that is aggravated by intercourse. Asking about intercourse is difficult, but questions such as 'Has this problem altered your relationship with your partner?' or 'Can you tell me about it?' will often lead to a discussion if relevant.

## Past obstetric history

Every pregnancy is very important. A useful structure to help you think clearly about each pregnancy is to ask about pre-conception planning, conception (treatments for infertility), the pregnancy itself (first, second and third trimesters), labour, delivery, the puerperium (including feeding) and plans for subsequent pregnancies.

- Establish how many babies were born after 24 weeks' gestation, and ask if they are alive and well; include the names of children. Document the parity; this is the total number of pregnancies that a woman has had, including those that did not produce a live infant, for example para 1 + 1 signifies one live infant and one miscarriage.
- Ask details of pregnancies that did not go past 24 weeks' gestation. Include details of miscarriage, ectopic pregnancy and termination of pregnancy. Rather than using the term 'abortion', it is better to ask, 'Did you have any pregnancies that you chose to interrupt?' Give the patient time to describe the detail of pregnancy loss, as this is always going to jog painful memories, which may be difficult.

## Past medical history

Enquire about previous gynaecological surgery and outpatient investigations, including ultrasound scans, blood tests for hormones and hysteroscopy (looking into the uterus with a endoscope). Enquire about abdominal surgery, as previous pelvic surgery alters the risks of future laparoscopic surgery.

**Breasts** Ask about the history of benign or malignant breast disease and the treatments used.

**Bowel and bladder** Enquire about bowel and bladder function, structuring your history to include intake, storage and emptying. Document the intake of fluids, particularly coffee, tea, cola and other caffeine-rich products. Ask about accidents of urine control. The loss of urine with sneezing, or even just standing from a chair (stress incontinence), is a highly distressing but common problem for which there are successful treatments. Having to run to the toilet but not making it in time (urge incontinence) is characteristic of unstable detrusor muscle contractions. Ask also about problems with voiding urine. A large vaginal prolapse, for example, will often cause an intermittent and slow flow of urine.

Bowel habit is important. Ask about constipation and diarrhoea. Difficulty with evacuating stools may need help with perineal pressure or even digitation with a finger in the anal canal if there is a large posterior vaginal prolapse.

## Family history and treatment history

- **Family history:** ask about a family history of osteoporosis and cancers of the breast, colon or ovary. Having a first-degree relative who had heart disease or thrombosis at a young age may well alter a patient's choice of contraception.
- **Treatment history:** many drugs can affect the menstrual cycle, so make sure all treatments are listed. Also ask about vitamin supplements, complementary medicine and other alternative treatments as these are frequently tried for problems that conventional medicine does not readily help.

## Additional history taking in pregnant women

The first visit during a pregnancy is called the 'booking'. Subsequent antenatal visits are short and are focused on changes since the last antenatal check. Although students see patients in undergraduate examinations during the third trimester, the full history must be taken as if it were the booking visit.

- Ask about a family history for both parents of abnormality, including Down's syndrome, as well as conditions known to have a link to specific social groups. Sickle cell anaemia is a useful example, but there are many others. Specifically ask about cystic fibrosis, as there is a test available to identify affected babies *in utero*.

- A general discussion about the plans for the pregnancy is important. There are options to discuss about which practitioner will carry out most of the antenatal visits and where the patient would like to deliver. Ask where the patient has been receiving most information, and whether she has attended antenatal classes. Establish which antenatal tests have been done and if the patient knows her results. Particularly important are the screening tests for fetal normality.
- In the third trimester, ask about the symptoms caused by pre-eclampsia. Headaches, visual disturbances, epigastric pain (often more on the right) and irritability are the most dramatic.

## Examination of the patient

### General observations

Gynaecological examination includes the breasts, abdomen and pelvis. Also check the height, weight and blood pressure. It can be a terrifying time for women. To help make things easier, the examination room should be warm and a chaperone should be present; it helps enormously if support is provided by female doctors.

### Examination of the abdomen

The patient should be examined in the supine position after emptying her bladder. After measuring the blood pressure and checking the breasts (see page 269), examine the abdomen. Expose the whole abdomen to just above the symphysis pubis. Observe for scars and distension, particularly distension arising from the pelvis. Check for splenic and hepatic enlargement on deep inspiration as you would in an examination of the abdomen in any other patient. Check the epigastric area for tenderness and any evidence of a mass. Next, examine the lower abdomen. Start at the umbilicus and, with the left hand working down towards the pubic bone, feel for suprapubic masses. Check for tenderness in both iliac fossae. Examine the groins for lymphadenopathy and hernias (see Chapter 8).

## BOX 7.3 PELVIC EXAMINATION

Check whether or not you will need to do a cervical smear, and think about whether or not you should take endocervical or high vaginal swabs if infection is suspected. Make sure that you have a light available, a warm Cusco speculum and the materials for a smear or a swab. Remember that this examination is embarrassing and uncomfortable for the patient, so keep her covered with a sheet until you have washed your hands.

- Always wear gloves for this examination. Put on gloves and assemble the warmed Cusco speculum (**Fig. 7.1**) (run the speculum under warm water from a tap, but take care that it does not get too hot). Roll back the sheets to the level of the upper thighs, and then ask the patient to bend her knees. Many doctors ask patients to put their feet together and flop the legs out to the side, but it may be easier and more natural for the patients to bend their knees and keep the feet 20 cm apart. Before using the speculum, look closely at the vulval skin, perineal skin and perianal skin. Identify whether there are any scars (including episiotomy), and see if the vulval skin has lost its normal outlines (which is one of the characteristic findings of vulval dystrophy).
- To place the speculum in the vagina, hold it in your dominant hand, while holding the labia apart with your non-dominant hand. Insert the speculum with the handle to the patient's right initially and, as it slides in, rotate the handle anteriorly (**Fig. 7.2**). Put the thumb and first finger of your dominant hand on the posterior lip of the speculum to push it sufficiently far in to see the cervix when the speculum is opened. Squeeze the handles of the speculum slowly. If you are unable to see the cervix after a slight adjustment, do not struggle. Remove the speculum and check the position of the cervix with a gentle one-finger examination of the vagina, using your dominant hand. To withdraw the speculum, pull slowly on the posterior blade with your dominant hand, while keeping your non-dominant hand on the handles with gentle pressure so that the blades are slightly open. This ensures that no vaginal skin is trapped. As you withdraw the speculum, use this opportunity to look at the vagina carefully so as not miss warts, polyps, etc.

*(Continued)*

**BOX 7.3 (*Continued*)  PELVIC EXAMINATION**

- After removing the speculum, stand on the right side of the patient, and perform a bimanual examination (**Fig. 7.3**). The lubricated and gloved first and second fingers of the right hand are introduced into the vagina. Identify the cervix. Place your left hand on the patient's abdomen suprapubically and gently push down towards the pelvis. The size and position of the uterus can be determined by pushing gently on the cervix and feeling the uterus with your left hand. In approximately two-thirds of women the uterus is anteverted, while in one-third it is retroverted (**Fig. 7.4**). A retroverted uterus is felt by moving the fingers from the cervix to the posterior fornix of the vagina and pressing gently on the abdomen with the left hand.
- To feel the right ovary, move the fingers of your right hand to the right of the cervix. Pushing cranially, your fingers are now in the top of the vagina next to the cervix (the lateral fornix). Simultaneously move your left hand to the right iliac fossa and sweep your fingers towards the fingers of your right hand as if you are trying to make your fingertips touch. The ovary will be palpable if it is enlarged. It is sometimes possible to feel a normal ovary in a slim premenopausal woman.

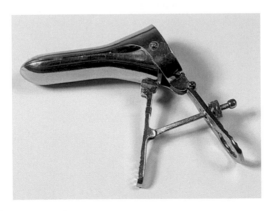

Fig. 7.1  A Cusco speculum.

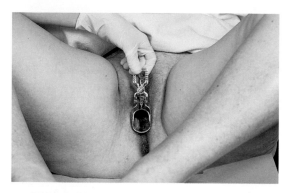

Fig. 7.2 A speculum examination of the vagina.

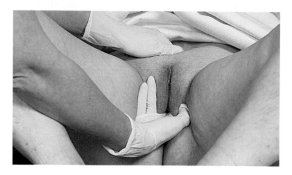

Fig. 7.3 Bimanual vaginal examination.

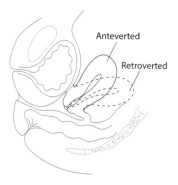

Fig. 7.4 Diagram of an anteverted and a retroverted uterus.

## BOX 7.4 EXAMINING FOR PROLAPSE

After completing the bimanual examination, the patient can be examined for prolapse. This is not necessary in a young patient who has not had symptoms of 'something coming down'. It is, however, necessary for all women who have urinary incontinence and for those with symptoms of prolapse.

- Ask the patient to lie on her left side and draw her knees up to her abdomen. Ask her to cough, and observe any descent of the vagina walls.
- Using a warmed Simm's speculum (**Fig. 7.5**), gently introduce the speculum in the line of the vagina, and apply a little pressure posteriorly to expose the anterior wall.
- Ask the patient to cough again and/or bear down, as if trying to push everything out. Observe at this time the descent of the cervix. In order to do this, you need to allow the speculum to gently slide halfway down the vagina (**Fig. 7.6**). If there is no chance for the speculum to come out with the patient's attempts to push the cervix down, the speculum itself will hold the cervix in.
- Posterior vaginal descent can be observed by replacing the speculum in the vagina and then, with a sponge holder holding the anterior vagina wall away, observing the descent of the posterior vagina with the patient bearing down.

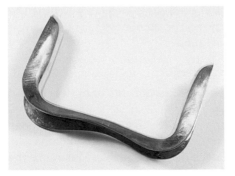

Fig. 7.5  A Simms speculum, used in examination for vaginal prolapse.

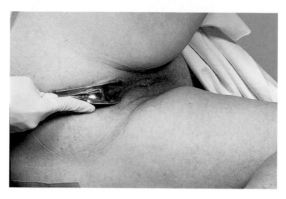

Fig. 7.6 Examination for vaginal prolapse.

### Rectal examination

Rectal examination is not needed unless there are symptoms of pelvic floor dysfunction. Assess whether the pudendo-anal reflex is intact. As you touch the perianal skin, the external anal tissues will contract in a reflex fashion. Also assess the integrity of the resting tone of the anal canal and the integrity of the external anal sphincter in response to a cough and/or voluntary contraction. Pushing the finger anteriorly into the lower rectum will demonstrate the extent of a rectocele. Do this gently, as rectal examination is extremely uncomfortable in the presence of uterovaginal prolapse.

### Neurological examination

Simple neurological assessment includes watching the patient walk and asking if any weakness or numbness has been identified in the saddle area and/or lower limbs.

### Obstetric examination

Antenatal visits include assessments of both the mother and the baby or babies.

At the booking visit in the first trimester, a standard gynaecological examination is carried out. This need not include a pelvic examination if an ultrasound assessment is available. Make sure that the uterine size is consistent with the gestation, and do a cervical smear if this has not been done within the previous 2 years. If there is a history of recurrent miscarriage (more than three consecutive pregnancies lost before 24 weeks' gestation), take vaginal and endocervical swabs to look for infections including bacterial vaginosis and chlamydial infection. While you are performing the examination, consider two objectives:

- Documentation of the baseline values.
- Identification of undiagnosed medical or surgical problems, and documentation of the extent of pre-existing illness.

If a problem is identified, consider the management under two headings:

- The effect of the illness on the pregnancy.
- The effect of the pregnancy on the illness.

### BOX 7.5 ASSESSMENT AT STAGES OF PREGNANCY

Assessment of the pregnant uterus/baby varies at different stages in pregnancy (**Fig. 7.7**). The mother should be semi-recumbent, leaning slightly away from you (never flat on her back after 28 weeks' gestation, as pressure on the vena cava can cause fainting). Before touching the patient, ask if there are any tender areas, and spend a few moments looking for scars.

- After 24 weeks, look for fetal movement. Establish that the size of the uterus is consistent with the gestation. Using your left hand, feel down from the xiphisternum to the fundus. The medial side and top of your index finger will feel the top of the uterus. Measure the distance from the highest point of the uterus to the top of the symphysis pubis in centimetres, and document this as the fundal height.
- After 28 weeks' gestation, feel for the lie of the baby. This will be longitudinal, oblique or transverse. There is no easy way to do this, but using both hands, predominantly the finger-tips, feel once on the left side of the abdomen, and then on the right side. Do not persist if you are unsure, but move on to identify the presenting part, as this may help.

*(Continued)*

## BOX 7.5 (*Continued*) ASSESSMENT AT STAGES OF PREGNANCY

- The presenting part is most frequently cephalic or breech. Other presentations are possible, including shoulder, arm, foot and cord, but these cannot be felt abdominally. Before doing this part of the examination, ask where the baby has been kicking: a baby that is breech kicks 'just where my bladder is', whereas if the baby is cephalic, the movements are felt at the level of the fundus on the side opposite to the baby's back. Put your hands on the abdomen above the symphysis pubis, one each side of the midline with the fingers together, pointing medially. To do this, turn your shoulders so that your back is towards the mother's face. A head shape is hard, whereas a bottom is soft!

- Listen to the fetal heart. You can use a Doppler fetal monitor to hear the heart from 11 weeks' gestation. Listen over the baby's anterior shoulder using gentle pressure. Always feel the mother's pulse at the same time as listening to the baby. This ensures that you have not picked up a maternal tachycardia, thinking that it was the baby. It is sensible to record the fetal heart rate, as abnormalities can be an indication of fetal compromise.

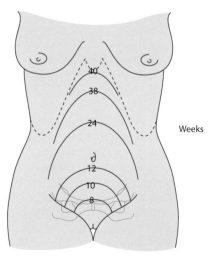

Weeks

Fig. 7.7 The uterus at different stages of pregnancy.

At the subsequent antenatal visits, examination of the mother is limited:

- Check the blood pressure with the woman in a semi-recumbent position. The diastolic pressure is measured at the point that the sounds disappear.
- Check for swelling of the fingers, and look for swelling in the lower limbs by gently pressing laterally on the tibia 8 cm above the medial malleolus for 5 seconds.
- Listen carefully to the mother's concerns and ask about symptoms of pain, tiredness, heartburn and alterations in fetal movement patterns. Mothers have a 'sixth sense', and it is a foolish obstetrician who ignores this.

## Therapeutic and technical skills

The technique for the urinary catheterisation of a female patient is shown in **Video 7.1** and collecting and testing urine in **Video 7.2**.

▶ VIDEO 7.1 Inserting a female catheter

https://www.crcpress.com/cw/kopelman

▶ VIDEO 7.2 Collecting and testing urine

https://www.crcpress.com/cw/kopelman

The following figures illustrate features of gynaecological disease: ectopic pregnancy (**Fig. 7.8**), ovarian carcinoma (**Fig. 7.9**), endometriosis (**Fig. 7.10**) and pre-eclampsia (**Fig. 7.11**).

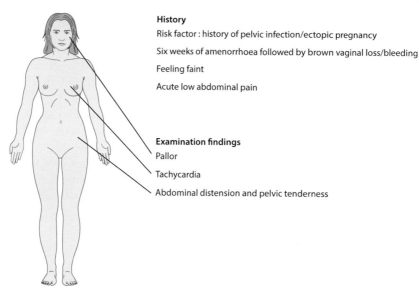

**History**

Risk factor : history of pelvic infection/ectopic pregnancy

Six weeks of amenorrhoea followed by brown vaginal loss/bleeding

Feeling faint

Acute low abdominal pain

**Examination findings**

Pallor

Tachycardia

Abdominal distension and pelvic tenderness

Fig. 7.8 Ectopic pregnancy.

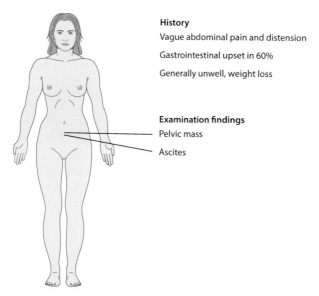

**History**

Vague abdominal pain and distension

Gastrointestinal upset in 60%

Generally unwell, weight loss

**Examination findings**

Pelvic mass

Ascites

Fig. 7.9 Ovarian carcinoma.

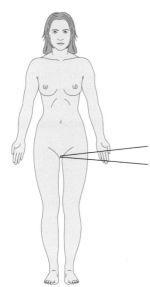

**History**

Heavy/painful periods

Pelvic pain for several days before period – onset often with ovulation

Pain with intercourse

**Examination findings**

Pelvic tenderness during vaginal examination

Nodules palpable on the uterosacral ligaments

Fig. 7.10 Endometriosis.

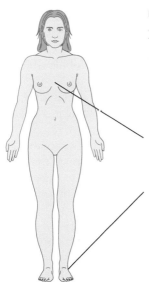

**History**

Any gestation in pregnancy, but most common in the last month and in the first week after delivery

Headache

Epigastric pain

**Examination findings**

Hypertension – blood pressure >140/90 mmHg

Proteinuria

Signs of cerebral irritation/hyper-reflexia (before eclamptic fit)

Swollen ankles – 6–8 cm above the medial malleolus

Fig. 7.11 Pre-eclampsia.

## THE BREASTS

Women usually consult doctors about their breasts because of discomfort, because they have found a lump or, more rarely, because of nipple discharge. Breast symptoms in men are much less common, but glandular development of the male breast forming a lump behind the areola (gynaecomastia) and, rarely, carcinoma of the male breast (less than 1% of all breast cancers) may occur.

Discomfort in the breasts is almost invariably benign, although breast carcinomas occasionally present with pain. Breast discomfort chiefly affects women of reproductive age and may be cyclical – occurring for a week or 10 days before the menstrual period – or non-cyclical. It may be associated with fibrocystic disease of the breast and is hormone dependent.

### Applied anatomy of the breasts and axillae

The breast is a highly developed sweat gland, which has acquired a specialised function. Although there are usually two breasts in humans, accessory breasts occasionally develop along the 'milk line', which extends from the axilla to the inner surfaces of the thigh. Occasionally, a breast fails to develop – a condition known as amazia.

The breast has a lobular structure, each glandular lobule draining via a main duct whose opening is on the nipple.

During reproductive life, the breast has a rubbery consistency, and nodules of glandular tissue may be felt within it. After the menopause, it becomes softer and more homogeneous.

Lymphatic drainage from the medial portion of the breast is to internal mammary nodes, which are inaccessible to clinical examination. The central and lateral portions of the breast drain to the axillary lymph nodes, which may be palpable if enlarged due to inflammatory reaction or malignant infiltration.

Involvement of supraclavicular lymph nodes in breast cancer is uncommon but, if it occurs, it does so via the internal mammary or axillary lymphatic channels (**Fig. 7.12**).

The axillary lymph nodes are said to constitute five named groups, but the number of nodes present and their distribution are

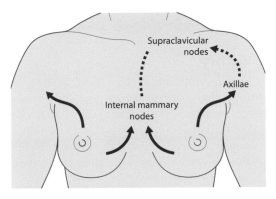

Fig. 7.12 Lymphatic drainage of the breast.

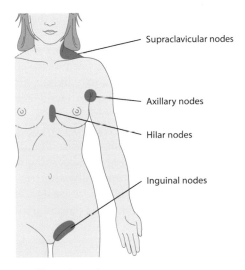

Fig. 7.13 Location of lymph nodes.

in fact highly variable. Examination of the axilla for nodes needs to be systematic, extending from the lower limit to the apex, and feeling anteriorly and posteriorly as well as medially (**Fig. 7.13**). In breast cancer, the lower axillary nodes are likely to become involved first.

## Assessment and diagnosis of breast disease

### Taking the history

Women with breast symptoms, even young women, always wonder whether they might have breast cancer, and some become extremely anxious as a result. Even though the vast majority do not have cancer, the anxiety – and also the embarrassment – associated with breast symptoms should be borne in mind when taking the history. Men with gynaecomastia are also likely to be anxious about their breast development.

### The presenting complaint

The presenting symptom – whether pain, lump or discharge – determines what questions are appropriate when taking the history, as does the patient's age. The patient sometimes has more than one of these symptoms.

**Breast pain (*Table 7.1*)** Severe breast pain of a few days' duration suggests infection (mastitis), which may progress to abscess formation. The patient may be breast-feeding or may have a history of previous similar episodes. Physical examination will reveal tenderness, induration, heat and redness of the overlying skin.

More persistent breast pain (mastalgia) may develop at any time during reproductive life, and may also remit. The duration of symptoms, their severity and whether they are becoming more or less troublesome should be determined – especially whether they are cyclical or persistent. Cyclical mastalgia is always benign, and non-cyclical mastalgia usually so. Is it certain that the pain is arising in the breast?

### Table 7.1 Causes of breast pain

- Infection
  - Mastitis
  - Breast abscess
- Hormonally-mediated pain
  - Mastalgia
  - Cyclic mastalgia
- Rarely
  - Fibroadenosis/cysts
  - Malignancy

Chest wall pain is sometimes confused with breast pain. Questions asked of the patient might include:

'Have you noticed anything that makes the pain more severe?'

'How disabling is the pain, and do analgesics ease it?'

'Did the pain first begin when you underwent any change in life-style, diet or medication?'

'Are you taking the oral contraceptive pill?'

Cyclical mastalgia may be associated with lumpiness of the breasts or with a dominant lump, which may be an area of fibroadenosis or a cyst. These findings become more common as the menopause approaches.

**Breast lumps** (*Table 7.2*) The differential diagnosis is usually between a fibroadenoma, fibroadenosis, a cyst and a carcinoma, but rarer conditions should be borne in mind. In cases of fat necrosis, there will be a clear history of a blow to the breast. Skin lesions may masquerade as breast lumps. Sarcomas, cold abscesses and other lesions are exceedingly rare. The time the lump has been present is a good starting point.

'Does the lump remain a constant size, or is it slowly enlarging?'

'Does it fluctuate in size with the menstrual cycle?' (in which case it is likely to be benign).

'Is it painful, tender or completely painless?'

'Have you had breast lumps before, and if so, were they biopsied and what were the findings?'

## Table 7.2  Causes of breast lumps

- Fibroadenoma (breast mouse) (see page 272)
- Fibroadenosis (background of nodularity)
- Cysts (can be aspirated)
- Carcinoma (poorly defined edge, merges into breast tissue)
- Fat necrosis (clear history of trauma)
- Sarcoma (rare)

## Table 7.3  Risk factors for breast cancer

- Early menarche (before 12 years of age)
- Late menopause
- Nulliparity
- Not having breast-fed
- Breast cancer in a first-degree relative
- A previous (ipsilateral or contralateral) breast cancer

At this stage, the patient should also be questioned relating to the risk factors for breast cancer (*Table 7.3*).

It is extremely unusual for patients with breast cancer to have symptoms of distant metastatic spread at presentation. Symptoms that might cause concern are a recent onset of localised bone pain or shortness of breath.

As the patient may require surgical treatment, suitability for anaesthesia and day-case surgery should be assessed.

Gynaecomastia in men is usually drug related (cimetidine, hormones and drugs affecting hormone metabolism). It is normal in boys in early puberty, and occasionally occurs in old age as testosterone levels fall. It may be the presenting feature of a feminising endocrine tumour, but this is very rare. The patient should be asked about drug and hormone treatment, and the genitalia should be examined.

**Nipple discharge** The discharge may be white, yellow, clear or bloody. Unless bloody, the discharge can be considered to be a glandular secretion; in other words, milk.

Galactorrhoea (abnormal secretion of milk) may persist for some months after the end of lactation, and the obstetric history should be obtained. Galactorrhoea as the presenting symptom of a prolactin-secreting pituitary adenoma is very rare, but it is prudent to ask about headaches and visual disturbance, and to check the visual fields. Galactorrhoea is usually mild, unexplained and self-limiting. If the patient also has a lump or mastalgia, questioning should be along the lines outlined above.

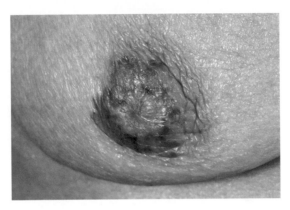

Fig. 7.14 Paget's disease of the nipple.

Bloody discharge usually indicates the presence of an intraductal papilloma, rather than a carcinoma. The patient should be asked if she is sure that the blood is coming from within the breast. Paget's disease of the nipple – a form of carcinoma – presents with a cracked or eroded nipple, which may bleed (**Fig. 7.14**).

## Examination of the patient

Male examiners should insist on a chaperone. The patient should be undressed to the waist. The examination must include both breasts, both axillae and the supraclavicular fossae.

Inspection of the breasts should begin with the patient sitting facing the examiner, with her arms at her sides. Look for any colour change in the skin, asymmetry of the breasts and unusual contour (although the normal right and left breasts are not always of equal size). Look in particular for any dimpling or tethering of the skin, and check that the nipples and areolae are healthy. Local oedema in the skin over a breast carcinoma may produce an appearance likened to the skin of an orange ('*peau d'orange*'), but this is an unusual finding.

Ask the patient to raise her arms above her head, and repeat the inspection. Tethering of the skin by an underlying carcinoma is likely to be made more obvious by this manoeuvre. **Figure 7.15** shows advanced carcinoma of the breast.

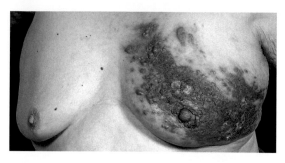

Fig. 7.15 Advanced fungating carcinoma of the breast.

## Care of the patient with breast symptoms

- Provide appropriate reassurance – most breast symptoms are not related to carcinomas.
- Aspirating the fluid in a breast cyst may make the cyst disappear – and reassures the patient that it is benign.
- Solid lumps need aspiration cytology.
- Patients aged over 35 years need mammography.
- Patients with malignant or equivocal lumps require surgical excision.

A carcinoma of the breast with nipple retraction is shown in **Fig. 7.16**.

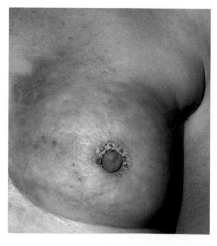

Fig. 7.16 Carcinoma of the breast with nipple retraction and *peau d'orange* skin changes.

## BOX 7.6 PALPATION OF THE BREASTS

Palpation of the breasts is best done with the patient lying on an examination couch. If the breasts are large, it is helpful to ask the patient to place her hand on the side being examined behind her head and to roll slightly to the opposite side, so as to flatten out the breast on the chest wall. It is usual to begin the examination on the asymptomatic side (if any) so as to gain an impression of the texture of the normal breast, which may range from quite smooth to decidedly nodular. Always examine both sides, and ask the patient to point out any areas of tenderness before beginning to palpate (**Fig. 7.17**).

The breasts are palpated by rolling the substance of the breast against the underlying chest wall with your flattened fingers. The entire breast should be examined systematically. A good method is to start below the areola and to work circumferentially, ensuring that all quadrants have been examined. Note that the axillary tail of the breast extends to the anterior border of the axilla and is a common site for breast pathology.

*(Continued)*

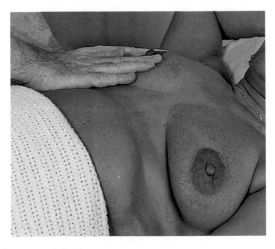

Fig. 7.17 Palpation of the breast.

## BOX 7.6 (*Continued*)  PALPATION OF THE BREASTS

Areas of tenderness are likely to be due to sepsis (look for heat, redness and induration) or, more commonly, fibroadenosis or cysts. Tenderness is not of undue concern unless there is an associated lump or there are signs of inflammation. Palpation may identify a discrete lump, less distinct lumpiness or an area of thickening. Thickening and lumpiness may be accepted as normal if they are present in both breasts and there are no other worrying features. A firm lump in a young patient that slips around under the examining fingers is likely to be a fibroadenoma (a 'breast mouse'). Cysts and carcinomas both give rise to firm or hard lumps that move with the breast, but not separately from it. Beware of an underlying rib giving undue prominence to an area of the breast, and simulating a lump.

Cysts may feel relatively smooth and carcinomas more diffuse, but it is difficult to distinguish the two clinically. It is not usually possible to demonstrate the sign of fluctuance in a breast cyst. Large carcinomas may be tethered to the skin or the chest wall. Check that the skin moves freely over the lump, and that the lump does not become fixed when the patient pushes against her hip (which tenses the pectoralis major muscle).

# Chapter 8
# The male reproductive system and hernias

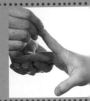

## THE MALE EXTERNAL GENITALIA

The male external genitalia comprise the penis, scrotum and scrotal contents. Media publicity has heightened awareness among young men of the potentially sinister significance of testicular swellings. Most swellings within the scrotum can be convincingly shown to be benign by clinical examination alone, but special investigations are sometimes necessary. The most common penile condition is phimosis (narrowing of the prepucial orifice), which may be caused by, and predispose to, infection, and may cause pain on erection and difficulty with micturition. A wide range of skin disorders may affect the penis, including squamous carcinoma (see below).

### BOX 8.1 CONDITIONS AFFECTING THE MALE GENITALIA

**Painless scrotal swellings**
- Hydrocoele
- Epididymal cyst
- Inguinoscrotal hernias
- Lesions of the scrotal skin
- Idiopathic scrotal oedema (young boys)
- Testicular tumours

*(Continued)*

## BOX 8.1 (*Continued*) CONDITIONS AFFECTING THE MALE GENITALIA

**Scrotal pain**
- Testicular torsion
- Torsion of a testicular appendage
- Epididymitis (localised or generalised)
- Orchitis, epididymo-orchitis
- Trauma

**Prepucial lesions**
- Phimosis ± balanitis xerotica obliterans
- Prepucial adhesion (normal up to 9 years of age)
- Paraphimosis
- Balanitis
- Viral warts, herpes, chancre
- Other skin lesions
- Squamous carcinoma

**Other penile conditions**
- Hypospadias (minor or major)
- Peyronie's disease
- Urethral discharge (gonorrhoea, non-specific urethritis)

## Applied anatomy and physiology

The **penis** comprises the paired corpora cavernosa and the corpus spongiosum, which surrounds the urethra and is expanded distally as the glans. Along the shaft of the penis, these structures are contained within a fibrous sheath and covered by freely mobile and very elastic skin, which is prolonged distally as the prepuce or foreskin. The corpora are attached proximally to the inferior pubic rami (**Fig. 8.1**).

The **testes** descend from the abdomen through the inguinal canal to reach the scrotum by approximately 38 weeks' gestation. The vas deferens and testicular vessels thus run through the inguinal canal within the spermatic cord, which takes a covering from each of the layers through which the testicle has passed, namely the transversalis fascia (internal spermatic fascia), the conjoined tendon (cremasteric fascia) and the external oblique aponeurosis (external spermatic fascia).

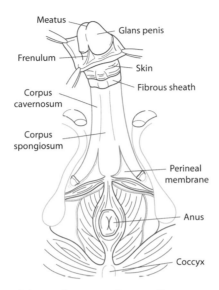

Fig. 8.1 Anatomy of the male external genitalia.

The **cremasteric fascia** is muscular, and contraction of this muscle may cause the testicles to retract into the groins, especially in children. This may lead to a mistaken diagnosis of undescended testicle. So long as the testes can be manipulated to the bottom of the scrotum, they will come to lie there permanently after puberty. During descent, the testicle draws with it a tube of peritoneum, the processus vaginalis, which usually closes during the first 1–2 years of life, except for the portion that covers the testicle itself. Here, it persists as a serous cavity surrounding three-quarters of the testicle (excepting the part which is in contact with the epididymis), known as the tunica vaginalis.

The **epididymis** is applied to the whole of the posterior aspect of the testicle, and is a specialised part of the collecting apparatus, where spermatozoa are matured and stored before travelling up the vas deferens to the seminal vesicles. The epididymis is not usually enclosed within the tunica vaginalis, its posterior surface adhering to the back of the scrotum. Occasionally, the epididymis is enclosed within the tunica vaginalis. This 'bell-clapper deformity' predisposes to the testicle twisting on its vascular pedicle, cutting off the testicular blood supply (torsion of the testicle).

The **appendix testis**, or hydatid of Morgagni, is probably an embryological remnant of the müllerian duct that gives rise to the fallopian tube in the female. It is a small pedunculated structure that is attached to the upper pole of the testis immediately in front of the epididymis. It may undergo torsion, giving rise to acute scrotal pain that may simulate torsion of the testicle itself.

## Assessment and diagnosis

### Taking the history

Patients often feel embarrassed about problems with their genitalia. Thus, questions should be asked sensitively.

#### The presenting complaint

**Painless swellings** Painless scrotal swellings in infants may be hernias or hydrocoeles. Hydrocoeles occur when partial closure of the processus vaginalis leads to its becoming valvular, so that peritoneal fluid can track down to surround the testicle, but cannot readily return to the abdomen. The swelling may vary in degree, and may be less marked after a night in bed. Infantile hydrocoele can appear at any time between birth and 18 months of age, and commonly resolves spontaneously before the age of 2 years, as closure of the processus vaginalis progresses to completion. If it persists beyond this age, surgical ligation of the processus is indicated.

The parents of a child with an inguinal hernia will report seeing a lump in the groin (occasionally both groins) that comes and goes and that may extend to the scrotum. The lump does not cause pain, but is more likely to appear when the child is distressed, as crying raises intra-abdominal pressure. It is often impossible to make the hernia appear in the clinic, but the condition may be confidently diagnosed on the basis of the history alone. Inguinal hernia is more common in boys than girls. Femoral hernia is rare in children (less than 1% of all hernias in children).

Adult hydrocoeles and epididymal cysts develop over months to years and present as painless scrotal swellings. The patient is concerned either that the swelling may be sinister or by the inconvenience it causes. There may be a history of previous ipsilateral groin surgery, but there are usually no predisposing factors. Unlike inguinal hernias, hydrocoeles and epididymal cysts do not change in size from day to day.

Patients with a varicocoele (**Fig. 8.2**) may complain of a swelling in the upper part of the scrotum (on the left side in 95% of cases). This may be associated with mild aching, although patients are often asymptomatic. Varicocoele is of concern chiefly because it may be associated with reduced fertility.

A lump in the testicle itself is likely to be malignant, usually a non-seminomatous germ cell tumour (in the past often referred to as a teratoma) or a seminoma (**Fig. 8.3**). Unlike most solid malignancies,

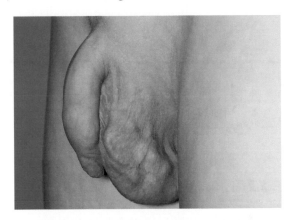

Fig. 8.2 Varicocoele.

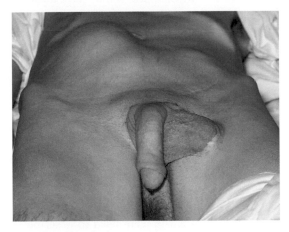

Fig. 8.3 Lump in the testicle. The most likely diagnosis is malignancy.

testicular tumours occur in the young, non-seminomatous germ cell tumour having its peak incidence between the ages of 20 and 30 years, and seminoma a decade later (with a second peak in the 60s and 70s). There is usually no associated pain, although there may be mild aching. A history of trauma to the scrotum is not reassuring, as this may occasionally draw attention to a pre-existing lump. It is unusual for there to be symptoms of disseminated malignancy at presentation.

**Scrotal pain** Testicular pain in the absence of any discernible physical abnormality is common, has a wide differential diagnosis, is almost invariably benign and often defies diagnosis (non-specific testicular pain). Torsion of a testicle gives rise to severe unilateral pain that begins suddenly and usually leads the patient to seek medical attention within hours. There may be a history of similar, milder episodes that have resolved spontaneously. Torsion affects almost exclusively teenage boys. It is a clinical diagnosis: imaging is unhelpful and merely delays emergency surgery. Unilateral scrotal pain may also be due to torsion of a testicular appendage or to trauma, although traumatic pain resolves quickly in all but the most severe cases.

In older men, persistent testicular pain is usually due to epididymo-orchitis, with associated swelling, tenderness and possibly fever. There may have been recent urinary frequency and dysuria, suggestive of urinary tract infection, and the patient may have more long-standing symptoms of frequency, nocturia, poor stream and terminal dribbling, suggestive of bladder outflow obstruction.

**Prepucial lesions** It is not abnormal for the foreskin to be unretractable until early adolescence. Before the early teens, non-retractability, ballooning on micturition and mild intermittent soreness around the prepucial opening are not indications for circumcision, which should only be recommended if there is a clear history of infection with purulent discharge from beneath the foreskin, combined with scarring (fibrous phimosis) or evidence of balanitis xerotica obliterans (lichen sclerosis of the foreskin). In adults, inability to retract the foreskin is abnormal, leads to problems with hygiene, commonly interferes with sexual activity and is an indication for circumcision.

Paraphimosis (**Fig. 8.4**) is the term used to describe gross oedema developing distal to a foreskin that has been left retracted. It is painful,

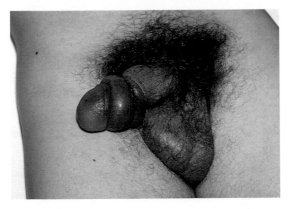

Fig. 8.4 Paraphimosis. Note the retracted foreskin and swollen glans.

as well as embarrassing, and may progress to ulceration. If the foreskin cannot be reduced after milking the oedema fluid proximally, emergency circumcision may be unavoidable.

All common skin lesions may occur on the penis. In cases of warts or possible syphilitic chancre, a sexual history should be taken. Carcinoma of the penis usually originates in the sulcus between the glans and the foreskin. It is rare in developed countries and in circumcised men. It may present as a lump or as bloody or offensive discharge from beneath the foreskin. The foreskin is commonly unretractable, but this is more likely to be a cause than a complication of the condition.

**Other penile lesions** Enquiry about penile lesions needs to be done in a sensitive manner, as the patient is often very embarrassed.

**Hypospadias** is a congenital anomaly in which the urethra opens more proximally than normal. Minor degrees of hypospadias may cause no problems or may be associated with spraying of urine. Openings on the shaft of the penis, or even on the scrotum, cause serious difficulties with micturition and sexual function. There is associated chordee (curvature of the penis). Patients with hypospadias commonly have an abnormal 'dorsal' foreskin, but should never be circumcised as the foreskin may be required for use in reconstructive surgery.

**Peyronie's disease** is a localised fibromatosis affecting the shaft of the penis. It leads to curvature of the penis on erection, and may therefore cause sexual difficulty. There is an association with Dupuytren's contracture, but no causal factors are known.

**Urethral discharge** is usually associated with **dysuria** and is usually due to chlamydial infection or gonorrhoea. A sexual history should be obtained, and the patient should be referred to a clinic for sexually transmitted diseases.

## Examination of the patient

The patient should be examined supine, with the abdomen and genitalia exposed.

### Inspection

This should take in the abdomen (masses or a distended bladder) and the groins (hernias and lymph nodes), as well as the penis and scrotum. The condition of which the patient complains will often be immediately recognised. In adults and adolescents, the foreskin should be retracted to check that there is no phimosis and no underlying pathology. If there is a phimosis preventing retraction, circumcision is warranted.

### Palpation

Palpation of the penis may identify areas of fibrosis in the shaft in Peyronie's disease, but is of little value in most conditions.

Palpation of the scrotal contents aims to identify the normal structures and the relationship of any abnormality to these. Using both hands, each testicle is picked up in turn. The testicle itself is sensitive and requires gentle handling. It should have a uniform, rubbery consistency with no discrete lumps or areas of induration that might suggest a tumour. Diffuse enlargement and extreme tenderness of the testicle in an older man suggest orchitis, while a testicle that is very tender, drawn up towards the neck of the scrotum and lying transversely in an adolescent is likely to be torted.

The epididymis should be palpable behind the testicle. It is usually soft, but may be swollen, indurated and tender in epididymitis.

These changes may be localised if mild. A tender nodule at the upper pole of the epididymis is likely to be a twisted testicular appendage.

In patients with hydrocoele, fluid within the tunica vaginalis may make it impossible to feel the testicle itself. A normal epididymis should nonetheless be palpable posteriorly. Epididymal cysts necessarily arise behind the testicle, and may make it difficult to feel the rest of the epididymis, but a normal testicle should be palpable anteriorly. Both conditions may initially be confused with an inguinoscrotal hernia, but may be differentiated from this by palpation of the spermatic cord. It is impossible to 'get above' the swelling produced by an inguinoscrotal hernia, whereas a normal spermatic cord can always be felt between finger and thumb above hydrocoeles and epididymal cysts.

In addition to palpation, scrotal swellings should be examined by transillumination (**Fig. 8.5**) using a pen light in a darkened room. Both hydrocoeles and epididymal cysts light up brilliantly when the light is placed behind them. This test proves that the swellings are fluid filled, and enables them to be differentiated from the adjacent normal testicle. It also differentiates them from hernias (although this should already

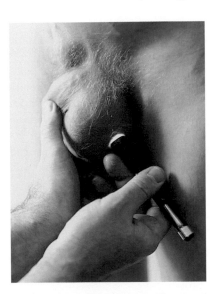

Fig. 8.5 Examining a scrotal swelling by transillumination.

have been achieved by palpation), except in infants, whose hernias may transilluminate because of their relatively small volume.

In cases of suspected testicular torsion, it may be useful to re-examine the patient when he is standing. This will not only confirm that the affected testicle is drawn up, but may also show that the contralateral one exhibits a transverse lie, suggesting a bell-clapper deformity predisposing to torsion.

The inguinal lymph nodes should always be palpated as part of the examination of the male genitalia. It is usual for one of two 'shotty' lymph nodes to be palpable in each groin, but more generalised enlargement may occur in inflammatory conditions and in the rare penile carcinoma. Testicular tumours metastasise to the aorto-iliac nodes, not the groins, and the abdomen should be palpated if a testicular tumour is suspected. Examination of the prostate per rectum is indicated if the patient has symptoms of bladder outlet obstruction.

## Therapeutic and interventional skills

### Male bladder catheterisation

Bladder catheterisation may be required for monitoring of fluid balance or for relief of acute retention of urine. The typical patient with retention is an elderly man who may have a history of urinary frequency, hesitancy and a poor stream. Patients requiring an emergency catheterisation are likely to be in acute discomfort, so you need to remember this and approach them with compassion.

Always introduce yourself and explain what you are going to do and why. Outline how you will perform the procedure, and ask if the patient has any questions. Make sure that you have the patient's verbal consent.

Before beginning any procedure, ensure that all the necessary equipment is there, and check the trolley.

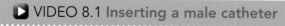

▶ VIDEO 8.1 Inserting a male catheter

https://www.crcpress.com/cw/kopelman

**Always remember** to *replace the foreskin* in its normal, unretracted position in an uncircumcised patient. Failure to do so will result in the development of a painful paraphimosis.

## HERNIAS (MALES AND FEMALES)

A hernia is a defect in the wall of a body cavity through which the contents of the cavity may protrude. Although the protrusion is usually towards the exterior, it may also occur from one body cavity to another (diaphragmatic hernia and hiatus hernia) and, occasionally, between different compartments within the same major cavity ('internal hernia', resulting from intra-abdominal adhesions or a defect in a mesentery).

External hernias usually occur at sites of intrinsic weakness of the body wall, principally the inguinal and femoral canals and the umbilicus, but their onset results, to a greater or lesser degree, in degeneration of the surrounding connective tissues. The weakness is occasionally due to surgery (incisional hernia). In adults, hernias are more likely to develop if the intra-abdominal pressure is chronically high. This may be the result of obesity. Chronic cough, constipation and chronic retention of urine have also been held to be contributory causes.

Hernias may be painless, but many cause a variable degree of discomfort and disability. Only a small minority cause more serious complications, such as obstruction or strangulation of intestine. A hernia whose contents cannot be pushed back into the abdomen is termed 'irreducible'. Intestine trapped within a hernia may become compressed and obstructed at the neck of the hernia, leading to the clinical picture of intestinal obstruction (colicky abdominal pain, abdominal distension, vomiting and absolute constipation). Obstructed bowel tends to become oedematous. This may result in a rise in the pressure within the hernia sufficient to cut off the blood supply and bring about infarction of the trapped bowel ('strangulation'). Hernias generally get larger, and the symptoms worsen, with the passage of time. For this reason, and also to eliminate the small risk of intestinal obstruction or strangulation, hernias should generally be repaired electively unless the patient is very frail or has severe co-morbidities.

## Types of abdominal wall hernia

### Applied anatomy

**Diaphragmatic hernia** may be a congenital anomaly, presenting in the neonatal period with respiratory distress, or may result from blunt trauma to the trunk later in life.

**Hiatus hernia**, which allows the gastro-oesophageal junction to herniate into the chest, is of concern chiefly because of the reflux oesophagitis that may complicate it. These conditions are not discussed further.

**Inguinal hernia** This is the most common type of hernia. Two variations occur, which are anatomically distinct but difficult to distinguish clinically. These are known as 'direct' and 'indirect' inguinal hernias.

Failure of the processus vaginalis to close leaves an incipient indirect inguinal hernia sac, which may become evident in infancy, or may remain collapsed until weakening and stretching of connective tissues in the groin in later life allows it to dilate.

- An **indirect inguinal** hernia follows the line of descent of the testicle, passing through the internal (deep) inguinal ring, along the inguinal canal, through the external ring and, in some cases, reaching the scrotum (**Fig. 8.6**).
- A **direct inguinal** hernia, by contrast, results from an acquired weakness of the posterior wall of the inguinal canal. It therefore arises medial to the internal inguinal ring, usually remains confined within the canal and never extends to the scrotum. Direct hernias often have wide necks and are much less likely to trap, obstruct or strangulate intestine than indirect hernias, whose necks are often narrow. Unfortunately, it is impossible reliably to distinguish a direct hernia from a small indirect hernia clinically.

**Femoral hernias** These pass through the femoral canal medial to the femoral vessels (**Fig. 8.7**). The femoral canal has tough, unyielding margins around most of its circumference (the inguinal ligament, periosteum overlying the superior pubic ramus). Femoral hernias thus have tight necks, and the risk of strangulation of small bowel entering them is relatively high.

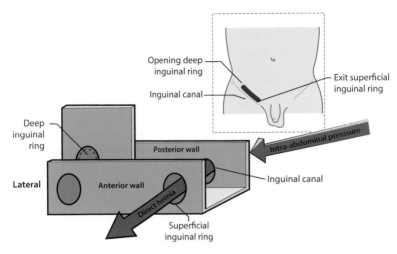

Fig. 8.6 The inguinal canal (posterior wall).

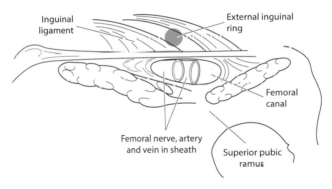

Fig. 8.7 The femoral canal.

### Umbilical/para-umbilical, epigastric and other ventral hernias

- An **umbilical hernia** is a congenital abnormality resulting from failure of the umbilicus to close in early life. Umbilical hernias in children do not cause pain and never strangulate; most close spontaneously by the age of 3–6 years. The main cause for concern is parental anxiety over the peculiar appearance and surgical closure if the hernia persists beyond the age of 3 may be justified for this reason.

Umbilical hernias in adults rarely cause complications but may be uncomfortable and should be repaired if symptomatic.

- **Para-umbilical hernias** are congenital or acquired defects immediately superior to the umbilicus that are most often seen in obese adults. These hernias are liable to enlarge with the passage of time and may cause complications. Elective repair should be undertaken unless the patient is very unfit.

- An **epigastric hernia** may present in childhood as a small tender lump in the midline. Occasionally, the hernia cannot be felt at all, and the child complains only of epigastric pain, which is commonly made worse by exercise. Epigastric hernias are small congenital defects in the linea alba through which preperitoneal fat protrudes. Surgical repair is justified by the symptoms.

- Adults may also develop **midline (ventral) abdominal hernias**, although the bulge that the patient has noticed is often due to separation of the rectus abdominis muscles and attenuation of the linea alba ('divarication of the recti'). A midline hernia with a distinct neck that has fibrous margins should be repaired, as these hernias tend to enlarge, may become massive and may strangulate the intestine. Divarication of the recti is a harmless condition, however, and the results of surgical treatment are often poor.

- **Incisional hernias** are most common following long midline abdominal incisions, although they may occur at other sites. Postoperative wound infection and obesity are the main predisposing causes (along with poor surgical technique). Herniation is due to separation or attenuation of the musculofascial layer at the site of the previous incision. Incisional hernias tend to enlarge, sometimes to massive proportions, and may strangulate. Early surgical repair should therefore be undertaken.

**Rare types of abdominal wall hernia (Fig. 8.8)** include:

- Obturator hernia – through the obturator foramen.
- Spigelian hernia – through the lower part of the sheath of the rectus abdominis muscle (which is deficient posteriorly).
- Lumbar hernia – through the inferior lumbar triangle.
- Gluteal hernia – through the greater sciatic notch.

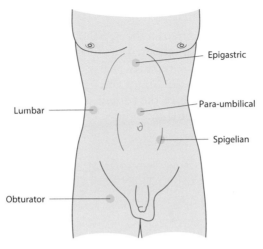

Fig. 8.8 Rare abdominal wall hernias.

## Assessment and diagnosis of groin hernias

### Taking the history

#### Presenting complaint

A patient with a groin hernia usually reports a lump or bulge in the groin that appears or enlarges on standing or coughing and disappears on lying. There may be associated discomfort, especially on exertion. The patient occasionally reports hearing gurgling noises (borborygmi) coming from the bulge.

#### Past medical history

As the patient may require surgical treatment, enquiry should be made about concurrent and previous illnesses and current drug treatment, all of which affect perioperative risk and anaesthetic technique. Some patients will have recurrent hernias, having undergone a previous repair at the same site. This will affect the choice of surgical technique, favouring laparoscopic over open surgery.

## Personal and social history

Occupation should be enquired about, although patients should be able to return to all forms of employment following groin hernia repair. Most groin hernias can be repaired as day cases, but the availability of a relative or friend who can escort the patient home, and accommodation that does not require the patient to climb numerous flights of stairs, is a prerequisite for this.

---

**BOX 8.2 EXAMINATION FOR GROIN HERNIAS**

The cardiovascular and respiratory systems should be examined to detect conditions that may affect suitability for anaesthesia.

Most patients with groin hernias are ambulant and are assessed in GPs' surgeries or hospital outpatient clinics. This usually makes it most convenient to start the examination with the patient standing, and a hernia is more likely to be visible when the patient is upright. The patient's abdomen and groins need to be exposed but, at this stage, the genitalia do not.

- Look at the site of the bulge that the patient indicates and compare it with the same site on the opposite side. Is a bulge visible? In acute cases, look for any inflammation of the overlying skin that would suggest the presence of strangulated bowel within.
- Palpate the site gently to assess the size of the bulge and any tenderness. Gently try to push the bulge back into the abdominal cavity (i.e. test for reducibility). Apply gentle pressure to the bulge and ask the patient to cough. In patients with hernias, an expansile cough impulse will generally be felt. Beware, however, only an *expansile* impulse is of significance. A *non-expansile* impulse is commonly felt in the region of the inguinal canal on coughing in healthy individuals.

---

*(Continued)*

## BOX 8.2 (*Continued*) EXAMINATION FOR GROIN HERNIAS

- Examine the asymptomatic groin similarly to check that there is not a small, asymptomatic hernia on that side.
- It is not possible to determine reliably whether a groin hernia is inguinal or femoral with the patient standing. After examining the patient standing, ask them to lie on the examination couch. Locate the pubic tubercle and determine the relationship of the hernia to this. Femoral hernias emerge below the inguinal ligament, and therefore below and lateral to the pubic tubercle. Inguinal hernias originate in the inguinal canal, above the inguinal ligament and pubic tubercle, and, if they extend to or beyond the neck of the scrotum, they pass above and then medial to the tubercle. Note that the inguinal ligament, which runs from the anterior superior iliac spine to the pubic tubercle, lies approximately 3 cm above the groin crease. Femoral hernias therefore present above the groin crease, although below the inguinal ligament.

Despite statements to the contrary, it is not possible to reliably distinguish a direct from an indirect inguinal hernia by clinical examination, unless the hernia extends to the scrotum (when it must be indirect). This does not matter as the precise anatomy can be determined intraoperatively.

In men, examination of a groin hernia finishes with an examination of the external genitalia.

Occasionally in adults – and often in children – it may not be possible to demonstrate the hernia in the clinic, however much the patient coughs and strains. A history of a lump in the groin that appears on standing and straining and disappears on lying is virtually diagnostic of a hernia. The only other condition that may give rise to a similar history is a saphena varix. A typical history combined with exclusion of a saphena varix therefore justifies surgical treatment, especially in children. Ultrasound scanning is of limited value in the diagnosis of groin hernias as it has a substantial false-positive rate.

## Assessment and diagnosis of other abdominal hernias (**Fig. 8.9**)

Once again, the cardiovascular and respiratory systems should be examined. Begin the examination with the patient standing.

- Inspect and palpate the site indicated by the patient to determine the site and size of the bulge. Test for reducibility and a cough impulse.
- Ask the patient to lie on the examination couch. Look to see whether the hernia is apparent with the patient supine and inspect for surgical scars, which may suggest an underlying incisional hernia. If the hernia is not apparent, ask the patient to raise their head and shoulders off the pillow. This tenses the muscles, raises the intra-abdominal pressure and usually makes the hernia protrude.
- Palpate the hernia gently to detect tenderness, and then try gently to reduce it. Feel for the fibrous margins of the defect, which may barely admit a fingertip in an infantile umbilical hernia, but may be very wide in incisional and some other ventral hernias. A general abdominal examination should then be completed.

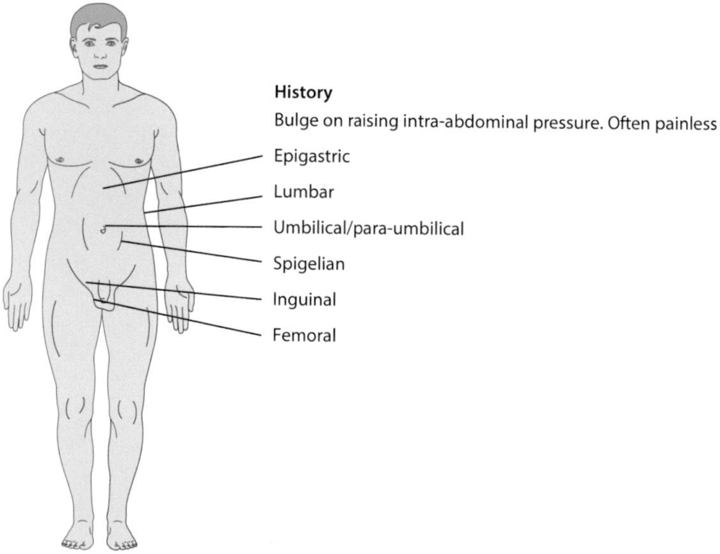

**History**

Bulge on raising intra-abdominal pressure. Often painless

Epigastric

Lumbar

Umbilical/para-umbilical

Spigelian

Inguinal

Femoral

Fig. 8.9 Assessment of external abdominal hernias.

## Illustrated physical signs

The two photographs illustrate hernial defects: large **bilateral inguinal hernias (Fig. 8.10)** and an **incisional hernia (Fig. 8.11)**.

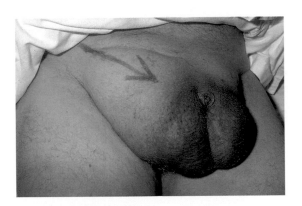

Fig. 8.10 Bilateral inguinal hernias.

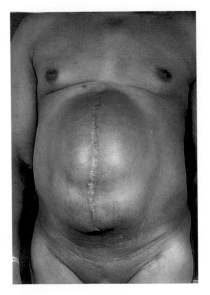

Fig. 8.11 Incisional hernia.

## Care of the patient with a hernia

- Adult patients, other than the very frail and those with severe co-morbidities, should generally be advised to undergo repair of ventral or groin hernias, except perhaps a wide-necked direct inguinal hernia.
- Hernias may be repaired by open surgery or laparoscopically, the choice depending on the preference of the surgeon and the patient.
- Most uncomplicated hernias can be repaired as day cases.
- A truss may relieve pain but may not prevent strangulation.
- A hernia causing intestinal obstruction or strangulation is a surgical emergency.

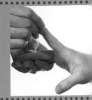

Disorders of endocrine function, which are not uncommon in clinical practice, tend to present with non-specific symptoms. As a consequence, the unwary clinician may overlook the possibility that either a deficiency (hypo-function) or excess (hyper-function) of a particular hormone or hormones may be the underlying problem. This emphasises the importance of always taking a comprehensive history and applying the clues provided when performing the general examination. Remember that hormonal deficiency may affect the function of several different organs.

## Applied anatomy and physiology of the endocrine system

The hypothalamus contains many vital centres for functions such as appetite, thirst, thermal regulation and sleep/waking. It also plays a role in circadian rhythm, the menstrual cycle, stress and mood. Releasing factors produced in the hypothalamus reach the pituitary via the portal system and run down the pituitary stalk. These releasing factors stimulate or inhibit the production of hormones by the anterior pituitary, which, in turn, stimulates or inhibits the peripheral glands or tissues.

The posterior pituitary acts as a storage organ for antidiuretic hormone (arginine-vasopressin) and oxytocin, which are synthesised in the supraoptic and paraventricular nuclei in the anterior hypothalamus and pass to the posterior pituitary via an axon within the pituitary stalk. Endocrine abnormalities result from either a primary or secondary abnormality, causing either excess or deficiency of pituitary hormone. Examples of the former are hyper- and hypothyroidism. An example of the latter is the production of excessive adrenocorticotropic hormone (ACTH) in Cushing's (pituitary-dependent) disease. Partial degrees of excess or deficiency may be difficult to detect unless a clinician is wary in relation to the likely presenting features. In contrast, absolute deficiency or marked excess usually presents with characteristics symptoms and signs.

## The thyroid gland

Disease of the thyroid gland most commonly presents with swelling, which may affect the whole gland (a goitre), or may be localised within it. Less often, the patient may present with signs of over- or under-secretion of thyroid hormones (with or without swelling). Pain arising in the thyroid gland is rare.

Clinical assessment of thyroid disease involves an assessment of the gland itself, related structures in the neck and 'thyroid status' (the quantity of hormone being produced). It is easy to neglect one or more of these aspects, and a methodical and practised approach is required in order to ensure that the assessment is thorough.

### Applied anatomy and physiology of the thyroid

The thyroid gland consists of two lobes, joined by the isthmus just below the cricoid cartilage. The gland develops as a downgrowth (the thyroglossal duct) from the primitive pharynx.

This section will focus on the clinical pointers and indicate the possibility of an underlying endocrine abnormality. Readers should refer to a specific textbook for more detailed information about the causes of the various hormonal deficiencies and excesses.

## Assessment and diagnosis of endocrine disease

A high index of suspicion is necessary for the diagnosis of endocrine disease, as a hormonal problem may affect any of the body systems.

## Taking the history

Areas of general health must be covered in the history. Endocrine dysfunction often manifests with non-specific symptoms that will be missed unless a full review of systems is completed. Particular enquiries that should be made are outlined in the following section.

### The presenting complaint

**Body weight** Hypothyroidism is commonly associated with weight gain; Cushing's syndrome may be accompanied by weight gain, particularly in the upper body ('truncal obesity'). Hypoadrenalism and hyperthyroidism are associated with weight loss. The patient might be asked:

'How has your weight been recently?'

**Appetite** An increase in appetite is a frequent association with hyperthyroidism and, less commonly, with Cushing's syndrome. In hyperthyroidism, the increased appetite is frequently associated with weight loss. By contrast, hypoadrenalism frequently presents with anorexia and malaise.

**Fatigue** Many patients with diabetes mellitus confess to a having had a feeling of profound fatigue for many months before the diagnosis, as a result of unsuspected hyperglycaemia. Similarly, fatigue may be a feature of Cushing's syndrome, hypoadrenalism, hypothyroidism or hypercalcaemia.

**Thirst** Increased thirst is a common presenting feature of diabetes mellitus, but it may also be seen in hypercalcaemia and diabetes insipidus. In the latter condition, the thirst is so severe that patients frequently report that they drink a jug of water during the night.

**Frequency of micturition** Diabetes mellitus and diabetes insipidus are both accompanied by an increased frequency of urination and the passage of moderate to large volumes of urine. Both conditions are associated with both daytime and nocturnal frequency, although patients with diabetes insipidus tend to pass greater volumes of pale (diluted) urine. Prostatism is usually differentiated by its association with a complaint of urinary hesitancy and the passage of small volumes of urine. Polyuria is also seen in patients who are hypercalcaemic. Remember that patients with Cushing's syndrome may also develop diabetes mellitus.

**Disturbances of bowel function** Patients with hypothyroidism may complain of constipation, while diarrhoea may result in the referral of a hyperthyroid patient to a gastroenterologist. A patient with an elevated plasma calcium level may present with abdominal pain, either as a consequence of constipation or due to pancreatitis (a sequela to hypercalcaemia).

**Sexual function** An early symptom that is suggestive of pituitary dysfunction in women is the development of altered menstrual function and, ultimately, amenorrhoea. A delay in menarche (onset of periods) may be the presenting complaint in a girl who is prepubertal. In men, hypogonadism presents with loss of sexual drive or libido and failure to achieve or sustain an erection.

**Headache** Although this is a non-specific symptom and one which accompanies many disease processes, it should be regarded with seriousness in a patient who appears to have an endocrine dysfunction. An expanding pituitary tumour or hypothalamic mass may lead to an endocrine dysfunction and/or may cause pressure symptoms that present as a headache.

**Alteration in growth** Hypopituitarism and growth hormone deficiency in children may present with short stature. In contrast, excess of growth hormone causes gigantism in children and acromegaly in adults (as it occurs after fusion of the epiphyses). The latter condition may lead to patients complaining of an increase in hand size or, more commonly, shoe size.

**Neck lump** Patients with thyroid disease may present with a swelling in the neck, although this is usually painless.

# Examination of the patient

## Specific points on examination

An examination of the endocrine system is performed as part of a general physical examination, at which time a large number of endocrine signs can be noticed. The thyroid gland, however, is examined separately.

### General observations

Some features of thyroid disease may be immediately detectable. These include the eye signs of Graves' disease, the goitre itself and hoarseness. This should not dissuade the examiner from carrying out a full and systematic assessment. The examination is best approached in two stages as described below.

### The gland and its surroundings

The neck should be inspected from the front. If a swelling is visible and lies in the region of the thyroid gland, ask the patient to swallow. (It is traditional, not always essential, to offer a glass of water.) A lump in the thyroid will move up on swallowing. Metastases to cervical lymph nodes may result in visible lumps lateral to the thyroid gland itself.

The gland is best palpated with the patient sitting and the examiner standing behind (**Fig. 9.1**). The left hand can be used to retract the left sternomastoid muscle laterally, enabling the right hand to explore the left lobe. The roles of the two hands are reversed to examine the right lobe. The aim is to define the overall size and consistency of the swelling,

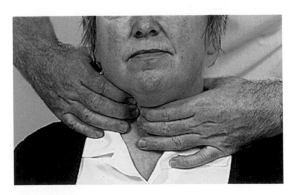

Fig. 9.1 Palpation of the thyroid.

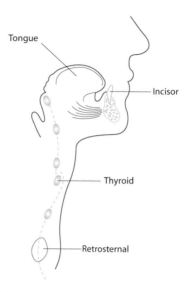

Fig. 9.2 Descent of the thyroid.

and of the normal part of the gland if any. Can you 'get below' the gland, or does it appear to extend retrosternally (**Fig. 9.2**)?

Diffuse nodular swelling suggests a multinodular goitre. A localised swelling may be a prominent nodule in a multinodular goitre, but it also raises the possibility of a cyst, adenoma or malignant tumour. The fact that the swelling arises in the gland may be confirmed by asking the patient to swallow once again.

It is usual to palpate the regional lymph nodes and the trachea at this stage. The deep cervical lymph nodes lie adjacent to the carotid sheath, behind the anterior border of the sternomastoid muscle.

Supraclavicular lymph nodes and those in the posterior triangle of the neck (behind the sternomastoid muscle) should also be palpated. It is easiest to palpate the trachea when standing in front of the patient (see Chapter 3). Deviation to one side or other suggests a large retrosternal extension of the goitre. Percussion over the sternum may be performed, but it is not a reliable way of detecting retrosternal extension. Auscultation of the gland may reveal a bruit in patients with Graves' disease, but beware of transmitted cardiac murmurs or carotid bruits.

## Other endocrine examinations

The common symptoms and signs associated with alterations in hormonal function are shown on in **Box 9.1**. These are intended as a guide and not as a comprehensive account of endocrinology.

### BOX 9.1  HORMONAL DYSFUNCTION SYMPTOMS AND SIGNS

| Hormonal abnormality | Symptoms | Specific physical signs |
|---|---|---|
| *Gonadotropin deficiency* | | |
| Male | Fatigue, muscle weakness, loss of libido/sex drive; failure to sustain an erection | Delayed puberty. In adult: loss of facial, body and pubertal hair; small and soft testes |
| Female | Irregular menses, amenorrhoea | Delayed menarche. In adult: often no specific signs |
| *Growth hormone deficiency* | | |
| Children | Delayed growth | Short stature with obesity |
| Adults | Symptoms of associated pituitary hormone deficiencies | Obesity |
| *Growth hormone excess* | | |
| Pre-fusion of the epiphysis: gigantism | Tallness with rapid increase in height | Excessive height |

*(Continued)*

### BOX 9.1 (*Continued*) HORMONAL DYSFUNCTION SYMPTOMS AND SIGNS

| Hormonal abnormality | Symptoms | Specific physical signs |
|---|---|---|
| *Growth hormone excess (continued)* | | |
| Post-fusion: acromegaly | Change in appearance, increase in size of hands and feet, headaches, weight gain. Excessive perspiration, joint pains | Characteristic acromegalic facies, large tongue, prominent supraorbital ridge, broad (wide) nose, prognathism of lower jaw, thick greasy skin, spade-like hands, carpal tunnel syndrome |
| *Thyroid hormone* | | |
| Thyroid deficiency (hypothyroidism) | Tiredness, malaise, weight gain, cold intolerance, change in appearance, dry skin, constipation | Mental slowness, dry thin hair, hypothermia, puffy eyes, loss of outer third of eyebrows, deep voice, obesity, slow relaxing reflexes; in primary thyroid failure, goitre |
| Thyroid excess (hyperthydroidism) | Weight loss, increased appetite, irritability, restlessness, tremor, palpitations, heat intolerance, diarrhoea, eye complaints, oligomenorrhoea | Exophthalmos, ophthalmoplegia, goitre with overlying bruit, weight loss, myopathy, brisk tendon reflexes, wide tachycardia pulse pressure |

(Continued)

## BOX 9.1 (*Continued*) HORMONAL DYSFUNCTION SYMPTOMS AND SIGNS

| Hormonal abnormality | Symptoms | Specific physical signs |
|---|---|---|
| *Glucocorticoid axis* | | |
| Hyperadrenalism: Cushing's syndrome | Weight gain (upper body), change in appearance, thin skin with easy bruising, poor libido/menstrual abnormalities, hirsutism, acne, muscle weakness | Thin skin and bruising, moon face, plethora (ruddy complexion), buffalo hump, centripetal obesity, hypertension, proximal myopathy |
| Hypoadrenalism: Addison's disease | Weight loss, anorexia, impotence/amenorrhoea, nausea and vomiting, dizziness on standing, abdominal pain | Buccal and skin pigmentation, general wasting and loss of weight, postural hypotension, vitiligo may be associated |
| *Arginine-vasopressin* | | |
| AVP/ADH excess: syndrome of SIADH | Symptoms resulting from hyponatraemia: headache, anorexia, irritability, lethargy. Extreme levels of hyponatraemia ($Na^+$ <110 mmol/l) may be associated with drowsiness and fits | There may be no specific signs but may be accompanied by mental confusion and altered level of consciousness |

*(Continued)*

## BOX 9.1 (Continued) HORMONAL DYSFUNCTION SYMPTOMS AND SIGNS

| Hormonal abnormality | Symptoms | Specific physical signs |
|---|---|---|
| *Arginine-vasopressin (continued)* | | |
| AVP/ADH deficiency | Excessive thirst and polyuria with passage of large volumes of urine; patients often relate how they require a jug of water by the bedside at night. Rarely presents with severe hypernatraemia and associated neurological confusion, fits and coma | No specific features but may be accompanied by signs of pituitary failure. Occasionally presents with dehydration with evidence of hypovolaemia (low blood pressure with postural fall) |
| *Parathyroid hormone* | | |
| Hyperparathyroidism | Personality change (often associated with depression), abdominal pain – constipation and/or dyspepsia, polyuria and polydipsia | Severe and prolonged hypercalcaemia, may be accompanied by corneal calcification, associated hypertension, haematuria if associated with renal calculi |
| Hypoparathyroidism | Paraesthesia, cramps, alterations in personality (occasionally psychosis), epilepsy | Carpopedal spasm (positive Trousseau's sign), positive Chvostek's sign (twitching of facial muscle on tapping), cataract formation |

(Continued)

## BOX 9.1 (*Continued*) HORMONAL DYSFUNCTION SYMPTOMS AND SIGNS

| Hormonal abnormality | Symptoms | Specific physical signs |
|---|---|---|
| *Insulin* | | |
| Insulin deficiency: diabetes mellitus | May present in any age group. Symptoms resulting from hyperglycaemia include thirst, polyuria, weight loss and intense fatigue, recurrent skin infections. Patients may also have related complaints: impotence, paraesthesia/hypoaesthesia of hands/feet, visual disturbances, foot ulcers | Look for signs of complications: examine the fundi to look for retinal changes, examine the feet to detect any loss of sensation (light touch, pin-prick and vibration sense). Examine pulses in lower limbs and test urine for protein and glucose |
| Insulin excess: hypoglycaemia | Patient may present in a coma. Symptoms suggestive of hypoglycaemia include hunger, cold perspiration, tremor, pallor and agitation. Generalised convulsion may accompany profound hypoglycaemia | Severe hypoglycaemia may present with focal neurological signs (reversible if glucose quickly restored to normal). Usually, the patient is cold and clammy with a 'bounding' pulse and a moderately elevated blood pressure |

ADH = antidiuretic hormone; AVP = arginine-vasopressin; SIADH = syndrome of inappropriate ADH secretion.

## Illustrated physical signs

The following photographs illustrate some common endocrine physical signs: a large, multinodular **goitre** (**Fig. 9.3**), Cushing's syndrome (**Fig. 9.4**), thyrotoxicosis (**Fig. 9.5**), Addison's disease (**Fig. 9.6**) and acromegaly (**Fig. 9.7**).

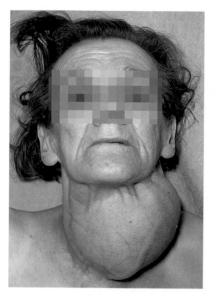

Fig. 9.3  A large multinodular goitre.

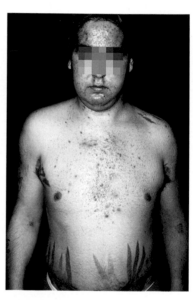

Fig. 9.4  Cushing's syndrome with central obesity, acne and striae.

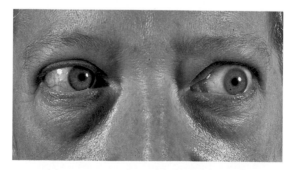

Fig. 9.5  Thyrotoxicosis causing lid retraction and dysconjugate gaze from thyroid eye disease.

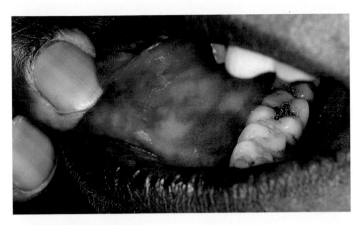

Fig. 9.6 Buccal pigmentation in Addison's disease.

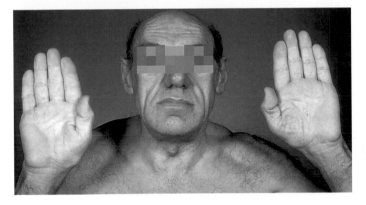

Fig. 9.7 Acromegaly. Note the lantern jaw and wide hands.

**Fig. 9.8** and **Fig. 9.9** highlight common findings in hyper- and hypo-thyroidism, respectively.

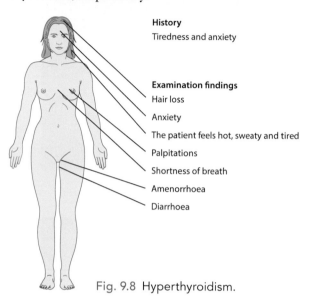

**History**
Tiredness and anxiety

**Examination findings**
Hair loss

Anxiety

The patient feels hot, sweaty and tired

Palpitations

Shortness of breath

Amenorrhoea

Diarrhoea

Fig. 9.8 Hyperthyroidism.

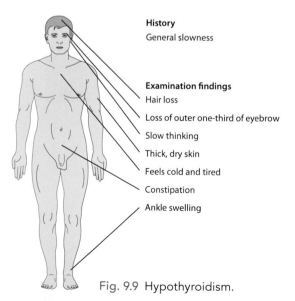

**History**
General slowness

**Examination findings**
Hair loss

Loss of outer one-third of eyebrow

Slow thinking

Thick, dry skin

Feels cold and tired

Constipation

Ankle swelling

Fig. 9.9 Hypothyroidism.

The skin is an important physiological structure. It also has a significant effect on a patient's psychological well-being, as dermatological diseases often cause blemishes and abnormalities that, although minor, may be a very large problem to the patient.

## Applied anatomy of the skin

The skin consists of two layers:

- An outer **epidermis**: this is composed of keratinised stratified squamous epithelium. Hair follicles, sweat glands, sebaceous glands and nails are modifications of the epidermis.
- An inner **dermis**: this is vascular connective tissue, containing tubular sweat ducts opening on to the skin's surface and sebaceous glands opening on the hair follicles. The roots of hair and sweat glands are present in the subcutaneous tissue.

The anatomy of skin is illustrated in **Fig. 10.1**.

## Assessment and diagnosis

The structure of the dermatological history is the same as for any other system, but dermatological conditions frequently have a pattern recognition element, and spot diagnoses can be made.

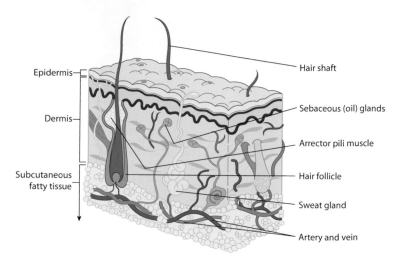

Fig. 10.1 Anatomy of the skin.

## Taking the history

### The presenting complaint

The patient may complain of a 'rash', 'spots', 'itching', an 'ulcer' or a 'growth'. It is important to ask them to describe exactly what they are worried about, and also to describe the distribution of the abnormality. Also ask about provoking and alleviating factors such as hot, cold, warm or dry conditions. Ask:

'Is the condition spreading or does it look as though it is gradually improving?'

Although often quite difficult, it is important to find out how long a rash or skin problem has been present. This is particularly true of skin tumours. It is also important to find out what has happened to a lesion since it started. Has it spread from the centre or from the edge, or has it come in crops and occasionally disappeared?

Finally, any other symptoms such as fever or malaise that appear to be associated with the rash should be ascertained. It is also useful to ask about treatments, whether over-the-counter or prescribed, that have already been tried, and the response to these.

## Past medical history

It is worthwhile asking whether the patient has had previous skin problems, as these may have been present since birth. Other conditions to consider screening for include inflammatory arthritides, diabetes and inflammatory bowel disease, as these can all have dermatological manifestations.

## Social history

An occupational history is very important in skin disease, as several chemicals used in industry can irritate the skin or give rise to allergy. Remember that skin allergies can also be provoked by hobbies and rashes can be provoked by plant antigens, and it is also important to ask about sunlight. Short-term exposure to the sun can precipitate photosensitive rashes, sometimes associated with drug reactions. In addition, repeated exposure over several years that includes the frequent use of sun beds predisposes to basal cell carcinomas, squamous cell carcinomas and malignant melanomas.

## Family history

It is important to establish whether there is a family history of atopy (eczema, hay fever or asthma) in patients with a rash classical of eczema, and of psoriasis in patients suspected of having this type of eruption. Skin cancers can also be familial, and thus a family history of these should be enquired about at this stage.

## Drug history

It is essential to establish what drugs patients are taking, and how long they have been taking them for. Drugs are an important cause of a large number of eruptions. Remember that some drugs, for example amiodarone for the treatment of arrhythmias, may have been taken for some months before a rash appears.

# Examination of the patient

Examination of the skin is largely based on inspection. The lesions should be identified and described. Any secondary changes such as excoriation should be established and documented. The shape, size, colour and consistency of any lesions should also be clearly documented, and their distribution over the skin noted. In addition, it is important to carry out a general examination, as skin conditions are often a component of a multisystem disorder.

## Key features of skin disease

It is particularly important not to miss the changes in a mole that may suggest malignant transformation. These are: a change in size, a change in shape; variability in colour; size ≥7 mm; inflammation; oozing, crusting or bleeding; and a change in sensation. The 7-point weighted checklist (*Table 10.1*) is a useful tool to apply to help to identify suspicious lesions.

Lesions to look for especially include benign pigmented naevus (**Fig. 10.2**), atypical mole (**Fig. 10.3**), malignant melanoma (**Fig. 10.4**) and basal cell carcinoma (**Fig. 10.5**).

### Table 10.1 Weighted 7-point checklist for assessment of skin lesions (suspicion great for lesions scoring 3 or more)

| Major features (score 2 points each) | Minor features (score 1 point each) |
| --- | --- |
| Change in size | Largest diameter 7 mm or more |
| Irregularly shaped border | Inflammation |
| Irregular colour | Oozing or crusting of the lesion |
| | Change in sensation (including itch) |

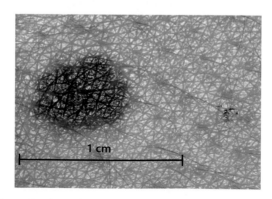

Fig. 10.2 Pigmented naevus.

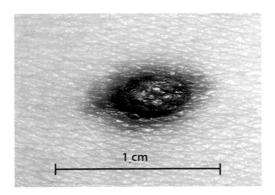

Fig. 10.3 Atypical mole.

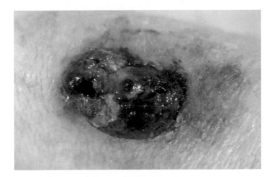

Fig. 10.4 Malignant melanoma.

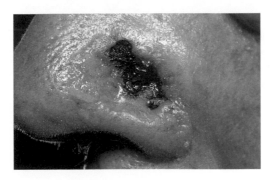

Fig. 10.5 Basal cell carcinoma.

## Illustrated physical signs

This section includes clinical photographs of common dermatological conditions: vitiligo (**Fig. 10.6**), atopic eczema (**Fig. 10.7**), psoriasis of the elbow (**Fig. 10.8**), psoriasis of the sole of the foot (**Fig. 10.9**), acne (**Fig. 10.10**), xanthelasma (**Fig. 10.11**), butterfly rash of systemic lupus erythematosus (**Fig. 10.12**) and vasculitic rash (**Fig. 10.13**).

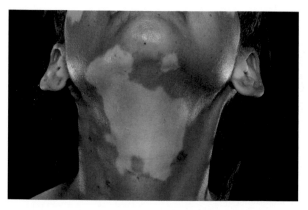

Fig. 10.6  Vitiligo.

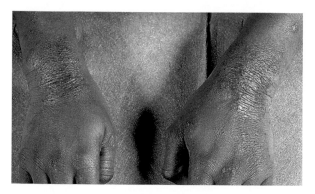

Fig. 10.7  Atopic eczema.

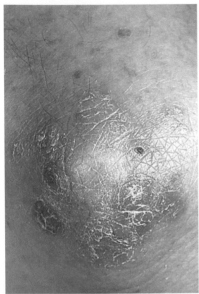

Fig. 10.8 Psoriasis of the elbow.

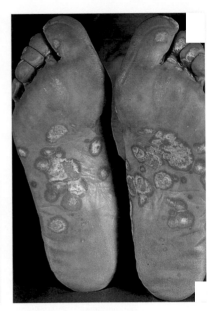

Fig. 10.9 Psoriasis of the soles of the feet.

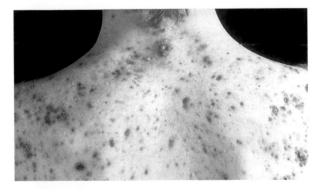

Fig. 10.10 Acne.

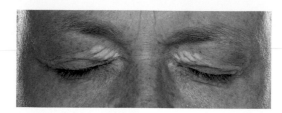

Fig. 10.11 Xanthelasma, resulting from a high level of cholesterol in the blood.

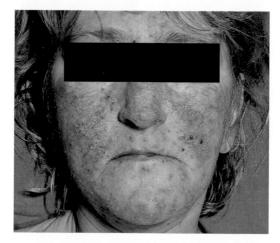

Fig. 10.12 Butterfly rash in systemic lupus erythematosus.

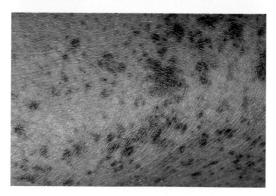

Fig. 10.13 Vasculitic rash.

## BOX 10.1  COMMON DEFINITIONS IN SKIN CONDITIONS

Dermatology, as with any other speciality, has its own group of descriptive terms. Fortunately, these are few and easy to remember:

**A Erythema** – redness.

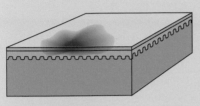

**B Macule** – a flat spot of a different colour from the surrounding skin (e.g. freckles).

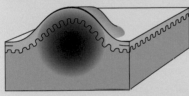

**C Papule** – a raised spot on the surface of the skin. **Nodule** – a raised spot on the skin which is ≥0.5 cm in diameter.

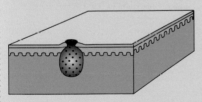

**D Comedone** – a blocked hair follicle containing keratin and sebum.

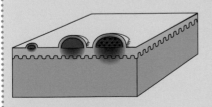

**E Vesicle** – a small fluid-filled lesion <0.5 cm in diameter (e.g. herpes simplex). **Bulla** – a fluid-filled lesion ≥0.5 cm in diameter. It may be subepidermal (e.g. pemphigoid or dermatitis herpetiformis) or intra-epidermal (e.g. pemphigus or eczema).

*(Continued)*

## BOX 10.1 (*Continued*) COMMON DEFINITIONS IN SKIN CONDITIONS

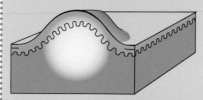

**F Pustule** – a pus-filled lesion.

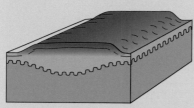

**G Plaque** – an elevated area of skin with a well-defined edge and a flat or rough surface (e.g. psoriasis).

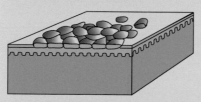

**H Scale** – visible flakes of skin that are fragments of the stratum corneum; usually indicates an epidermal disorder.

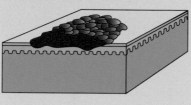

**I Crust** – varying colours of liquid debris (serum, pus, blood) that have dried on the surface of the skin; usually results from trauma to vesicles, bullae or pustules.

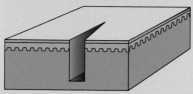

**J Fissure** – a crack or split.

(*Continued*)

## BOX 10.1 (*Continued*) COMMON DEFINITIONS IN SKIN CONDITIONS

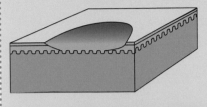

**K Erosion** – an area of partial loss of the epidermis of the skin or mucous membrane.

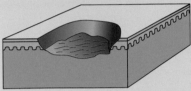

**L Ulcer** – an area of total loss of the epidermis of the skin or mucous membrane.

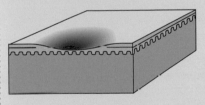

**M Atrophy** – loss of thickness of the skin due to a reduction in the underlying tissue.

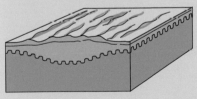

**N Lichenification** – thickening of the skin commonly caused by rubbing.

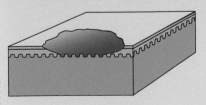

**O Excoriation** – a break in the skin caused by scratching.

The following illustrations highlight the distribution of lesions in common skin conditions: psoriasis (**Fig. 10.14**), acne (**Fig. 10.15**) and seborrhoeic dermatitis (**Fig. 10.16**).

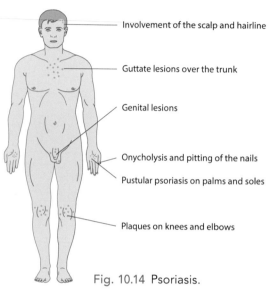

Involvement of the scalp and hairline

Guttate lesions over the trunk

Genital lesions

Onycholysis and pitting of the nails

Pustular psoriasis on palms and soles

Plaques on knees and elbows

Fig. 10.14  Psoriasis.

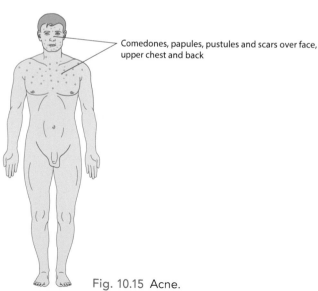

Comedones, papules, pustules and scars over face, upper chest and back

Fig. 10.15  Acne.

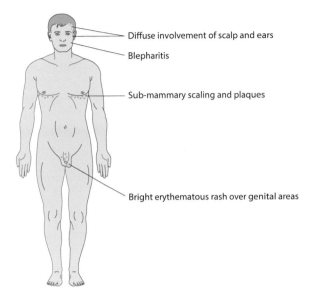

Diffuse involvement of scalp and ears

Blepharitis

Sub-mammary scaling and plaques

Bright erythematous rash over genital areas

Fig. 10.16 Seborrhoeic dermatitis.

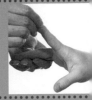

The general practice consultation shares the consulting structures and behaviours outlined in this book so far. It is an encounter between the doctor and a patient relating to either a new problem or the follow-up of an existing one; it can take place either in the general practitioner (GP) surgery or at the patient's home. To ensure optimal patient outcomes, it must adopt a patient-centred approach underpinned by a good structure, systematic clinical reasoning and, most importantly, a strong rapport between the doctor and patient.

Previous chapters have already summarised a systems-based approach to the diagnostic process. In a 'typical' week, a GP will see a range of presenting conditions including, for example, those with a potential cardiac, respiratory, gastrointestinal, musculoskeletal or psychological origin. Therefore, what has already been covered is firmly applicable to the general practice setting. There are, however, some key differences, and these will be outlined in this chapter.

## The general practice setting

### Familiarity and continuity of patient care

General practice sits firmly within a community of people, and thus frequently cares not only for the individual, but also for whole families and indeed, over time, multiple generations within these families. During their career, a GP may care for the great-grandparents, grandparents, parents and children. Although this can contribute to challenges in terms of respecting and maintaining an individual's right to confidentiality, the knowledge of such dynamics can help in understanding a patient's presentation and ability to cope with illness. For this reason, the psychosocial aspects of a consultation are of paramount importance in general practice.

The UK's general practice system also has the benefit of holding a patient's entire medical record. Since 2004 these have been held electronically, with SystmOne, EMIS Web and Vision as the most common computer programmes used. These records are a rich source of information about a patient's history, previous medical problems and consultations, investigations and treatment. Each patient consultation represents a single step on this healthcare journey and should be considered in this context.

Finally, with the benefit of proximity and availability, time can be used as a useful tool to aid diagnosis. This requires careful follow-up and safety-netting to ensure that if patients are not getting better (or are indeed getting worse), they will come back for a review during which the history and differential diagnosis can be re-evaluated.

## The presenting complaint

The problems presenting to general practice are similar to those of hospital medicine, with some important distinctions. The breadth of patient concerns in general practice is 'unfiltered' and the variety of conditions wide-ranging; the potential list of differential diagnoses is therefore long. Many patients presenting to general practice have mild, short-lived and self-limiting illnesses, and/or simply need reassurance. A normality-orientated approach model ('common things are common') is typically adopted, which contrasts with the usual disease-orientated approach of hospital medicine. Serious illness and pathology will, however, often first present to the GP, and a robust system for screening for the presence or absence of serious conditions is essential to ensure safe clinical practice. The adoption of the 'red flag' approach, described below, will facilitate this.

## The clinical consultation in general practice

The fundamental importance of adopting a patient-centred approach in general practice has already been identified. The skill comes in applying such an approach to the necessarily abbreviated consultation time, commonly no more than 10 minutes owing to the number of patients to be seen. This requires both efficient and effective consultation skills.

A number of different consultation models have been created to facilitate this. The Calgary–Cambridge Observation Guide is one such tool.[1–3] This offers a basic framework to guide both the structure and the content of a doctor–patient consultation. A modified version is displayed in **Fig. 11.1**. The figure summarises the five main steps to a consultation in general practice. Steps 1 and 2 focus on the generation of a diagnostic hypothesis, step 3 involves a targeted examination to confirm or refute this hypothesis, and steps 4 and 5 are for explanation and planning and closing the session. These stages complement the scheme outlined in **Fig. 1.7** (page 21).

## The five steps of the Calgary–Cambridge Observation Guide

Step 1, the initiation of the session, starts before the patient has entered the consultation room. Time should be taken to look at the patient's record and note any signficant past medical history, recent consultations and medication. This can help to build a picture of the patient you are about to see and offer potential clues to their current presentation.

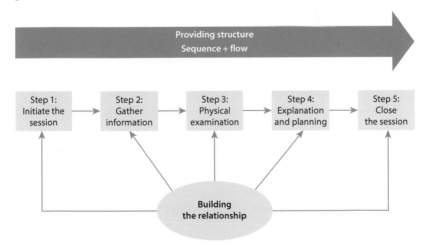

Fig. 11.1 The Cambridge–Calgary Observation Guide (1996).

Once the patient is in the room, introductions should be made and an open question offered to identify the reasons for the patient coming in:

'How can I help you today?'

Steps 2 and 3 of the consultation involve the process of the medical interview and examination as introduced in Chapter 1. The key difference in these when consulting in general practice is that time pressures necessitate a more focused approach. An **open-to-closed question funnel** can help to guide this and enable key symptoms and signs of concern, the so-called 'red flags' (see below), to be directly asked about and identified early. The physical examination performed in step 3 often needs to be focused and guided by the information identified in the history.

Once the history has been taken and the patient examined, the consultation moves on to the explanation and planning stage (step 4). This involves giving the **correct amount** of information to the patient in a way that they can **understand**. Care should also be taken to avoid medical jargon. This step must include the patient's perspective so that joint decision making and planning, the ultimate outcome of this step, can be facilitated.

The consultation ends with step 5, 'Closing the session'. During this stage, the next aspect of care is identified, a summary provided and a final check made that the patient is content. It is also imperative at this stage that care is taken to set up a 'safety net'. As most patients are being sent home, they *must* know what to do if their symptoms worsen. This includes identifying any symptoms or signs that warrant immediate re-presentation, and providing empowerment to make sure patients feel they can come back sooner if they have any concerns.

By respecting these five steps and using a logical flow through them, consultations naturally gain structure and organisation. **Summarising** and **signposting** are useful techniques to apply at the end of each of the five steps to offer clarification of what has been discussed (and also demonstrate that you have been listening) and to highlight the next stage of the consultation. Combining these will facilitate good time management, effective consultation and improved doctor and patient satisfaction.

**Figure 11.2** demonstrates a worked example of how this model can be applied to a typical patient encounter.

**Providing structure**
Sequence + flow
Signpost and summarise between steps

| Step 1: Initiate the session | Step 2: Gather information | Step 3: Physical examination | Step 4: Explanation and planning | Step 5: Close the session |
|---|---|---|---|---|
| Dr B checks the electronic medical record. He notes a lack of significant medical history and that the patient is an infrequent attender<br><br>Dr B introduces himself and checks the patient's details: Jess Smith (JS), date of birth 16 February 1985<br><br>Dr B asks 'How can I help you today?' | JS reports 3 weeks of diarrhoea<br><br>OPEN QUESTION 'Have you any other symptoms?' This reveals associated crampy pain<br><br>OPEN QUESTION 'How did it start?' JS says she had thought it was food poisoning after a takeaway meal. Very bad at the start, with bowels open 10/day. Now when she eats she gets pain + diarrhoea<br><br>CLOSED QUESTIONS: 'Is there any associated nausea or vomiting?', 'Any blood or mucus in your motions?', 'Any change in your appetite or weight?', 'Any fevers?', 'Any urinary symptoms?' Check last menstrual period/family h story/ previous episodes<br><br>ICE: JS is worried it is an infection and thinks she may need antibiotics | Temperature: 36.5°C<br><br>Pulse: 55/min and regular<br><br>Blood pressure: 100/50 mmHg<br><br>Abdomen soft and non-tender, with normal active bowel sounds | Dr B advises that this is probably post-infectious irritable bowel syndrome and reassures JS it should settle with time<br><br>Discusses dietary changes that can help and prescribes hyoscine butylbromide (Buscopan®)<br><br>He acknowledges her concerns about infection and suggests testing a stool sample<br><br>He discusses other possibilities (e.g. coeliac disease) and arranges a blood test screening (full blood count, ferritin, tissue transglutaminase, C-reactive protein, urea + electrolytes, liver function tests) | Dr B summarises what has been discussed. He checks whether JS has understood and has further questions<br><br>He advises JS how to take a stool sample and how to book the blood tests<br><br>Dr B arranges a review in 2 weeks with the test results<br><br>SAFETY NET: JS should return to the surgery before this if she has new or worsening symptoms<br><br>He checks JS is happy with the consultation |
| Good eye contact<br>Open body language<br>Active listening | Explains reasons for questions<br>Addresses ICE | Obtains permission | Shares thinking with patient | Encourages patient's involvement |

**Building the relationship**

Fig. 11.2 An illustrated example of a 10-minute consultation.

## Building the relationship

Establishing a good rapport wth a patient is undoubtedly one of the most important aspects of any doctor–patient encounter in general practice, and is key to ensuring ongoing patient-centred care. As the 'family doctor', you are likely to be the first port of call for an individual who has concerns about their health or that of a family member. It is thus important that the inidividual feels listened to and respected, and has opportunities to voice their Ideas, Concerns and Expectations (ICE) so that explanations and management plans can be tailored to these. This will also improve the patient's adherence to the advice and treatment given, and enable a long and successful mutual partnership.

Various techniques can be applied within the Calgary–Cambridge model to aid this. Ascertaining a patient's ICE forms an important aspect of step 2 of the model and this should be recognised, acknowledged and validated. In addition, active listening methods ('listening with all senses') that include body language and gestures to convey your continuing attention should be used throughout the five steps, and you should show an attentiveness and appreciation for the patient's expressions and responses. These techniques are summarised in *Table 11.1*; it may also be helpful to refer to Chapter 1 (pages 9 and 10).

### Table 11.1  Non-verbal and verbal communication techniques

| Non-verbal techniques | Verbal techniques |
|---|---|
| Eye contact | Checking ICE |
| Facial expression | Recognising, acknowledging and validating feelings |
| Posture and positioning | Clarifying statements |
| Touch | Using concise, easily understood language |
| Vocal cues – rate, volume and tone | Avoiding medical jargon |
| General appearance (e.g. clothing) | |

# Red flags in general practice

Red flags are a set of alerting symptoms and signs that indicate the potential for there to be a more serious underlying pathology to account for a patient's presentation. Some red flags, for example the thunderclap onset of the headache accompanying a subarachnoid haemorrhage, are highly diagnostic, whereas others are less specific; nevertheless they all help to risk-stratify the patients we see in general practice. This is especially important, given the time restraints and the usual application of a normality-orientated approach, to help us to identify at an early stage patients who may need further investigations, more immediate treatment and potentially specialist referral and management.

*Table 11.2* lists some of the more common red flags, by body system, that are used for adults, but this is by no means an exhaustive list; it may also be helpful to refer to *Table 1.5* (page 14). Although unexplained weight loss appears as a 'general' symptom, it is important to

## Table 11.2 Red flags by system: adults

| System | Symptom | Sign |
|---|---|---|
| General | Unexplained loss of appetite<br>Unexplained weight loss<br>Night sweats<br>Persistent fever | Looks unwell |
| Cardiovascular | **Hypertension *with*:**<br>• Headaches<br>• Visual disturbance<br>• Encephalopathy: altered level of consciousness, fits, coma<br>• Pregnancy | • Blood pressure ≥220/120 mmHg<br>• Retinal haemorrhage<br>• Papilloedema<br>• Signs of end-organ damage: left ventricular hypertrophy, left ventricular failure, reduced renal function, retinopathy |

*(Continued)*

## Table 11.2 (*Continued*)  Red flags by system: adults

| System | Symptom | Sign |
|---|---|---|
| Cardiovascular (*continued*) | **Palpitations *with:*** <br> • Chest pain <br> • Shortness of breath <br> • Acute dizziness/ syncope <br> • Exertion <br> • Family history of sudden death | • Irregular pulse <br> • Pulse rate <40/>100 beats/min <br> • Hypotension |
| | **Chest pain:** <br> • Exertional, progressive, at rest <br> • Central, crushing <br> • Radiation to the jaw, neck or arm(s) <br> • Asssociated breathlessness, nausea or sweating | • Hypertension |
| | **Shortness of breath:** <br> • On exertion <br> • Nocturnal <br> • Orthopnoea <br> • Peripheral oedema | • Raised jugular venous pressure <br> • Gallop rhythm <br> • Pitting oedema <br> • Basal chest crackles |
| Respiratory | Unexplained/persistent cough <br><br> Unexplained/persistent shortness of breath | Dyspnoea affecting speech <br><br> Use of accessory muscles <br><br> Cyanosis |

(*Continued*)

## Table 11.2 (*Continued*)  Red flags by system: adults

| System | Symptom | Sign |
|---|---|---|
| Respiratory (*continued*) | Pleuritic chest pain | Tachycardia |
| | | Raised respiratory rate |
| | Haemoptysis | Reduced oxygen saturations |
| | Hoarseness | |
| | Persistent or recurrent chest infections | Unilateral wheeze |
| | | Focal chest signs on auscultation |
| | Significant smoking history | |
| | Significant asbestos exposure | |
| Gastrointestinal | Constant/severe abdominal pain | Pallor |
| | | Jaundice |
| | Persistent/unexplained dyspepsia | |
| | Dysphagia | Localised tenderness with guarding |
| | | Generalised peritonism |
| | Persistent/unexplained vomiting | |
| | Blood in vomitus | Organomegaly |
| | | Palpable mass |
| | | Ascites |
| | Change in bowel habit | |
| | Prolonged diarrhoea | |
| | Blood mixed in with motions | |
| | Melena | |
| Locomotor | Joint pain improving *with* activity or *with* the day | Symmetrical joint involvement |
| | | 'Boggy' swelling |
| | Nocturnal pain | Swelling associated with redness or heat |

(*Continued*)

## Table 11.2 (*Continued*) Red flags by system: adults

| System | Symptom | Sign |
|---|---|---|
| Locomotor (*continued*) | Morning stiffness ≥1–2 hours | Joint deformity |
| | Associated constitutional symptoms | |
| | Back pain *and*:<br>• Focal neurological symptoms<br>• Bladder or bowel dysfunction<br>• Past medical history of cancer or corticosteroid use | • Focal neurological signs<br>• Saddle anaesthesia: loss of sensation in the area of the buttocks, perineum and inner surfaces of the thigh<br>• Reduced anal tone |
| Nervous system | Headaches *and*:<br>• New onset, progressive<br>• Thunderclap start<br>• Association with sleep disturbance<br>• Worse in the mornings<br>• Provoked by coughing or exertion<br>• Association with persistent vomiting<br>• Association with focal neurological symptoms | • Fever<br>• Neck stiffness<br>• Photophobia<br>• Papilloedema<br>• Temporal artery tenderness<br>• Focal neurological signs: focal seizures/ status epilepticus |
| | Fits/blackouts:<br>• Tongue biting<br>• Urinary or faecal incontinence | |

screen for this specifically alongside each of the system-based red flags as an important presenting feature of any serious disease. Children are considered separately within this approach (*Table 11.3*), as serious illnesses typically presents very differently in this patient group.

## Table 11.3 Red flags: children

|  | Symptom | Sign |
| --- | --- | --- |
| Febrile child | Fever for >5 days despite regular antipyretics | 'Appears ill' |
|  |  | Pale, mottled, ashen, blue |
|  |  | Weak, high-pitched cry |
|  | Reduced fluid intake | Floppy |
|  | Reduced urine output | Reduced response to social cues |
|  | Irritability |  |
|  | Reduced responsiveness | Cool peripheries |
|  |  | Reduced skin turgor |
|  |  | Prolonged capillary refill |
|  | Seizures |  |
|  | Non-blanching rash | Tachycardia |
|  |  | Tachypnoea |
|  |  | Grunting |
|  |  | Moderate to severe recession of the chest |
|  |  | Bulging fontanelle |
|  |  | Non-blanching petechial rash |
|  |  | Neck stiffness |
|  |  | Focal neurological signs |
|  |  | Focal seizures or status epilepticus |

*(Continued)*

## Table 11.3 (*Continued*) Red flags: children

|  | Symptom | Sign |
|---|---|---|
| Non-febrile child | Unexplained weight loss | Lymphadenopathy for ≥6 weeks |
|  | Persistent night sweats |  |
|  | Bloody diarrhoea | Abdominal mass |
|  | New-onset headaches with or without neurological symptoms | Focal neurological signs |
|  | New-onset seizures |  |
|  | New-onset back pain | Swelling of a limb or joint |
|  | New-onset joint swelling or pain |  |
|  | New-onset limp |  |

When a 'red flag' sign or symptom is detected within a consultation, care must be taken to fully evaluate the patient, including ascertaining the speed with which any treatment is needed. In some circumstances, for example a severe headache with a thunderclap onset, this may necessitate immediate transfer and admission to hospital. In other situations, the detection could trigger further investigation involving screening blood tests and X-rays. The National Institute for Health and Care Excellence has produced a set of urgent referral pathways into secondary care, the '2-week wait' guidances.[4] These can be used for patients presenting with any of the specified symptoms or signs within the guidance chosen as key indicators of a possible underlying malignancy; this approach will streamline access to the necessary investigations and specialism they require.

## Investigating the patient in general practice

### Recording vital signs: an objective measure of health and disease

The importance of a basic set of observations cannot be overstated. These need to be documented and dated clearly and accurately in the patient's medical record. For an adult patient, basic signs that should be recorded include body temperature, pulse, blood pressure and oxygen saturation; for a child, readings should cover temperature, colour and alertness, heart rate, respiratory rate and capillary refill time (central and peripheral). It may also be helpful to document in the records an overall impression of the patient's general appearance in observational, non-judgemental terms.

Recording these signs provides an immediate, objective measure to quantify the severity of an underlying illness (whether acute or chronic). In addition, abnormal values can also serve as an early warning for the doctor about the evolution of a potentially serious underlying medical problem and the need for further investigations. For example, although a patient with acute diarrhoea may seemingly appear generally well in themself, a persistent tachycardia may signify possible dehydration or underlying sepsis, and thus a need to take further action.

### Investigations: choice, interpretation and application

General practice has access to a wide range of investigations to aid patients' diagnosis and management. Some of these tests, for example basic urinalysis, electrocardiograms (ECGs) and spirometry, can be performed 'in house', with the results immediately available. There may, however, be an inevitable delay in obtaining the results of other tests. This can range from approximately 24 hours for basic blood tests to 6–12 weeks for routine computed tomography (CT) and magnetic resonance imaging (MRI) scans. This contrasts markedly with the speed of accessing results for inpatients in an acute hospital setting, and must be acknowledged by the requesting doctor at booking. Once again, careful safety-netting and signposting helps to keep the patient safe during this time period.

Not all patients presenting to general practice require investigations, and the importance of a thorough history and examination cannot be emphasised enough. It may be entirely appropriate to initially manage a patient with some self-care advice and then proceed to further tests only if they are not improving as anticipated. A good example of this is the use of a chest X-ray for patients presenting with a cough. Individuals with no pre-existing illness who are well and have a short history of a cough and no localised signs can initially be safely managed by observation. However, if the cough persists for longer than 3 weeks, especially if there is a significant smoking history, a chest X-ray should be requested.

**Figure 11.3** expands **Fig. 1.1** by summarising the range of investigations and tests commonly available in UK general practice.

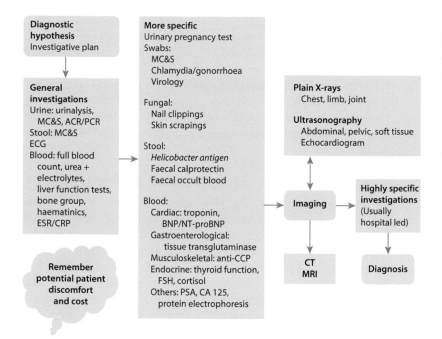

ACR/PCR = albumin:creatinine ratio/protein:creatinine ratio; CRP = C-reactive protein; ESR = erythrocyte sedimentation rate; FSH = follicle-stimulating hormone; MC&S = microscopy, culture and sensitivity.

Fig. 11.3 The investigative plan in general practice.

GPs must be selective in the investigations they use given the fundamental importance of not putting patients through unnecessary investigations and the finite resources available to healthcare around the world. **Figure 11.4** demonstrates a worked example of this for a patient presenting with diarrhoea.

It must be understood that the responsibility for interpreting test results always lies with the requester. Thus tests and procedures should only be ordered if the requesting doctor feels confident and competent enough to interpret the results. A good question to ask oneself before ordering any test is therefore 'How will the results of this affect my management of this patient?'

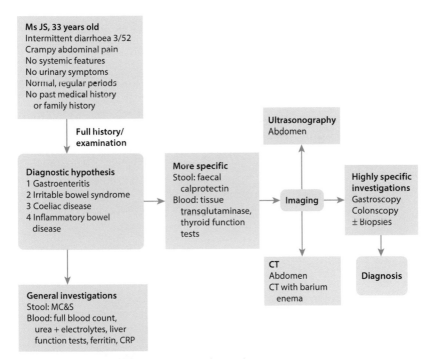

CRP = C-reactive protein; MC&S = microscopy, culture and sensitivity.

Fig. 11.4 The investigative plan in general practice: a worked example.

## Biomarkers of disease and their use in general practice

**Figure 11.3** also highlights a series of ever-expanding system-specific biochemical markers that can aid the diagnosis of a patient in primary care. These include:

- **Faecal calprotectin** and **faecal occult blood** test as a screen for gastrointestinal disease.
- **Serum natriuretic peptides** (B-type natriuretic peptide [BNP] or N-terminal pro-B-type natriuretic peptide [NT-proBNP]) for heart failure.
- **Cardiac troponins** for cardiac ischaemia.
- Antibodies to citrullinated proteins (**anti-CCP**) for rheumatological disease.
- **Prostate-specific antigen** (PSA) and **CA 125** as potential cancer markers.

Further information about these markers is provided in *Table 11.4*.

## Table 11.4  Biomarkers of disease

| Biomarker | Use | Limitations |
|---|---|---|
| **Faecal calprotectin** (Stool specimen) | To detect possible inflammatory bowel disease | Gastrointestinal infection invalidates results |
| Substance released into the intestine when inflammation is present | | Stool sample must be sent for MC&S at same time |
| **Faecal occult blood** Stool specimen – to detect blood in faeces | To screen for colorectal cancer in asymptomatic patients[a] | *False-positive* results can occur due to: <br>• Other sources of gastrointestinal bleeding <br>• Dietary factors |

(Continued)

## Table 11.4 (*Continued*)  Biomarkers of disease

| Biomarker | Use | Limitations |
|---|---|---|
| | Possible role in the diagnosis of colorectal cancer in some symptomatic patients | ***False-negative*** results can occur due to:<br>• Tumour present but not bleeding<br>• High vitamin C consumption |
| **Serum natriuretic peptides**<br>(Blood test)<br><br>BNP and NT-proBNP<br><br>Released from the ventricles in response to stretching | To look for the presence of heart failure<br><br>Raised levels should prompt a request for an echocardiogram | Other factors can increase their levels (e.g. atrial fibrillation) |
| **Cardiac troponin**<br>(Blood test)<br><br>Protein released from the myocardium when it has been damaged | To look for evidence of cardiac ischaemia | Role in general practice is controversial as there is a possible delay in receiving results, placing patients at potential risk |
| **Anti-CCP**<br>(Blood test)<br><br>Antibody present in most cases of RA | Increasingly used instead of rheumatoid factor for the early detection of RA as it has a higher sensitivity<br><br>Rises prior to the clinical manifestations of RA | |

(Continued)

## Table 11.4 (*Continued*) Biomarkers of disease

| Biomarker | Use | Limitations |
|---|---|---|
| **PSA** (Blood test)<br><br>Protein produced by both normal prostate cells and prostate cancer cells | Used **with a digital rectal examination** to look for possible prostate cancer | Raised levels not specific to prostate cancer<br><br>Prostate cancer may occur with a 'normal' PSA |
| **CA 125** (Blood test)<br><br>A protein found in higher concentrations in tumour cells | Used **with a pelvic ultrasound** to look for possible ovarian cancer<br><br>Has a role in monitoring of patients after treatment for ovarian cancer | Other cancers can produce CA 125<br><br>Some benign conditions can cause a high level (e.g. ovarian cyst)<br><br>Some women naturally have raised levels in the absence of pathology |

[a] The UK has an established screening programme for the over-60s.
MC&S = microscopy, culture and sensitivity; RA = rheumatoid arthritis.

## Referring on: the structure and contents of an effective referral letter

When a decision is made to refer a patient to hospital, whether as an emergency admission or for an outpatient review, a letter must accompany that referral to provide the reviewing doctor with enough information to allow them to start making a comprehensive assessment of the patient. In certain settings, the letter may also aid with triaging the patient and determining the priority with which they should be seen. If a patient has consented to the sharing of their summary care record (an electronic patient medical record available to UK hospitals via the National Health Service [NHS] spine), it may be accessible to the hospital doctor at the time of review. Currently, however, this usually contains only very basic information about the patient, such as date of birth, NHS number, medications and allergies, and therefore must not be seen as a replacement for a comprehensive referral letter.

Learning to write a good referral letter takes time and requires practice. It is ideal to start this process as a student when direct and immediate feedback can be sought from your supervisors to help develop and refine your skills. It is important to make a referral letter as clear and concise as possible. It should not be so long and rambling that it becomes too tedious to read, but it is vital that all the important points are included. A worked example of a typical referral to a hospital consultant from a GP is demonstrated in **Fig. 11.5**.

A referral letter should always start with a clear identification of the patient's details, including name, date of birth, address and NHS number. The first paragraph of the letter should then be a statement indicating **why the referral is being made** and **what it is hoped the specialist will provide**.

Next the **presenting problem** should be highlighted, and a **brief summary of the history** of this outlined. It is important that this section only highlights key points rather than detailing a long list of negative findings. Within this section, treatments tried already should also be listed, together with the investigations undertaken or pending and the salient examination findings. The results of the most recent investigations should ideally be attached to the letter.

The next section of the letter should be a summary of the patient's significant **past medical history** and the **drugs** that they are taking. A printed copy of this information from the patient's electronic medical record may also be included. It is also useful at this point to include important aspects of the patient's **social history** and their **ICE**.

The letter ends with the referring doctor's **differential diagnosis** and a final closing statement such as, 'I would be grateful for your opinion and guidance with this patient.'

---

GP Surgery
[*Details inserted here*]

Referring department/hospital
[*Details inserted here*]

[*Date*]

Dear Dr Jones,

**Re: Patient Jess Smith, DOB 16/2/95, Address xxxx, NHS No. xxxx**

I would be very grateful for your advice and guidance with regard to the ongoing management of the above 33-year-old woman with persistent diarrhoea.

She initially presented to the surgery in May with a 3-week history of intermittent diarrhoea associated with colicky abdominal pain. There was no history of any change in her appetite or weight, and she denied any blood or mucus in the stools. A full abdominal examination was unremarkable, and an initial stool culture was negative for infection. We subsequently sent blood samples for full blood count, ferritin, CRP and tissue transglutaminase, and all were unremarkable. We also sent a stool specimen for faecal calprotectin, which was within the normal range. Despite adopting a bland diet and trying both over-the-counter probiotic products and buscopan, she has failed to improve.

She is otherwise well with no significant past medical history of family history of note. Her only regular medication is the oral contraceptive pill.

Given the normal investigation results obtained so far, I wonder whether this is an irritable bowel syndrome. However, I would be grateful for your review and advice with regard to the need to investigate this further, and also in terms of alternative management options.

With many thanks in advance,
Yours sincerely,

General Practitioner

---

Fig. 11.5 A worked example of a referral letter.

## Safe prescribing in general practice

For many consultations in general practice, all that is required is reassurance and/or the recommendation of a self-management plan. This may include the use of readily available over-the-counter medication. At times, however, it may be necessary to prescribe a short course of treatment, for example antibiotics, or start a new regular long-term medication, such as antihypertensives.

Before starting any new medication, it is important to review the patient's medical history, including previous allergies and intolerances.

Factors such as renal impairment or hepatic dysfuntion must be taken into account as they can increase an individual's susceptibility to a drug and necessitate either a dose reduction or an alternative medication to be considered. In addition, other medication that the patient is taking should be checked for potential interactions. It is also a good opportunity to assess a patient's compliance with the current medication regimen and to stop treatments that are not being taken or are no longer felt to benefit the individual.

A patient must be given enough information in order to be able to make a fully informed decision on whether or not to start a drug. This should include not only the benefits of taking the medication, but also any potential side effects or risks. In addition, some drugs require more specific monitoring processes, and these must also be covered at this stage. A fully informed patient is more likely not only to comply with the regimen being prescribed, but also to adhere to subsequent follow-up. Finally, for medico-legal purposes, this conversation should be documented in the notes in a clear and concise fashion.

## References

1   Kurtz SM, Silverman JD, Draper J (2005). *Teaching and Learning Communication Skills in Medicine*, 2nd edn. Oxford: Radcliffe Publishing.
2   Silverman JD, Kurtz SM, Draper J (2013). *Skills for Communicating with Patients*, 3rd edn. Oxford: Radcliffe Publishing.
3   Kurtz S, Silverman J, Benson J, Draper J (2003). Marrying content and process in clinical method teaching: enhancing the Calgary-Cambridge Guides. *Academic Medicine* **78**:802–809.
4   National Institute for Health and Care Excellence (2005). Suspected cancer: recognition and referral. NICE Guideline NG12. Available at: https://www.nice.org.uk/guidance/ng12 (accessed 4 October 2017).

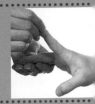

Psychiatry is concerned with the study and management of patients suffering from disorders of various mental functions. Like many conditions, these are recognised as resulting from a combination of biological, psychological and social factors. Although people often place a greater emphasis on the psychological and social aspects where psychiatric diagnosis is concerned, vital to an understanding of this is the physiology that underpins the disorders central to it. These may be primary and 'functional', representing a disorder of function, or secondary to another diagnosis or prescribed medication. These possibilities are central to formulating a differential diagnosis. However, rather than being based on an established aetiology, such as one that might be confirmed by specific clinical investigations, psychiatric diagnosis relies on the recognition of groups of symptoms that cluster together as syndromes, and which occur consistently and to a certain degree predict the response to both pharmacological and psychological treatments.

This chapter will focus on the clinical skills relevant to the assessment of patients with a mental disorder. As with any branch of medicine, the accuracy of diagnosis necessarily depends on an understanding and knowledge of the symptoms that may arise within a given psychiatric disorder, but also of their overlap. There is often a lack of specificity in psychiatric diagnosis, which means that there is a large overlap in symptoms occurring between disorders. In the absence of clinical investigation, the interview skills necessary to obtain an accurate history and the ability to collect information in a systematic manner are of the greatest importance in the assessment of these disorders.

Subjective distress and disability, or some degree of impairment of function, are central to mental disorders and are indeed the reason why individuals frequently seek help. However, they are often recognised not by the individual suffering from them, but rather by those around them. Changes in behaviour may put the individual or others at risk, and this may be the reason that your assessment is called upon.

Historically, psychiatric diagnoses were separated into 'neurotic disorders' and 'psychotic disorders'. The neuroses are representative of symptoms that reflect normal human experience but vary in degree such that, at their worst, they are severely disabling. Examples of neurotic symptoms include low mood and anxiety. By contrast, 'psychotic disorders' include symptoms that are less easily understood, by virtue of being far removed in quality from normal human experience. Examples of such symptoms include delusions and hallucinations (see page 357 'Mental state examination'). These symptoms are associated not only with the prototypical psychosis, schizophrenia, but also with disorders such as delirium that are commonly encountered on general medical and surgical wards. This distinction is reflected in the various classifications of psychiatric disorders, based on what are believed to be the central symptoms. A hierarchy is implied, whereby certain diagnoses take precedence if symptoms are evident to suggest more than one diagnosis. For example, if symptoms are present that are suggestive of a diagnosis of schizophrenia, but significant symptoms of anxiety coexist, the primary diagnosis is schizophrenia.

There is no ideal system of classification in the absence of biological markers of disease (*Table 12.1*). Although some symptoms may suggest certain disorders, others are far less specific and occur across a range of diagnoses. In addition, variations exist within each diagnostic category. For example, mood disorders may be mild, moderate or severe, each with different numbers and types of symptoms. Psychotic disorders, such as schizophrenia, might better be considered as a heterogeneous group of disorders with a variable presentation and each with potentially different responses to treatment.

## Table 12.1 Examples of different types of psychiatric disorder

**Main adult psychiatric diagnoses**

- Organic mental disorders
  - Acute (delirium)
  - Chronic (dementia)
- Psychoactive substance use disorders
- Schizophrenic and related disorders
- Affective (mood) disorders
  - Depressive disorders
  - Mania
- Neurotic disorders
  - Anxiety disorders
  - Phobic disorders
  - Reactions to stress
  - Obsessive compulsive disorder
  - Dissociative disorders
  - Somatoform disorders (e.g. pain syndromes, unexplained physical symptoms)
  - Eating disorders
  - Sexual disorders
- Personality disorders
- Learning disabilities

### BOX 12.1 THE PRESENTING COMPLAINT

It is useful to start by explaining the **purpose of the interview** and how it will proceed, and by addressing any initial questions that the patient may have. Begin with **open general questions** to identify the most significant concerns:

'Could you tell me about some of the problems that led to your coming to see me?'
'How have you been feeling?'

*(Continued)*

## BOX 12.1 (*Continued*) THE PRESENTING COMPLAINT

Try to allow the patient to talk freely and without interruption for a few minutes. If the patient appears unaware of any specific problems or finds talking difficult, refer to other available information, for example:

'I have a letter from your GP which says you've been having some difficulties concerning ... Could you tell me some more about this?'

Identify each complaint, and record it in the patient's own words. For each, attempt to clarify:

- **Time of onset:** be as specific as possible. 'When did you first become aware of this problem?' or 'When were you last reasonably well?'
- **Antecedents or precipitants:** 'Did anything happen or change just before this problem began?' The patient can be given some examples. 'Were you feeling physically unwell? ... Were you under a lot of stress? ... Were there any difficulties at home or work?' Establish whether any such difficulties preceded, or may have resulted from, psychological symptoms.
- **Mode of onset and time course:** determine whether the symptoms developed suddenly or gradually and have remained persistent. Enquire about any periods of respite, reduction or intensification, and if anything is associated with relief or exacerbation.
- **Time relations between different symptoms:** ask about the sequence of events from the time the patient reported last being well, in order to identify which symptoms came first, and which may have subsequently arisen. If there are a number of complaints, their time of onset in relation to each other can be important for diagnosis (e.g. anxiety symptoms or persecutory feelings following other symptoms of depression).
- **Associated symptoms:** the patient's initial complaints may indicate other areas of enquiry. In most cases, it is appropriate to ask direct brief screening questions for symptoms of anxiety, depression, suicidal ideas, hostile feelings toward others or psychotic phenomena (see page 357, 'Mental state examination'), but this will depend on the individual case.

(*Continued*)

> ### BOX 12.1 (*Continued*) THE PRESENTING COMPLAINT
>
> - **Effects on usual level of functioning:** symptoms of psychiatric disorders often impair an individual's functioning, which in turn reflects the severity of the condition. Enquiring about sleep pattern, appetite, weight change, sexual function and self-care often reveals abnormalities that can support certain diagnoses. Waking earlier than usual, reduced appetite and weight, decreased libido and diurnal variation in mood (lower in the morning) suggests depression of at least moderate severity. These symptoms are often called biological. In mania, in which the mood is elevated, sleeping time is reduced without tiredness, and libido may increase.

## Assessment and diagnosis of psychiatric disorders

### Taking the history

#### The psychiatric interview

A good interview technique takes time to develop but is central to good psychiatric practice. The clinical interview is used for the following purposes:

- Establishing trust.
- Gathering information.
- Making a diagnosis.
- Therapeutic reasons, as many patients find it helpful to talk their problems through.

**Setting** Interviews should be carried out in circumstances that allow privacy. This will preferably be in a room free from interruptions or distractions. Chairs should be arranged at an angle, and interviewing across a desk avoided.

**Personal safety** Personal safety should always be considered, although overall it is unusual for patients with mental illness to be violent. If you have any concerns, other members of staff should be within earshot, or should accompany you. Ideally, there should be a panic button to hand,

and you should sit between the patient and the exit to the room. If it is felt that a patient will be violent, it is advisable politely to terminate the interview, leave and summon help.

**Assessment** The process of assessment begins from the moment the patient is first encountered, at which stage important observations can be made before any verbal exchanges. Information collected should be clear, and recorded systematically (*Table 12.2*).

**Informants** Although the patient is the main source of information, it is always helpful to have information from other individuals whose knowledge will add to an understanding of the patient's difficulties. Such corroborating informants include other professionals, family and friends. This information should preferably be sought with the patient's consent, and is particularly important if the patient denies any problem, if the patient is electively mute or if the assessment has been arranged in response to concerns expressed by others. Such information should be identified clearly and recorded separately. The information that follows should be sought and recorded.

**Source and reason for referral** This provides clues to the nature of the difficulties – which may not be initially apparent from the patient's account. There may be a conflict between why the patient believes they are seeking help and the thoughts of others, including family members and referring health professionals.

You should also ask about the effects on work, family commitments (e.g. childcare), relationships and social activities. It is helpful to ask the patient to describe the activities of a typical day at present, and then describe a typical day prior to the onset of their difficulties.

**Previous help** Ask about any other treatment during the course of the individual's current problems and their response to this. Record current

## Table 12.2 Important areas of inquiry

| | |
|---|---|
| • Main concerns | • Delusions |
| • Mood symptoms | • Hallucinations |

## BOX 12.2 FAMILY HISTORY

The purpose of this section of the history is to identify significant predisposing factors and to assess current support or family stresses. There is evidence for a significant genetic contribution to some of the major mental illnesses, and intrafamilial childhood relationships can predispose to later problems. Ask about:

- Father and mother: for each, ask about their age, occupation, physical and psychiatric health (including alcohol or other substance misuse), temperament, nature of the relationship with the patient in the past and currently, and the quality of the parents' own inter-relationship. Try to assess the validity of the answers given by reflecting the patient's feelings and asking open, exploratory questions.
- Siblings: ask about ages, order of birth, occupations, marital status, nature of relationships in the past and present, and their physical and psychiatric health.
- Separations or disruptions (e.g. marital break-up or relationship with a step-parent).
- Adverse recollections and attitude to childhood.
- Atmosphere in the family home.
- Important adult figures (e.g. a teacher or doctor).

and recently taken medication. Record previously prescribed medications, maximum doses prescribed, length of prescription, positive and adverse effects experienced, and the reason for the drug being stopped or withdrawn. It is also important to ask about other forms of treatment, such as psychological interventions. If psychotherapy has previously been used, it is important to record the number of sessions completed, the outcome and whether the patient considered it to be a helpful treatment.

Social support and community treatment are also central to the management of and rehabilitation from a mental disorder – what has been previously employed (successfully or otherwise) should be noted, as should the local community mental health team involvement with the patient and the name of a key worker or community psychiatric nurse. These contacts may prove vital sources of additional information where history is concerned.

## Past psychiatric history

Establish whether the patient has ever previously had psychiatric problems, and ask about previous diagnoses or treatments and their nature, response and duration. Determine the similarity to current symptoms and the extent of recovery from previous episodes. Always ask about episodes of self-harm, suicidal thoughts and suicide attempts.

Previous history should also include:

- Episodes for which no assistance was sought.
- General practitioner consultations.
- Psychiatric assessments and admissions. Try to obtain previous records and ask about regular medication, for example depot antipsychotic preparations. If there have been admissions, investigate the number, length of stay and whether they were voluntary admissions or involved detention under the Mental Health Act.

## Past medical history

Medical conditions and their treatments can give rise to psychiatric disorders, and possible drug interactions must be considered when prescribing psychotropic medication. Enquiries should be made concerning:

- Acute and chronic medical illness, for example epilepsy, diabetes and cancer.
- Medication, both prescribed (e.g. corticosteroids) and self-administered (including over-the-counter medications and slimming pills).
- Major surgery and head injuries.

## Background history

Before beginning a detailed enquiry, it helps to explain to patients that background information can contribute to an understanding of their current difficulties. Although the majority of patients are able to talk about personal details of their lives without too much difficulty, some may be uncomfortable during the first interview. The areas covered are slightly different from the usual areas in a medical or surgical history, and include both family and personal sexual histories, a forensic history, details of any substance misuse and personality.

**Childhood abuse** The relevance of adverse childhood experiences on physiological responses to stress are recognised as potentially providing a biological predisposition to the development of a mental disorder, rather than a purely 'psychological' one.

Childhood abuse is difficult to discuss. You may find that it is not appropriate to breach this subject at an initial assessment. It may be an uncomfortable aspect of the history for the patient to cover, and this should not be forced as it may adversely affect the rapport necessary for obtaining a satisfactory history and upon which a therapeutic relationship can be built.

### BOX 12.3  PERSONAL HISTORY

A chronological account of the important events from birth to the present should be obtained, covering the following:

- **Childhood:** enquiries may reveal causes and evidence of learning disabilities or long-standing behaviour problems.
- **Birth and neonatal history:** including health, injuries, infections, convulsions and developmental milestones (e.g. walking and talking).
- **Education:** this gives an indication of intelligence and development, both social and emotional, against which you can compare current functioning. In particular, relevant enquiries may cover the patient's schooling – 'Were there disruptions? ... Was there any special education? ... Were there conduct or emotional problems (e.g. school refusal)?' Also ask about relationships with peers and teachers, bullying, truancy, participation in social activities, academic performance-specific difficulties (e.g. reading) and general attitude to school. Determine the age at which the patient left school, their qualifications and further education.
- **Occupation:** the patient's work record can add to an understanding of their personality and capabilities, as well as to the onset and severity of mental health problems. Current work or unemployment may be a significant stress. Discrepancies between education and employment record, or a decline in responsibilities, may reflect functional impairment, suggesting repeated or chronic mental illness. Important information includes the duration of employment and reasons for termination, attitude to work, satisfaction, performance and relationships with employers and colleagues.

Open and non-specific questions relating to happiness during childhood are a sensible starting point. Should the patient volunteer unhappiness when growing up, it may be appropriate to explore further, allowing the patient to guide the conversation and the details disclosed. It may then be

## BOX 12.4 SEXUAL HISTORY

Enquiries about sexual behaviour should be approached with discretion. A more detailed account is required if there is a sexual problem. Establishing how comfortable the patient is with the questions and giving permission to decline to respond can put the patient more at ease.

'Do you mind if I ask about your sexual life and the physical side of your relationship?'

If it is explained that a number of psychiatric disorders (e.g. anxiety and depression) and their treatments are associated with alterations in libido and sexual function, most patients will appreciate the opportunity for discussion. Sexual problems can add considerably to the distress of psychiatric disorders, and can be an unexpressed reason for non-compliance with psychotropic medication.

'It's not uncommon for the problems you describe to affect a person's sexual life. Have you noticed any changes?'

'Have there been any difficulties on the physical side of the relationship?'

Areas covered may include:

- Sexual development and current practice.
- Satisfaction.
- Dysfunction.
- Contraceptive measures and safe sexual practice.
- Sexually transmissible diseases.
- Transgendering issues.

Mental ill health may be experienced in women at the time of childbirth, premenstrually and at the menopause. Such associations should be explored.

appropriate to expand further: 'When you were growing up, did anyone ever hurt or abuse you?' Remember that abuse can occur in many forms, including emotional, physical and sexual, and that it can be both active and passive, such as in the case of neglect.

**Relationships, marriage and children** The course, duration and quality of relationships can reflect personality and suggest areas of stress. Mental health problems may be caused by or impair relationships. It is important to ask about children and their problems. Enquiries include:

- **Current status:** for example married/cohabiting, duration of the relationship, partner's personality and occupation, quality and satisfaction, attitude toward partner, for example separations and the ability to confide in or communicate and give and receive support.
- **Previous relationships:** age of first significant relationship, subsequent relationships (details as above, focusing on the most important), longest within and outside the current relationship, any repeated patterns within relationships, reasons for ending relationships, for example divorce or death of spouse, with dates and the patient's response.
- **Children:** names, health, learning or behavioural problems, psychiatric help, ability of patient to provide care, attitudes to children, quality of the relationship, social services involvement and family composition.

**Current life circumstances** Ask which life circumstances, if any, cause undue stress. If none is identified, enquiries about money, housing, neighbours and support from family, friends or professional agencies may identify significant stresses or areas of need.

## Forensic history

This may be a sensitive area, and the purpose of questions should be explained clearly. Your questions may identify long-standing maladaptive behaviour or legal transgressions driven by symptoms of psychiatric illness.

'Have you had any difficulties that led to legal problems or contact with the police?'

Particularly note any violent or sexual offences, or other dangerous behaviour (e.g. arson).

This will have implications for management and for the safety of others, including those involved in the patient's care. Even if there has been no legal involvement, you should ask about previous aggressive behaviour in order to gain an impression of the level of dangerousness of which the patient has been capable. If this behaviour is episodic, consider whether this may reflect historical episodes of illness.

You should ask about arrests, convictions and, where relevant, detentions, the longest period of imprisonment, mental health detentions via the courts or prison, attitude to offending behaviour, probation and the probation officer, and outstanding charges.

**Substance misuse** The use of illicit drugs and alcohol bears a twofold relationship to mental disorders. They may be associated with the development of an illness or episode of illness, but are also frequently used as a form of 'self-medication' to help alleviate symptoms. Further considerations are the presence of a dependence syndrome or addiction and the effects of acute intoxication, which might include the new onset of psychiatric symptoms or alterations in behaviour.

Substances differ in their ability to cause dependence and withdrawal symptoms, and in their tendency to precipitate psychiatric symptoms. Patients may present with symptoms reflecting drug intoxication or withdrawal, or with psychiatric disorders triggered by the abuse of drugs. The acute effects of drugs may include psychotic symptoms (seen most often with amphetamine, cocaine and LSD). Alcohol abuse is associated with delirium tremens, chronic organic brain disorders and a chronic paranoid psychosis. If an abuse of a common drug is suspected, a simple urine dipstick may confirm recent use (typically opiates, benzodiazepines, cannabis and cocaine). Urine or serum toxicology may be required for other substances.

Enquiries should include:

- The substance used, the duration of first use, route of administration and (if intravenous use) safe injecting practice.
- The amount used. This is sometimes difficult to clarify. Ask how much was used in the previous day, and work backwards to build up an initial picture of use during the previous week. Ask how much money is spent and how the habit is funded.

- Evidence of dependence, the longest period of abstinence and withdrawal effects (e.g. alcohol – morning nausea or shaking, delirium tremens or fits).
- Adverse effects – psychological, physical and social (e.g. criminality and family or work problems).
- Treatments – for example outpatient/inpatient detoxification, rehabilitation or attendance at Alcoholics Anonymous or similar groups.

**Personality** This describes an individual's habitual pattern of behaviour. A personality disorder occurs when a person's consistent behaviour causes repeated suffering to themself or to other people. This disorder is different from a mental illness by there being no clear onset and by the long-standing nature of the problems, which usually started in childhood or adolescence. Personality may influence the expression of mental illness, while certain personality traits may predispose to particular types of illness. Furthermore, stresses that can precipitate illness can also exacerbate the maladaptive behaviour which characterises personality disorders.

In practice, an individual's personality is too complex a matter to be able to adequately and accurately appraise in a single assessment, especially in the absence of a collateral history. Personality traits may be evident from the history and from your experience of the patient during the assessment; remember that these are enduring aspects of an individual's behaviour and their means of contextualising and interacting with the world around them. As such, the personality traits exhibited during an interview, which the patient may find anxiety-provoking, are unlikely to represent a stable reflection of enduring behaviour.

It is important not to stereotype your patient or be judgemental about a patient's personality.

In assessing personality sources of information include:

- The patient's account – this may be coloured by the current illness, for example depressed patients may have difficulty saying anything positive about themselves. It may also be inaccurate: for example, antisocial behaviour may be understated or a report of being 'happy-go-lucky' given when this trait is not corroborated.
- Moods, stability and variability ('cyclothymia').
- Impulse control, for example self-harm (see *Table 12.3*) and verbal or physical aggression.

- Leisure, whether solitary or collective, hobbies and interests.
- Coping with stress and how previous difficulties were dealt with.
- Relationships and the ability to trust others, for example stable and long-term or short and fleeting relationships.
- Information from other parts of the history. This may provide a better indication of any problems, for example adversity, suffering, behavioural or emotional problems in early life, relationship or work difficulties and antisocial behaviour (e.g. criminality or substance misuse).
- Objective opinions of other informants, who know the patient well, which are often the most reliable sources of information. If possible, it is important to obtain the patient's consent first.

## Table 12.3 Assessment of deliberate self-harm

A common presentation. The aim is to identify mental illness and patients at risk of committing suicide. Factors associated with increased risk include the following:

*The patient*
- Socially isolated
- Male
- Older age (young males are also at higher risk)
- Unemployed

- Psychiatric diagnosis
- Previous attempt(s)
- Chronic painful illness
- Family history of mental illness/suicide
- Alcohol or drug misuse

*The attempt*
- Planning (e.g. taking care of affairs, leaving a note, and steps to avoid detection)
- Method (e.g. violent, severe [if overdose] or believed to be lethal)

*Mental state*
- Depressed mood
- Suicidal thoughts
- Hopelessness
- Delusions/hallucinations

*The history*
- Recent life event (e.g. bereavement, retirement or divorce)

## Table 12.4 Checklist for psychiatric history taking

- Demographic information
- Presenting complaints
- Past psychiatric history
- Past medical history
- Family history
- Personal background
  - Childhood
  - Education

- Occupation
- Sexual and relationships
- Current social circumstances
- Forensic history
- Substance misuse
- Personality

The following areas of enquiry may be relevant:

- Attitude to others and to self, for example friends and colleagues, the ability to trust and confide, self-esteem, confidence, self-consciousness and satisfaction with achievements.
- Standards, for example religious beliefs, obsessionality and perfectionism. Such questions may include: 'How would you describe yourself?', 'What do you feel are your strengths and weaknesses?' and 'Do you have a strong religious faith?'

A number of traits associated with defined personality disorders have been described. Examples include anankastic (obsessional), passive-dependent, passive aggressive, antisocial and paranoid. It is best to describe patients using dimensional measures (e.g. 'moderately passive aggressive') rather than categorical descriptions, as there is considerable overlap between personality traits and the severity of a disorder will determine its presentation. A checklist for psychiatric history taking is shown in *Table 12.4*.

## Examination of the patient

### Mental state examination

The mental state examination (MSE) is an assessment of the patient's behaviour and state of mind at the time of the interview (*Table 12.5*). It is analogous to, but not exclusive of, the medical physical examination. While the history can be expanded after the initial assessment, the MSE

## Table 12.5 Mental state examination

- Appearance and behaviour
- Speech
- Mood
- Thought content
- Perception
- Cognitive function
- Insight

is a once-only 'snapshot' taken at a particular time. Repeated examinations may be needed as part of the diagnostic process, so that a patient can explain and better communicate their internal world, as well as respond to changing thoughts and feelings. The MSE may be the only source of information on which to base the initial diagnosis and management, for example in the case of uncooperative or uncommunicative patients.

A good MSE depends on a good use of communication skills and knowledge of how key symptoms are defined (descriptive psychopathology), asking appropriate questions and the systematic collection of information under the headings outlined. Clear descriptions and quoted speech are preferable to subjective terms such as 'normal' or 'reasonable', which convey little information. Negative findings should be recorded if they contribute to the diagnosis or management, for example noting that there is no depressive affect or no suicidal ideas. Information from corroborative sources, for example nursing observations, may be included.

### Appearance and behaviour

This section of the examination can provide important clues to diagnosis, as a great deal of subjective mental experience can be reflected in the patient's appearance and behaviour. Once again, however, be careful not to be judgemental in your assessment.

Aspects to consider include general physical appearance, state of dress, facial appearance, posture and movement (gait) and socially interactive behaviour.

The attitude to the interviewer, rapport and level of cooperation will be variable and should be noted. Some of the observable features that may reflect psychiatric problems include:

- **Anxiety:** tension, apprehension, sensitivity to noise or light, vigilance, irritability, restlessness and tendency to fidget. Face – flushed or pale, sweating and lined due to tension in the facial muscles. Eyes – widened, with dilated pupils. Posture – stiff and tense, with elevated shoulders.

- **Depression:** poor self-care, signs of weight loss and difficult rapport. Face – sad, unanimated, reduced blinking, but there can be tears. Eyes – contact reduced and eyes downcast. Reduced or increased movement (retardation or agitation).

- **Mania:** overactivity, disinhibition, distractability, noisiness, irritability, arousal, over-friendliness or familiarity, hostility or truculence. Clothes – bright, inappropriate or neglected. Face – cheerful or irritated look. Eye contact: intense.

- **Hallucinating:** strange, seemingly purposeless behaviour, sudden changes in movements, reduced cooperation and attention, distracted and socially withdrawn. Face – preoccupied or perplexed, sudden intense change in gaze in response to extraneous stimuli, unusual movements of the facial muscles, subvocal movements of the mouth or tongue, talking to themself, or incongruous smiling or fear.

- **Delusions:** bizarre behaviour, arousal, hostility due to suspiciousness and verbal or physical aggression. Dress – bizarre or inappropriate. Face – fearful and wary. Eyes scanning the environment.

- **Delirium:** impaired attention, reduced cooperation, overactivity alternating with inactivity, repetitive purposeless movements (e.g. plucking at the bed clothes). Signs of anxiety, hallucinations and abnormal ideas.

- **Schizophrenia:** strange, inappropriate or socially awkward behaviour, and self neglect. Behaviour suggesting delusions or hallucinations. Blunted or absent affect. Uncommon specific motor abnormalities may be evident that include stereotypies (repeated regular movements without obvious purpose, e.g. rocking to and fro), mannerisms (regular movements with some functional significance, e.g. saluting), posturing (adopting bodily positions for long periods of time), negativism (a tendency to perform the opposite action to that which is asked while resisting efforts to encourage compliance), echopraxia (automatic imitation of the interviewer's movements) or ambitendence (seemingly purposeless alternation between opposite movements). There may be signs of the side effects of medication, for example akathisia, pseudo-Parkinson's syndrome or tardive dyskinesia (involuntary orofacial or bodily movements).

## Speech

This section deals with how the patient speaks, which is assessed with reference to tone, volume, spontaneity, rate, quantity (amount) and form (reflecting the form of thought).

- In **depression**, speech may be monotonous and softly delivered, hesitant or only in response to questions (reduced spontaneity). The rate may be reduced (retardation of speech), which, together with slow movement, is described as psychomotor retardation. Speech may be reduced in amount and monosyllabic (poverty of speech).
- In **mania**, speech may be loud, rapid and difficult to interrupt (pressure of speech). Speech may be disordered in the form of flight of ideas, which is characterised by frequent shifts of topic connected by sounds, puns, rhymes or word associations, which can be difficult to follow. Other abnormalities of the form of speech include circumstantial speech (inability to stick to the point), neologisms (new words created by patient) and perseveration (repetition of the previous verbal response).
- **Thought blocking** is an abrupt cessation in the flow of speech that can be experienced when anxious, but may be a manifestation of delusional experience (i.e. thought withdrawal – see below). If this occurs, ask why – 'Could you tell me what happened when you suddenly stopped talking?'
- **Disordered thinking** occurs with schizophrenia. The speech becomes difficult to understand or unintelligible, and the logical sequence of thoughts is difficult to follow. This is also referred to as 'loosening of associations' or 'knight's move thinking'. In its most severe form, speech becomes an incoherent mixture of words and phrases ('word salad').

## Mood/affect

Change in mood defines a mood disorder, but may also occur in other psychiatric disorders. Objective evidence of mood disturbance can be taken from the patient's appearance, behaviour and speech, and is termed their 'affect'. A patient will describe their mood and will feel an emotion. Examine for:

- **Congruity:** does the affect match the patient's described mood? Incongruity suggests loss of control over emotional responses and can be seen in schizophrenia and personality disorders.
- **Reactivity:** this refers to how the mood changes during the interview as a response to the social interaction.

---

### BOX 12.5 SPECIFIC MOOD DISTURBANCES

Initial, open questions might be:

- 'How are you feeling?'
- 'How do you feel in your mood?'

Closed questions might include:

- 'Have you been feeling particularly low or sad … happy or particularly cheerful?'

If the answer is yes, ask for elaboration.
In a mood disturbance, the individual may be:

- Depressed, whereby the mood is reported as sad, low, despondent, anhedonic (lacking enjoyment) or blue.
- Elevated, described as extraordinarily happy, high, elated, super-confident and full of energy – as seen in mania.
- Anxious, fearful, apprehensive or worrying repetitively.
- Irritable, with impatience, anger or hostility – as seen in both mania and depressive illness.
- Labile, where the mood rapidly changes from high to low and irritable, as seen in mania, mixed affective states (an uncommon mixture of depression and mania) and delirium.
- Blunted, where the mood is impassive or absent, as often seen in chronic schizophrenia.

The extent of the mood disturbance and the thoughts that may develop from it must be explored by asking about the following. Abnormalities may be evident even if mood disturbance is not conspicuous:

- **Biological features:** there may be changes in sleep, appetite, weight, sexual function, bowel habit and diurnal variation in mood – suggesting that depression may be identified from the history.

---

*(Continued)*

## BOX 12.5 (*Continued*) SPECIFIC MOOD DISTURBANCES

- **Motivation/interest:** if reduced and the patient has become less productive (depression), ask 'Have you found yourself motivated to do the things you usually do?' If increased – with overactivity, extravagant projects might be started, but not necessarily completed or done well (mania), enquire: 'Have you developed any new interests recently?' 'Are they finished and complete?'
- **Energy:** this can be reduced (depression) or increased (mania).
- **Ability to experience pleasure:** an inability to experience pleasure (anhedonia) is an important symptom, which suggests significant depression of mood. Look for a change in attitude to things that the patient previously enjoyed, taking examples from the history. 'Are you able to enjoy anything at the present time?'
- **Memory and concentration:** ask about subjective impairments that may be evident in depression. 'Do you have difficulty in remembering things?'
- **Helplessness or hopelessness:** loss of hope and pessimism indicates significantly depressed mood, and is a predictive factor for suicide. 'Do you see things improving?' ... 'How do you see the future?'
- **Suicidal feelings:** if a depressed mood is suspected, suicidal thoughts and any suicide plans made must be explored in detail. Asking about the subject does not put new ideas into patients' heads, nor does it increase the risk of an already suicidal patient taking their own life. Those with suicidal thoughts (the majority of patients with depressive illness) will find that it helps to talk about these feelings. Identifying them shows an understanding and acknowledgement of the patient's distress. 'How bad does it get?' ... 'Have you had any desperate thoughts?' ... 'Have you thought it would be better not to go on?' ... 'Have you had any suicidal thoughts or intent?' Although most typically associated with a depressed affect, suicide risk is increased in all mental disorders apart from obsessive compulsive disorder. It is, therefore a vital consideration when assessing any patient's mental state.

(*Continued*)

## BOX 12.5 (Continued)  SPECIFIC MOOD DISTURBANCES

- **Other mood-associated thoughts:** a negative attitude to themself, others and events, guilt, self-recrimination, worthlessness and low self-esteem are all associated with depression. Overconfidence and excessive optimism, expansive thinking and extravagant plans (see also delusions) are all associated with mania.

**Thought content** You should concentrate your enquiries on abnormalities suggesting diagnoses. These may include predominant concerns or morbid ideas. Record the patient's responses to questions such as 'What would you say are your main worries?' Subsequent questions may be guided by the history. Specific enquiries may be necessary concerning:

- Anxiety, panic (sudden-onset intense fear and apprehension associated with physical symptoms of anxiety and ideas of 'losing control'), phobias (morbid irrational fears of situations or objects that are then avoided): 'Have you been feeling anxious, tense or frightened? ... How often? ... In what circumstances?' 'Are you having these feelings now?'
- Attitude to health, bodily concern or body image disturbance: 'Have you any worries about your physical health?' 'Have you suffered from an eating disorder?'
- Obsessions (recurrent persistent thoughts, impulses or images present despite efforts to resist them). These ruminations are recognised as the patient's own, and often concern dirt or contamination. They are usually associated with compulsive behaviour in order to minimise the ruminations (e.g. repeated hand washing). Ask 'Have you been finding decisions difficult?' 'Have you been spending a lot of time washing yourself or checking things?'

## Delusions

**Definition** These are beliefs for which there are no rational grounds, which are unshakeable despite counter-argument or proof to the contrary, and which are inconsistent with the individual's cultural background.

Delusions are very helpful in making a diagnosis. Their presence defines the illness as a psychosis. Delusions may be detected when the patient is asked about their main worries, but closed questions are often required. A positive response to such a question should always be clarified with open questions. The firmness with which the belief is held, and its plausibility, should be established. Ask the patient about the feelings that are associated with the abnormal beliefs expressed, and whether they have any particular actions in mind. Delusional thinking may motivate behaviour, and detailed enquiries should be made considering the health and safety of the patient and that of other people. Delusions may be classified according to the following:

**Onset**

*Primary delusions* are uncommon but are highly suggestive of schizophrenia. They arise from a delusional mood and usually follow a delusional perception. A delusional mood is the feeling that something unusual and ill defined is happening that concerns the patient. A delusional perception is a normal perception followed by a delusional interpretation. For example, the sensation that something momentous is about to happen, followed by seeing the traffic lights turn green and suddenly realising that you are the Messiah, would represent delusional mood, a normal or mundane perception and an instantaneous delusional misinterpretation.

'Do you have a feeling that something strange is going on around you?'

'Do you feel that some of the things you see around you have a particular meaning for you?'

Clarification is always required.

*Secondary delusions* arise in the context of other disorders of mental state, such as mood, for example delusions of guilt following the onset of depression. One significant difference between primary and secondary delusions is their 'understandability'. Primary delusions are typically bizarre, and following the connections that the patient might make that led to them is difficult. Secondary delusions are easier to understand as they arise within a context – such as guilt within low mood in the example above.

**Theme**

*Persecutory delusions* are the most frequently encountered; they can occur in delirium and schizophrenia, but less often in affective disorders. They may arise in mania but usually occur secondary to other abnormal beliefs, such as believing that people are spying on you because of a particular special ability that you may have and which they want.

'Do you believe anyone is trying to harm you?'

*Grandiose delusions* relate to ideas of exaggerated self-importance and abilities. They are particularly associated with mania.

'Do you feel that you have any extraordinary abilities?'

'Do you think anyone could have reason to be envious of you?'

*Delusions of reference* are beliefs that aspects of the environment, for example objects, events, people or communications, have a particular significance to the patient. They are suggestive of schizophrenia. The appropriateness of this belief should be explored in order to distinguish from the self-consciousness which some have in social situations. Non-delusional thoughts of this type are termed 'ideas of reference'.

'Do you have the feeling that people are talking about you?'

'Do you think people mention you on radio, television or in the newspaper?'

**Passivity phenomena** These involve the belief that one is no longer in control of one's thoughts, desires or actions. They are usually separated into passivity or delusions of thought possession and of control.

*Delusions of thought possession* a number of delusional experiences are recognised in which the patient may lose the conviction that their thoughts are private experiences under their own control. These are highly suggestive of schizophrenia and include:

- **Thought insertion:** the patient believes that some of their thoughts have been put into their mind from outside.
- **Thought withdrawal:** the patient believes that some of their thoughts have been removed from their mind; this may be evident

objectively by a sudden cessation in the flow of speech that is known as thought blocking (see above).

- **Thought broadcasting:** this is the belief that thoughts, although unspoken, may become known to other people by various means, such as them directly hearing the thoughts; this must be distinguished from the common feeling that others can infer thoughts from a person's actions. 'Do you have difficulty thinking clearly?' … 'Have you had the feeling that perhaps your thoughts were not your own?'

*Delusion of control* is the belief that actions, impulses or volitions, or sensations (somatic passivity) are being controlled and caused by an outside agent. This can be distinguished from command hallucinations that the individual obeys. Delusions of control are sometimes referred to as passivity experiences, and are highly suggestive of schizophrenia. 'Do you ever feel that you are not completely in control of … some of your actions … thoughts … feelings … the functioning of your body?'

*Delusions of guilt and worthlessness* are associated with severe depressive illness.

'Do you feel you are to blame for anything?'

*Nihilistic delusions* are abnormal beliefs that the patient has ceased to exist, or that something inside has died. It is an unusual delusion, but can be seen in a depressive psychosis.

*Delusion of jealousy* is the conviction of an individual (usually male) about their partner's infidelity. Their presence is a matter for great concern, as dangerously aggressive behaviour can ensue. Morbid jealousy should be distinguished from less intense and less persistent preoccupations, which are relatively common.

Other delusional themes include *religious, hypochondriacal and sexual/amorous.*

### Perception
- *Déjà vu* phenomena are feelings of having seen or done something before when in fact the experience is novel. They are associated with complex partial seizures, although they occur in other disorders and can occur as a normal experience.

- **Depersonalisation and derealisation** are unpleasant feelings of an altered unreal sense of self or the external world. Objects seem less real and the sense of the passage of time is often altered (sped up or slowed down). Although they can occur in the absence of psychiatric illness, they are particularly associated with anxiety disorders.
- **Illusions** are abnormal perceptions of external stimuli. Visual illusions are associated with delirium, are more common in Parkinson's disease and are more likely when sensory stimulation is reduced, for example a poorly lit ward. They may also arise in the context of a normal mental state.

**Hallucinations** These are perceptions in the absence of an external stimulus. They have a similar quality to that of a true perception (i.e. they are perceived in objective space rather than inside the head). Their presence can be suggested by a patient's behaviour, for example auditory hallucinations by a patient speaking to themself. They can occur in any of the five senses. Brief hallucinations when falling asleep (hypnagogic) or while wakening (hypnopompic) are within the range of normal experience. Since some patients may conceal or are unable to express their hallucinations, enquiries should be tactful and sensitive.

Auditory hallucinations are most common and occur in all psychoses, although certain types are particularly associated with schizophrenia.

'Have you been having any strange or unusual experiences?'

'Do you sometimes hear noises or whispering that no one else seems to hear?'

'Do you sometimes hear someone is speaking to or about you when there is no one else around?'

Hallucinations can be considered in terms of their:

- Modality (auditory, visual, tactile, olfactory, gustatory).
- Nature (simple or complex).
- Content.

## Cognitive assessment (see also Chapter 6)

All patients should undergo cognitive screening, although this will vary in complexity depending on the presenting difficulties. If the patient can give a clear and accurate history, there is unlikely to be a cognitive impairment. The aim is to carry out a global assessment of intellectual functioning. Some patients may find the questions very easy, and it is useful to acknowledge this and explain the reason for them in order to avoid any possible offence being taken:

> 'I'd like to ask some questions to test your memory and thinking, which are part of the routine assessment; you may find them easy.'

**Orientation** Is the patient fully alert or is there an impairment of attention, suggesting an acute organic mental disorder (delirium)?

**Attention and concentration** In the digit span test (a test of registration or immediate memory), ask the patient to repeat a sequence of digits given slowly, both forwards and backwards. The average person should manage six numbers forwards and five backwards.

**Memory**
- **Short-term memory:** ask the patient to recall a name and address, learned accurately 5 minutes earlier. Make sure the patient can say it fully and accurately initially without prompting, otherwise the problem could be of registration rather than retention of new material.
- **Long-term memory:** test for current affairs and well-known information, for example leaders of state.

**Intelligence** Simple arithmetic, meanings of words and reading (ask the patient to read a newspaper if there is one to hand).

**Tests of specific cortical areas** An example is of visuospatial awareness. Ask the patient to draw a clock, copy a three-dimensional object, put on an article of clothing (parietal lobe), name objects or perform abstract reasoning (frontal lobe).

**Insight** This is the patient's understanding of the nature of their problems. The degree of insight varies between patients and may change over time. Severely restricted insight is a poor prognostic sign that may lead to non-compliance with treatment and continuation or recurrence of the illness. It is the most consistent symptom in psychosis, affecting 98% of patients, although it is not defining in this regard. Attempts to improve insight are an important part of management.

Insight can be divided into three parts – recognising that something is wrong, being able to conceive of this as illness and recognising that treatment might be required. It can be assessed using a series of enquiries, the responses to which should be summarised.

'What do you think is wrong with you?'

'Is the cause within you or something outside?'

'Do you think you are ill?'

'What do think will help you?'

'Do you understand what this treatment is for?'

## Physical examination

When psychiatric admission is considered necessary, the responsibility for medical care is transferred to the psychiatric team, and a physical examination and relevant investigations are carried out. However, the possibility of an underlying physical cause should be considered in all psychiatric presentations, and physical examination and investigations performed as indicated.

## Key laboratory tests and investigations

Specific tests will be determined by the particular presentation. Commonly ordered investigations are listed in *Table 12.6*.

The following illustrations depict the key features found in anxiety (**Fig. 12.1**), schizophrenia (**Fig. 12.2**), depression (**Fig. 12.3**) and mania (**Fig. 12.4**).

## Table 12.6 Key laboratory tests/investigations

- Thyroid function tests
- Urea and electrolytes (calcium concentration)
- Liver function tests
- Full blood count, plasma viscosity
- Venereal Disease Reference Laboratory (VDRL)
- Hepatitis virus antibodies, HIV counselling and testing
- Therapeutic drug monitoring (lithium, anticonvulsant levels)
- Urine screen for illicit drugs
- Electroencephalography (EEG)
- Computed tomography (CT) and magnetic resonance imaging (MRI) scans for neuropsychiatric presentations

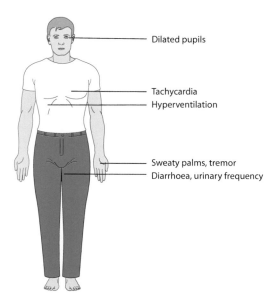

Fig. 12.1 Anxiety.

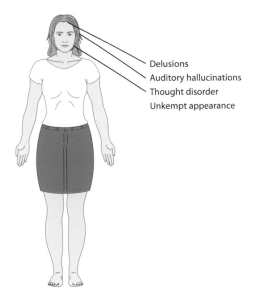

Delusions
Auditory hallucinations
Thought disorder
Unkempt appearance

Fig. 12.2 Schizophrenia.

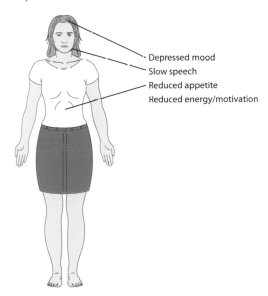

Depressed mood
Slow speech
Reduced appetite
Reduced energy/motivation

Fig. 12.3 Depression.

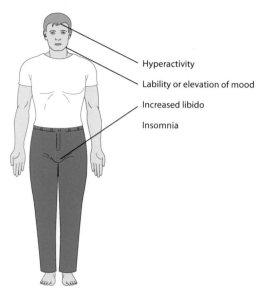

Hyperactivity

Lability or elevation of mood

Increased libido

Insomnia

Fig. 12.4 Mania.

# Chapter 13
## Paediatric history and examination

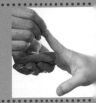

This chapter explores the key aspects of history taking and examination in children and young people. It both builds on some of the similarities that will be familiar from adult medicine and details some of the key additional areas that need a specific focus. It emphasises the importance of really listening to children, young people and their parents and carers, the value of observation and the role we all have in safeguarding the welfare of children.

There is no doubt that successfully taking a history from and examining a child is more an art than a science. However, in order to develop these skills, the same basic knowledge as applies to adults needs to be thoroughly learned and then adapted to the needs of the child in front of you. Children can get bored quickly and may have a particular order in which they feel most comfortable explaining things. Likewise, when observing and examining a child, one must seize the opportunities as they arise, while keeping in mind an orderly scheme so as not to miss any signs. There is also great value in serial observation of children to establish whether or not they are improving.

The approach taken to babies, toddlers, primary school-age children and young people needs to adapt depending on their cognitive and communication skills. The aim, wherever possible, is to give them space for their voice and opinions. For young people, this also means ensuring that they also have the opportunity to be seen without their parents.

## A scheme for history taking and examination of the child

Paediatric history taking and examination can be time-consuming. However, time can be minimised if you spend a few cursory minutes gaining the confidence of the child's parents and the child's confidence in you. A relaxed, friendly introduction is important, clearly stating your name, exactly who you are (and what that means) and your aims. Get everyone seated or at least comfortable. You quickly need to establish the baby's or child's given name, the name by which they like to be called and their age and sex. The latter is not always obvious, and it is better to avoid embarrassment later on. Never refer to a baby as 'it'. Next, determine the relationship of those in the room to the child. It is all too easy to assume the big sister is the mother, or that the grandmother is the mother and the real mother the child's sister!

Once you have engaged the parents, introduce yourself to the child – preferably using your given name and theirs. If the child is very young and unable to contribute much to the interview, aim to distract them with handily placed toys. If the child is older, try to start by talking with them in the initial history taking, with frequent, but gentle, affirmations of the parents' details. The more you can get children to talk from the beginning, the more you will learn from them – their parents can then add to the story afterwards. This does not always work but as a general rule is worth trying in all children who are in school (5 years old and above).

Watch how the child plays with toys, in particular how the hands and feet are used, the eyes and ears, and the way the child moves. Assess the child's level of anxiety: for example, are they happy to leave their mother or father to play or do they remain on their parent's lap? Are they altogether disinterested? If so, they may be feeling quite ill. All this visual information will also give you an indication of how best to examine the child later. Try to gauge the gravity of the problem and the parents' concerns early on so that you can behave appropriately. Tuning in to parental anxiety and matching it with appropriate listening, concern, empathy and advice is a key tenet of care in paediatrics.

## Taking the history

Overall, the information sought in a child's medical history is the same as that for an adult, but with a few important additions and changes of emphasis. You have already ascertained the name, age and sex of the child – now you need the date of birth, name of the school or nursery they attend, where they live (including the address and telephone number) and who lives with them. You may want to begin with these administrative details or leave them to the social history section; either way, try to develop your own system so as not to forget to ask for these details.

When you first begin history taking, you may feel the need to write at the same time as listening, speaking and looking, which is quite difficult. It is worth asking the child's or parents' permission, and stopping the interview to do this. Try not to let this interfere with the natural flow of the interview – if needs be, take no notes at this time. Experienced paediatricians often write up their notes when the consultation is over. The emergence of electronic health records has changed this dynamic further, the key point being self-awareness around what writing and looking at a screen may do to the quality of the interaction with a child and their family.

### The presenting complaint

Start by noting the child's or parents' main complaint(s), allowing them to recount this in their own way. Only then ask specific questions to clarify important points. It is often a very useful exercise to repeat back to the child or parents these points, to show your understanding of the situation. Try to ascertain the time interval and chronology of events. It can be useful to ask when was the last time the child was completely well. If the problem(s) have been going on for some time, determine how much school has been missed and whether sports and leisure activities have been affected. It is important to enquire about altered patterns of sleep, appetite and activity as these are often associated with serious illness in children. Ask about weight loss. Is the cry different from normal? With babies, ask what volume of milk is usually taken and is currently actually taken. Try and get a picture of what the child is like when not ill. Are they an active child? Do they have many friends? What do they like playing with?

Rather than use a rigid system-by-system barrage of questions, try to concentrate on presenting problems and ask about associated features. The key is to be taking a history around a 'differential diagnosis'. This means asking questions that make certain possible diagnoses more or less likely. Some examples of this are given below:

- **Abdominal pain** is a common complaint in babies and children. Babies tend to draw up their legs with abdominal pain, but it must be remembered that this pain may emanate from anywhere. Toddlers often say that they have 'tummy ache' when asked to localise pain. Enquire about the type of pain and its timing. What aggravates and what relieves it? Is it constant or intermittent? Where does it radiate to? Children with chest infections or pneumonia can present with abdominal pain, as can children with tonsillitis who get associated cervical and abdominal lymphadenopathy. 'Is there any diarrhoea, constipation, blood in the stools, vomiting or swelling?'
- **Abdominal distension.** Is it present or absent? Has it been present but now resolved?
- **Vomiting.** You need to determine the frequency of vomiting and the volumes each time. The consistency and colour (bile stained, clear or bloody) of the vomitus is important. Is it forceful or projectile? – possibly indicative of upper gastrointestinal obstruction (i.e. pyloric stenosis). Is it associated with screaming (intussusception), diarrhoea or pyrexia? In babies, it is important to distinguish normal posseting from true vomiting.
- **Bowel movements.** Ask about the frequency of bowel opening and the consistency of the stools, bearing in mind that babies often have semi-solid, mustard-coloured motions. Determine whether there is any accompanying mucus or blood. If there is blood, is it streaky or uniform? Is it dark (melena) or fresh? What colour are the stools (pale or dark)? Are they difficult to flush away? Is there an unusual odour? Is there pain on defecation? Does the child soil (encopresis)?
- **Sore throat.** Infants and toddlers are unable to localise pain well and rarely complain of sore throats, but in older children it can be much more of a feature.
- **Swallowing** may be painful in an upper respiratory tract infection or tonsillitis and lead to refusal to eat. An obstructive or neuromuscular cause usually permits the child to swallow, but shortly afterwards the food is regurgitated.

- **Thirst.** Enquire about the frequency and intensity of thirst (frequent drinking is called polydipsia). Is it accompanied by excess urine output (diabetes or renal disease)? What kinds of volume are involved? Might the thirst be something behavioural?
- **Micturition.** Is there frequency or urgency? Is this nocturnal or only during the day? Is there accompanying pain (crying or screaming)? What is the colour of the urine (red, dark or clear)? Is there an unusual odour? Is the child's urine concentrated first thing in the morning?
- **Bed wetting or day wetting** (enuresis). This is common in young children, especially in boys up to the age of 10 years. How much water are they drinking and at what times of the day or evening? If this is a new symptom, have there been any recent events in the child's life that may be connected? Is the child chastised for bed wetting?
- **Cough** is common. You need to determine its character; is it moist or dry, worse at night, paroxysmal or continuous? Is it associated with chest pain, an inspiratory 'whoop' or wheezing? Is the quality 'barking' (croup)? Is the sputum clear, mucopurulent or bloodstained?
- **Difficulty in breathing.** Is breathing noisy (wheeze or stridor)? Is it associated with exercise or present at rest? Are there any exacerbating factors? Is there an associated cough or cyanosis? Does the child snore or sleep with their mouth open or shut?
- **Cyanosis.** Is this central or confined to the peripheries? Is it intermittent or persistent?
- **Pallor.** Babies are often pale and can become mottled even when there is only mild illness.
- **Breath.** Does the breath smell of acetone (peardrops), or is there fetor?
- **Swelling.** Determine the exact size and position, and whether it is increasing or decreasing. Is it painful at rest or just to touch? Is it fluctuant? Is there any associated lymphadenopathy?
- **Rashes and skin lesions.** Ascertain the site and distribution. Where did it begin? How has it spread, and over what timescale? Ask the parents to describe the rash in terms of its colour and morphology – blistering (vesicular), ulcerative, papular (raised), macular (flat) or itchy (pruritic). Has the child remained well with it?
- **Jaundice.** How long has this been noted? When did it start? Has there been any change in the colour of the urine or stools?
- **Musculature.** Ask whether the parents have noted any abnormal movements or lack of movement. Was the infant floppy at birth?

Does the mother find it difficult to handle her child for fear of the child slipping through her fingers (hypotonia)? On the other hand, is the child stiff (hypertonic/spasticity)? Are there any involuntary movements? In infants, a good history of feeding can be helpful here.

- **Posture.** Is there anything unusual about the child's posture?
- **Coordination.** Is the child unduly clumsy when their age is taken into account? Has this always been the case or is this a new phenomenon?
- **Fits.** Fits, and episodes that look like fits, are relatively common in young children and need to be thoroughly investigated. Ask the parents or witness what they saw and to describe the type of movements (if any) involved. 'Was there generalised shaking or localised twitching? … If so, which limb? … Was the child unconscious? … Did they vomit or bite their tongue? …How long did the episode last? …How long was the child unconscious for after the fits ceased? …Has this ever happened before? …Did the child hit their head before the fit or as a consequence of it? …Was the child incontinent? …Was there any indication of a preceding aura or pyrexia?' Have the parents managed to video an episode?
- **Speech.** Was there any delay in onset of speech? Is there any residual language or speech articulation problem? Once speech was achieved, was there any subsequent loss of speech? Ask whether the child has ever had speech therapy?
- **Vision.** If the patient is a baby, have the parents noted whether they are able to follow an object held close up? In older children, is there any difficulty in reading or seeing the blackboard at school? Does the child bump into things in subdued light (night blindness)?
- **Hearing.** Are there any concerns about hearing?
- **Behaviour.** Is the child active or hyperactive, or are they quiet or apathetic? How would the parents describe the child: aggressive or placid, gregarious or a loner, obedient or disobedient? If they are a toddler, do they show frequent temper tantrums, nightmares, sleep walking or night-time waking? How does the rest of the household cope with these problems, and what has been done to improve them so far?

In this section, it is really important to very openly ask the parents what they think is causing the problem(s). It is a key way to *really* listen, and may save you a lot of unnecessary questions, examining and investigations.

## Past medical history

Try to collect information in some kind of order. A chronological order of events is the easiest to remember.

**Pregnancy and birth** Begin at the beginning with the mother's pregnancy (single or multiple) and labour. Were there any maternal infections or illnesses? Did the antenatal scans show anything up? Was the baby born at term (40 weeks) or preterm (usually, for example, written as '30/40' if the baby was born at 30 weeks)? Was the delivery vaginal or caesarean? If the latter, was it elective (why) or emergency (why)? Was the presentation normal vertex or breech, or assisted by forceps or ventouse (suction) extraction? What was the baby's condition at birth? (If the mother has the child's community record book to hand, check the Apgar scores.) What was the birth weight? What were the first few days of life like (e.g. jaundice or a need for special care)? Was the baby breast- or bottle-fed and when were they weaned? Were there any feeding problems?

**Apgar scoring** This is a validated scoring system for assessing the health of a neonate. The total score (maximum 10; *Table 13.1*) is usually assessed at 1 and 5 minutes after birth. A low score of less than 5 at 5 minutes is associated with long-term developmental problems.

**Drug history and allergies** Has the child received any medication for the current problems? Are they on any long-term drugs? State the

### Table 13.1  The Apgar score

| | Score | | |
|---|---|---|---|
| **Sign** | **1** | **2** | **3** |
| Colour | Blue/pale | Pink trunk, blue extremities | Pink all over |
| Heart rate | Absent | <100 beats/min | >100 beats/min |
| Reflex irritability | None | Grimace | Cry |
| Tone | Limp | Some limb flexion | Active movement |
| Respiratory effort | Absent | Slow, irregular | Strong cry |

generic name as well as the trade name in all cases. Record the dose and frequency of administration, and not just what was prescribed.

Does the child have any allergies to drugs, house dust mites, cats, dogs, fur, nuts or shellfish? What happens when they are exposed to the antigen? Is there any history of acute anaphylaxis or rash? It is important to focus on both the history of allergy as well as any skin-prick or blood tests that may have previously been done.

**Infections or illnesses** Which common childhood infections/exanthems has the child had? Have there been any hospital admissions? Where and what were the date and duration? Has there been any recent contact with infectious persons or animals (including birds)?

**Recent travel or residence abroad** Obtain details of which countries the child has lived in, and whether they were resident in a town or rural location (malaria, for example, is seldom found in large towns).

**Immunisations** An immunisation history must be sought, noting whether it is up to date with the current national schedule. This continues to move and adapt with the introduction of new immunisations and approaches (three recent examples being rotavirus as part of the primary immunisations, nasal annual flu vaccines in younger children, and human papillomavirus vaccine for teenage girls), so look up the latest schedule. It is worth specifically asking about measles, mumps and rubella (MMR) vaccination as, despite very strong evidence for its safety, there are still communities who are anxious about giving it to their children. Additionally, has the child had any inoculations related to foreign travel (e.g. cholera or typhoid)? The 'Green Book' is the definitive national guide to vaccines and communicable diseases in the UK and is a very useful resource for up-to-date information in this area.

## Family history

Determine the relationship of all members of the immediate family. Constructing a family tree will help in organising your questions and records. You should record the age and state of health of each sibling and parent. Is the parents' union consanguineous? If so, to what degree? Have there been any childhood deaths or stillbirths? Are there any hereditary disorders in the family? Ask about thalassaemia and sickle cell disease if the patient is not white. As insight into genomics expands, it is likely that this is an area of healthcare that will change dramatically.

## Social history

This is a sensitive part of the interview, and there is no way easy way of asking the relevant questions. Most people do not mind answering these if you explain their importance. You need to know which family members work. What are their occupations? Are there any hazards? Who smokes cigarettes, a pipe or cigars? What is the overall mood in the household? Are there any conflicts, separations or divorces? Who else lives in the house other than the immediate family (note their name and sex in cases where there may be safeguarding concerns)? Try and ascertain the size and condition of the home. Is there heating, running water and adequate sanitation?

Try and determine how well the child is doing at school. Are they reluctant to go to school in the morning? Is the child being bullied? The child may be happy to tell you, a stranger, about these problems which they might not mention to their own family.

## Developmental history

Developmental milestones are divided into four broad categories:

1 Social.
2 Hearing, speech and language.
3 Vision and fine motor skills.
4 Gross motor skills.

Try to learn at least two features from each category at key ages (i.e. 6 weeks, 6 months, 1 year, 18 months, 2 years, 3 years, 4 years and 5 years), as this will give you a broad framework for assessing a child's development.

In basic terms, developmental assessment is about exploring, through both the history (i.e. what is reported by the parent[s]) and direct observation (i.e. what is actually seen during the assessment), which milestones the child is able to achieve (baseline) and not quite achieve (ceiling) in each of these four categories.

## Examination of the child

How you approach the examination depends on their age. The approach for older children will be no different from that used with adults. However, younger children are not so straightforward. Approach the child with a quiet voice and warm hands. Next – and this is most important – get down to the child's level, even if this means on your hands and knees or sitting on the floor. The examination is just as daunting for the child as for you. Keep your examination equipment out of sight or you will rapidly lose a friend before you have even begun. Introduce the stethoscope and allow the child to play with it. Starting to examine their parent's hand or knee with the stethoscope can be another gentle way to start.

Babies aged 1–3 months are surprisingly cooperative if you remember to smile and speak quietly. The easiest age for examination is probably between 6 and 10 months, when almost all babies are friendly. By about 10 months, as part of their developmental progress, they have learned to be suspicious of strangers, and remain so throughout their time as a toddler. This age group is the most difficult, and they need to be distracted by making a game of the examination. Let them play with your stethoscope or pen torch. Toddlers do not like to be stared at, and will usually avoid direct eye contact.

From 5 years onwards, children usually become more cooperative again, and are less reluctant to leave their parents' side. Always try to build conversations with the child and not at them. Try to break the ice by talking about something topical in the child's life, such as a favourite toy, pop group, game, sports team or TV programme. If the patient is very young, ask the parents to help undress the child down to the underwear at first. The rest can come off in stages. Begin by touching the child's hands, and even play a game such as 'this little piggy' to win their confidence. Demonstrate auscultation, auroscopy or ophthalmoscopy on an adult or doll first. Leave the examination of the ears, nose and throat until the end.

Babies almost always dislike having their head circumference measured, so it may be wise to leave this until later.

## Physical measurements
Do these first, so as not to forget them.

- **Height/length:** obtain measurements of crown–rump length, as this is easier to perform and more reliable than crown–heel length. Use a measuring board if available. Children who can stand need to be measured against a wall-mounted rule, with their shoes removed. Plot the values on age- and sex-related charts, and note the nearest percentile. If you are worried about limb length or asymmetry, measure both limbs for comparison. For the upper limbs, measure from the tip of the acromion process to the tip of the middle finger. For the lower limbs, measure from the anterior superior iliac spine to the internal malleolus.

- **Weight (Fig. 13.1):** a newborn baby usually loses 10–15% of their birth weight within the first week of life. They should have regained their birth weight by 10 days. The average weight gain in the first 3 months is about 25 g (around 1 oz) per day. Infants usually double their birth weight by 5 months, and treble it by 1 year. A quick formula for roughly estimating the weight of a child between 1 and 9 years of age is:

$$\text{Weight (kg)} = (\text{Age [in years]} + 4) \times 2$$

Again, these values need to be plotted on standard charts, and the nearest percentile noted.

**Head circumference (occipital frontal circumference)** Measurements are made at the level of the supraorbital ridges and the occipital protuberance (**Fig. 13.2**). Plot these on standard charts.

**Heart and respiratory rates** These basic measurements are key to paediatric practice. Normal values are age dependent and take significant experience to learn and be comfortable with; it is therefore best to continue to look them up and double check them. Measurements outside normal limits should lead the doctor to question what might be going on and to re-review the child, potentially with a senior colleague. The emergence of Paediatric Early Warning Score (PEWS) charts have helped to develop a structured way to look at what is and is not normal, and to escalate intervention appropriately.

**Blood pressure** Historically, auscultatory blood pressure measurements were taken using a cuff and sphygmomanometer in children aged 3 years and older, while in younger children and babies palpatory methods were employed. This is still done in many paediatric renal clinics, but the accuracy of automated blood pressure machines has significantly improved so this is now the standard way of measuring blood pressure. The usual caveats of ensuring the correct size of cuff is used remain. In difficult cases, Doppler ultrasound blood pressure monitors can also have value.

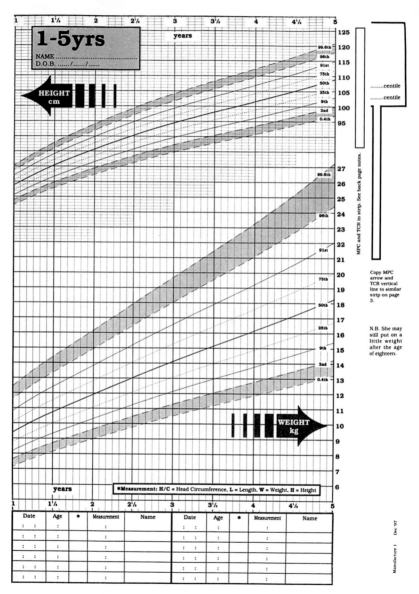

Fig. 13.1 Example of a growth chart for weight of girls aged 1–5 years.

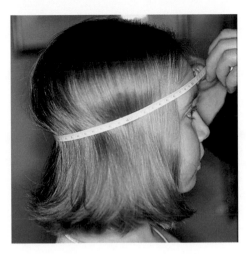

Fig. 13.2 Measuring the head circumference of a girl.

Normal blood pressure ranges are dependent on age, sex and height and so for accuracy should be looked up on centile charts. As a broad indicator, normal blood pressure values are:

- Newborn                     75/50 mmHg
- Infants                       80/55 mmHg (± 20%)
- Pre-school child           85/60 mmHg
- Primary school child     90/60 mmHg

It is important to point out that a low blood pressure in infants and children is a very late sign of circulatory compromise (occurring much later than in adults), so is a finding that requires immediate review and action.

**Temperature** In babies, a disposable thermometer may be placed in the groin crease or axilla. In older children, the axilla is preferred. Infrared devices have been developed in which an unobtrusive ear probe is placed in the external auditory meatus for 1 second to directly measure the reflected heat of the tympanic membrane. Many parents have one of these at home, but in clinics and wards the direct method still tends to be used as it is thought to be more accurate.

## BOX 13.1 EXAMINING THE CARDIOVASCULAR SYSTEM

- **Inspection.** Start with the peripheries and work your way centrally towards the heart. Note any cyanosis, clubbing, tachypnoea, pallor (anaemia) or polycythaemia. Watch for a visible precordial heave or lift due to heart enlargement (left ventricular hypertrophy– apical region; right ventricular hypertrophy – sternal/parasternal). The jugular venous pressure is very difficult to determine in young children due to the shortness of the neck, so, unlike in adults, this is not something that is routinely looked for.
- **Pulses.** Feel for the radial, brachial and femoral arteries bilaterally, using your fingertips and pressing lightly at first. It is easy to miss a pulse through total occlusion. The femoral pulses are often difficult to find, but persist in looking for them as a truly absent pulse may be indicative of coarctation of the aorta. Go on to look for radiofemoral delay. If you can feel a dorsalis pedis pulse in an infant, they do not have coarctation. Do not forget to place a hand over the scapulae if you suspect a coarctation – you may feel the pulsation of collateral vessels.

Determine whether the pulse volume is normal, large or small. Sinus arrhythmia (increased heart rate on inspiration and decreased rate on expiration) is accentuated but a normal finding in children. A large 'bounding' pulse may indicate a hyperdynamic circulation associated with shunting. A feeble, low-volume pulse may indicate left outflow tract restriction. A collapsing 'water-hammer' pulse is associated with aortic regurgitation.

## Examination by systems

A detailed description is provided here of the examination of an infant and older child. For details of the neonatal examination, the reader should refer to a textbook of neonatology. The general order for examination is as follows: inspection, percussion, palpation and auscultation. Perhaps even more so than in adults, there are significant opportunities for understanding what might be going on through observation and inspection, so these are really key phases not to rush.

## BOX 13.2 PRECORDIUM

The apex beat is best felt with the pulp tip of the third finger of the right hand lightly resting on the left fourth or fifth intercostal space between the mid-clavicular and mid-axillary lines (**Fig. 13.3**).

Precordial pulsations of left ventricular hypertrophy and right ventricular hypertrophy, and cardiac thrills, are best appreciated with the palm of the hand.

- **Percussion.** Unlike in the adult, percussion of the cardiac borders can be easily achieved in children due to the thinness of the thoracic cage. The right cardiac border should not extend beyond the right border of the sternum. The upper cardiac border should not be felt above the second intercostal space.
- **Auscultation.** It is acceptable to use the bell throughout the auscultatory examination of young children. However, in difficult situations the second heart sound is often best heard with the diaphragm over the pulmonary area. A systematic examination should begin by listening over the mitral area (apex), the pulmonary area (second left costal cartilage), the aortic area (in the first and second intercostal spaces at the right sternal edge) and the tricuspid area (along the left lower sternal edge at about the fourth intercostal space). Listen for radiation of murmurs: mitral systolic into the left axilla, aortic systolic into the neck. Physiological splitting of the second heart sound can often best be heard over the pulmonary area on inspiration in children and young adults. A third heart sound is also commonly heard, especially at the apex, and is entirely normal in young individuals. This should be differentiated from a pathological splitting of the second sound, which is more widely spaced (and quieter) than the physiological split. Other sounds to note are the presence of a gallop rhythm (heart failure) and a pericardial rub.

Examination for hepatosplenomegaly and other respiratory signs of heart failure is also an important part of a cardiovascular system examination.

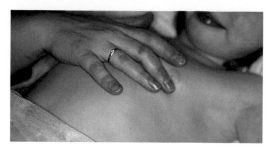

Fig. 13.3 Listening for the apex beat.

## BOX 13.3 EXAMINING THE RESPIRATORY SYSTEM

Look at the shape of the chest. Note the presence of any deformities such as pectus excavatum, pectus carinatum (pigeon chest), Harrison's sulci (chronic severe asthma), costochondral junction swelling (rickety rosary) or dinner-fork deformity (scurvy).

Is there prolonged expiration, as in virally induced wheeze or asthma? Is there any intercostal indrawing or costal recession indicative of airflow obstruction? Are there any upper airways noises such as stridor (inspiratory or expiratory), grunting (infants) or wheezing (expiratory)?

- **Percussion.** Chest percussion in the child is more resonant than in the adult, and it is relatively easy to determine dullness.
- **Auscultation.** Due to the equality of the inspiratory and expiratory phases, breath sounds in children are bronchovesicular. Breath sounds may be decreased in bronchiolitis, pneumothorax, severe asthma, pleural effusion, collapse or emphysema. They may be increased in consolidation of the lung and have a whistling quality of bronchial breathing, in which the inspiratory and expiratory phases are of equal length. The wheeze of asthma tends to be high-pitched and 'musical', and the expiratory phase is likely to be prolonged. Listen for a pleural rub.

Vocal resonance may be diminished in pleural effusion and increased in consolidation. Whispering pectoriloquy may be heard with consolidation. It is fair to say that neither of these, nor chest expansion, is routinely tested in respiratory examinations in children as the yield of useful information is very low.

## BOX 13.4 EXAMINING THE ABDOMEN

Begin with the hands, looking for signs of anaemia, clubbing, leu-conychia and spider naevi. Note any distension of the abdomen, and whether there is accompanying venous congestion indicative of liver disease (and ascites). Look for visible peristalsis, which may be associated with obstruction. Is there swelling at the hernial ori-fices (including the umbilicus – **Figs 13.4** and **13.5**)?

- **Palpation.** Make sure the child is lying flat on the couch or in their parent's arms. Before you begin palpitation, a really nice trick is to ask the patient to make their tummy as big or fat as their possibly can, and then to suck it in to make it as small and thin as they possibly can. This can be done with you standing at the end of the bed. If they are able to do this without pain, peritonitis, for example from a perforated appendicitis, is very unlikely.

  Kneel down so as to be on a level with the child's abdomen, and warm your hands. Begin by using your right hand with light palpation in all four quadrants to determine whether there are any areas of tenderness. If you ask a young child (e.g. a toddler) whether they have pain, they often invariably answer in the affir-mative – which may be unhelpful. Always watch the child's face. If there is tenderness, test for rebound tenderness by sudden withdrawal of the hand on deep palpation. If the pain is severe, there may be abdominal guarding or even board-like rigidity.

  If there is mild or no tenderness, proceed with deeper palpation of specific organs. We suggest beginning with the spleen. In young children the spleen enlarges into the left iliac fossa, whereas in older children and young adults it tends to enlarge across the midline to the right iliac fossa. Work your way up into the left hypochondrium until you can just tip the spleen on inspiration. Concomitant placement of your left hand in the child's left renal angle and lifting gently will facilitate identification of the spleen.

  Next, identify the sharp hepatic edge on inspiration, begin-ning in the right iliac fossa and working upwards towards the right costal margin. The liver edge is usually felt one finger-breadth below the costal margin in young children (**Fig. 13.6**).

*(Continued)*

## BOX 13.4 *(Continued)* EXAMINING THE ABDOMEN

The kidneys are best balloted between the examiner's hands, with the left hand placed behind the child in the renal angle and the right hand on the right hypochondrium (**Fig. 13.7**).

Palpate the suprapubic region for a distended bladder. A pyloric mass may be felt in the right hypochondrium close to the midline, and historically was best elicited with the child bottle-feeding. In reality, if this diagnosis is suspected, ultrasound is used to examine this area. An intussusception is sausage-shaped and can on occasions be felt in the right upper quadrant during abdominal relaxation. Again ultrasound is a key adjunct to clinical examination here. If ascites is suspected, try and elicit a fluid thrill.

- **Percussion.** This may be helpful in determining the borders of the liver. If there is a suspicion of free fluid in the abdomen, percuss for dullness in the flank with the patient supine. If dullness is present, turn the child onto their left side and percuss again to determine whether there is shifting dullness.
- **Auscultation.** Bowel sounds may be loud following a feed (borborygmi) or tinkling in partial obstruction. They are usually absent in complete obstruction or ileus.

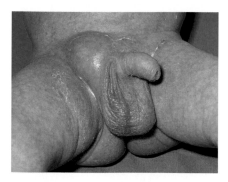

Fig. 13.4 Inguinal hernia.

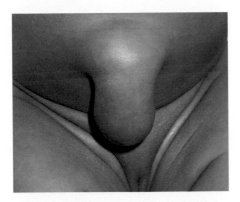

Fig. 13.5 Umbilical hernia.

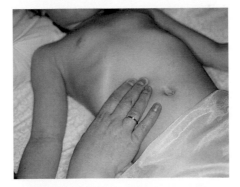

Fig. 13.6 Feeling the liver edge.

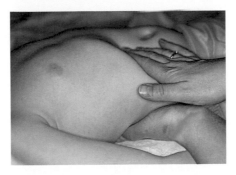

Fig. 13.7 Assessing the kidneys.

## BOX 13.5 EXAMINATION OF THE NERVOUS SYSTEM

A formal systematic examination of the nervous system is extremely difficult in the very young child, due partly to lack of cooperation but mainly to immaturity of the nervous system itself. Observation – particularly during certain activities – is the most useful form of examination and forms the basis of the developmental assessment. Examination is not very different from that in the adult, and some useful reminders are presented here under relevant headings.

- **Inspection.** Assess the level of consciousness of the child, and whether they are irritable or drowsy.

    Next, note the posture at rest and during movement. Are there any abnormal spontaneous movements such as writhing (choreoathetosis) of the upper limbs? Is purposeful, voluntary movement normal? Is there any tremor or clumsiness?

    Look at the posture while the child is sitting and standing. Are there any abnormalities of gait? Describe them: the broad-based walk of ataxia; the stiff, scissor-like movements of spasticity; or the high-stepping gait associated with foot drop.

    If the child is speaking, try to assess the level of speech. Is it appropriate for the child's age? Is articulation of speech normal? Is there monotony or stammering? Try and determine the child's use of language, as this gives an indication of intelligence.

- **Cranial nerves.** These are only partially examinable in the young. In older children, the same adult format should be followed.
    *Power:* the same grading for power is used as for adult medicine (see Chapter 6).
    *Sensation:* the dermatomal distribution in children is the same as that in adults (see Chapter 6).

- **Reflexes.** Primitive reflexes may be categorised by age as follows:
    *2 months* – palmar grasp lost; stepping reflex lost.
    *6 months* – Moro reflex lost; asymmetrical tonic neck reflex lost.
    *12 months* – Babinski response becomes flexor (down-going).
    *5 years* – loss of Galant response (stimulation along a paravertebral line leads to lateral spinal flexion towards the stimulated side).

    Other reflexes have the same root innervations as adults (see Chapter 6).

## BOX 13.6 EXAMINATION OF THE EXTERNAL GENITALIA

This examination is only done where potential findings support a clinical question. In girls, look for labial symmetry, clitoral enlargement, abnormalities of the introitus and position of the urethra. Note any bruising or unusual marks.

In boys, note the size of the penis, the position of the urethra (hypospadias) and the condition of the prepuce (phimosis or balanitis). Examine for the presence of testes in the scrotum. If they are not palpable, determine their position in the inguinal tract, noting whether or not they are retractable.

## BOX 13.7 RECTAL EXAMINATION

This is not performed in routine paediatric examination, the exception being by paediatric surgeons considering the possibility of pathology in the anus or lower rectum, such as Hirschsprung's disease.

## Child abuse

Everyone working in healthcare, whether or not they are a paediatrician, and however junior or senior they are, has a role to safeguard and promote the welfare of children. Within that duty is a responsibility to recognise and act on suspicions of possible child abuse.

The National Society for the Prevention of Cruelty to Children (NSPCC) defines child abuse as any action by another person – adult or child – that causes significant harm to a child. It can be physical, sexual or emotional, but can just as often be about a lack of love, care and attention. An abused child will often experience more than one type of abuse, as well as other difficulties in their lives. The abuse often happens over a period of time, rather than being a one-off event, and it can increasingly happen online. The NSPCC estimates that over half a million children are abused in the UK each year.

Internationally, the classification of child abuse is as follows:

- Physical abuse.
- Neglect.
- Emotional and psychological abuse.
- Sexual abuse.

Within this classification are situations around non-accidental injury, domestic violence, gang-related violence and - abuse, and fabricated and induced illness (which was historically labelled as Munchausen syndrome by proxy).

Every healthcare professional in the UK should have formal training relating to safeguarding children (and indeed safeguarding adults) that will provide them with the basic knowledge and skills to be able to recognise and respond appropriately to possible abuse. It is important make sure that you have had access to this training and feel comfortable that you would be able to recognise common presentations of abuse, and know what steps you would need to take to get appropriate senior and then multiagency input.

## Conclusions

Although thinking of children and young people as 'small adults' misses much of the nuance of the physical, physiological, emotional and functional development that occurs through childhood, there is much related to history taking and examination that can be taken from what you know from adult medicine and thoughtfully applied to paediatrics. This chapter has emphasised the importance of really listening to children, young people and their parents and carers, the value of observation, particularly repeated observations, and the role we all have in safeguarding the welfare of children.

# Index